Rheumatology for Nurses:
Patient Care

Rheumatology for Nurses: Patient Care

Edited by
Patricia le Gallez RGN, MPhil

Clinical Nurse Practitioner in Rheumatology
Dewsbury Health Care NHS Trust

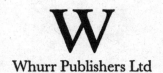

Whurr Publishers Ltd

British Library Cataloguing-in-Publication Data
A catalogue record for this book is available from the
British Library.

ISBN 1 86156 032 X

Contents

Contributors

Valerie Arthur RGN Clinical Nurse Specialist – Rheumatology, University Hospital (Selly Oak), Birmingham.

Elizabeth M Barrett RGN BA (Hons) RegHV Dist Nursing Cert, Cert Ed, Clinical Manager, Norfolk Arthritis Register, St Michael's Hospital, Aylsham, Norfolk.

Kay Henderson, Leeds, Yorkshire.

Patricia le Gallez RGN MPhil, Clinical Nurse Practitioner – Rheumatology, Dewsbury and District Hospital, Dewsbury, West Yorkshire.

Sarah Loukes RGN, Ward Sister Orthopaedics, St Michael's Hospital, Aylsham, Norfolk.

Sarah Ryan RGN Bsc (Hons) Msc (Distinction), Clinical Nurse Specialist – Rheumatology, The Hayward Hospital, Stoke on Trent.

Heather Smruti Riley MCSP SRP, Senior Physiotherapist – Rheumatology, Norfolk and Norwich Health Care Trust, Norwich, Norfolk.

Margaret Somerville RGN BA (Hons), Clinical Research Manager, Rheumatology, Norfolk and Norwich Health Care Trust, Norwich, Norfolk.

Susan Tromans DIP COT SROT, Occupational Therapist Team Leader, Musculo-Skeletal Team, Chapel Allerton Hospital, Leeds, Yorkshire.

Margaret-Ann Voyce RGN, Clinical Nurse Specialist – Rheumatology, Royal Cornwall Hospital, Truro, Cornwall.

Christine White RGN, Clinical Nurse Specialist-Rheumatology, Pinderfields Hospital Trust, Wakefield, West Yorkshire.

Clare Widdows BSc (Hons) SR Ch Dipod M, Senior Hospital Chiropodist – Rheumatology, Leeds General Infirmary, Leeds, Yorkshire.

Preface

The approach to nursing within rheumatology has progressed at an astonishing speed over the past 10 years and a new book focusing on the care of the patient with a rheumatic condition is most certainly required. The definitive book *Combined Care of the Rheumatic Patient*, by Bird, le Gallez and Hill, was written in 1985, and while much of what it contains is still relevant today, it is now out of print. While this new book does not cover a new topic, it does offer a new, comprehensive and holistic approach to an established speciality.

The book has been written mainly for nurses, though allied health professionals, i.e. occupational therapists, physiotherapists, social workers, podiatrists and dieticians, all of whom are fully involved in caring for the patient with a rheumatic condition, will also be interested, and even more so because a number of their professional colleagues have contributed to the book. The book will be a significant addition to the required reading list of all centres running ENB 983, Principles of Care and Rehabilitation of People with Rheumatic Disease and will also be of particular interest to all members of both the Rheumatology Nursing Forum and the British Health Professionals in Rheumatology.

Rheumatology is an expanding speciality, with new consultant rheumatologists being appointed at an increasing rate; also, more and more nurses are specialising in rheumatology. In addition, practice nurses are now acknowledging their responsibility for the care of such patients, and as a result see the urgent need to increase their knowledge, rather than leave the care of the patient to the staff in the local district or general hospital. Arthritis Care, the charity devoted solely to people with an arthritic condition, has a recommended reading list which is distributed to professionals and patients alike and hopefully this book will be a useful addition to this list.

Below are given the aims and objectives of this book:

- to stimulate an interest in rheumatology among nurses;
- to improve standards of nursing care in rheumatology;
- to fulfil the need for an up-to-date text book on rheumatology care for nurses, both nationally and internationally;
- to draw together the expertise of nurses and other professionals each with an interest in rheumatology, for the overall benefit of the patient.

When a nurse encounters a rheumatology patient for the first time the problem all too often arises whereby there is no one available with the required expertise to help, advise, direct and support him or her in providing adequate and specialised care. The situation can arise on a medical or surgical ward, in the community or in the out-patient department. Sadly, it can also happen on specialist rheumatology wards or more usually on wards which have only a small number of designated rheumatology beds.

The ultimate aim while editing this book has been to achieve a publication which is both an excellent resource and also an inspiration. One which will meet the needs of the nurse with little or no prior knowledge of rheumatology care and who has been thrust into the speciality with very little time to prepare for it. It will also meet the needs of the self-motivated nurse who is seeking to expand her or his knowledge of care in rheumatology and is fortunate enough to have the support and encouragement of management. It is a book to turn to in the short term and to keep as a permanent resource, a book in which the reader will find an immediate solution to a problem and a motivation to improve, in the long term, the standards of nursing for the patients in their care. It is a book which will provide a very interesting read at all these levels.

Each chapter in the book is complete in itself and is well cross-referenced. A chapter on osteoporosis has been included as this condition is rapidly becoming a major issue in which rheumatology nurses, both in hospital and in the community, are becoming involved.

Patricia le Gallez RGN MPhil,
January 1998

Chapter 1
The patient's perspective

KAY HENDERSON

One morning in May 1983 I got out of bed to find my toes feeling stiff and uncomfortable. I couldn't walk properly for an hour or so. The same happened every morning and I would shuffle about until the stiffness wore off. After a month my toes began to swell. I blamed the hot weather but my feet were unusually uncomfortable and I went to my doctor who did a blood test. I hadn't considered it being anything more serious than an allergy so when my doctor told me, a week later, that my blood test indicated rheumatoid arthritis (RA), I was stunned. He was very matter-of-fact, said he'd be referring me to the hospital and I was out of his surgery before anything had sunk in. Whilst walking home I suddenly thought of what having rheumatoid arthritis would mean. I was 33, married, with a son of nine and a daughter aged six. I was an infant teacher with everything going for me. A month earlier I had been appointed to a full-time job from my part-time one and was full of plans for the future. A terrible wave of panic came over me and I felt that nothing would ever be the same. I arrived home in tears to tell my husband, who fortunately was much calmer and convinced me that life was not going to stop there and then. He said there was no point in worrying unnecessarily when we knew so little about the disease. I didn't tell him that secretly I thought I'd be in a wheelchair by the next year.

Of course, that fear came from ignorance and during those early days I had little information about rheumatoid arthritis. It was October before I saw a rheumatologist and apart from stiff feet life was the same as usual. The rheumatologist advised against playing

1

badminton, which I did weekly, or anything else of a strenuous nature including knitting and crocheting! I could do my job but should rest completely in the evenings. I took his advice, put weight on and several weeks later could barely walk.

I was urged by my family to seek further help but at that time it was difficult. Rheumatologists were few and far between, and though my mother wanted to pay for me to go privately, when we made enquiries there were none within our reach. I visited the hospital regularly and took the drugs prescribed but felt unhappy about the situation. On every visit during the first two years I saw a different doctor and each one would ask the same questions as the previous one. I found it all deeply disappointing and came away after each visit feeling frustrated and no better informed.

I won't put all the blame on the medical people. I know that in those early months I was like the proverbial ostrich. I kept my head in the sand because I preferred not to think about the way things might develop. I probably didn't ask the right questions of the rheumatologist – perhaps I didn't ask any. Anyway, I hated the whole scene and I had anger in me. I hated sitting in the waiting room at the rheumatology clinic as it meant seeing others with RA. It reminded me of what might be still to come. It frightened me so much that I would creep round the corner and bury my head in a book.

The Effects of RA on My Family

Telling my family of the diagnosis was hard for me and for them, particularly as it was so unexpected. There was no history of anyone in the family having had RA so there was nothing we could put the blame on. Everyone was upset for me and I was upset for myself, and we were all trying not to upset one another. I didn't like to talk about it very much. I think my mother has found it the most difficult to come to terms with, and I know that even now she feels guilty that she is so fit and well when I am not. She has done her utmost to find me new cures and has treated me to every pill and potion on the market! She was always full of optimism and would ring every day to ask how I was feeling. I know she must have been longing to hear me say I felt better but optimism can be annoying when you are feeling sorry for yourself. I used to get irritable with her then, and I still do now when she asks me how I feel. I suppose I didn't want to be reminded about it.

At that time we read what literature was available. Someone lent us a book about a nurse who had RA so badly she couldn't walk.

Through diet and exercise she cured herself and led a normal life. We all hoped that my arthritis would burn out in the same way.

My husband has always taken things calmly. Although extremely concerned for me he has never treated me as an invalid or let my arthritis get too much in the way of things. Over the years he has developed a sensitivity to my needs and helps in such an unobtrusive way that often others don't notice that I am being helped.

'I'll get you out', other people say when we're in a car, or 'I'll help you with that', which draws more attention to your helplessness. My husband just gets on with it, without announcing it to the world first. I know I am still sensitive to what people say but I wish they would think before they speak. My husband knows that I will ask if I need help for anything; by not being asked I feel more independent.

I don't remember telling my children much about arthritis when I was first diagnosed. They knew my feet hurt and that I couldn't run about with them, but I don't remember ever discussing with them how it might develop. I don't think I wanted to face up to that myself. They have grown up accepting it as part of me. We had to plan things more carefully but I don't think the children ever missed out on anything because of my having RA. What I couldn't do with them their dad did instead, so we were no different from any busy family.

I think my being able to carry on working helped: it maintained the normality of life for them even though I couldn't do as much at home. That too, though, has brought its own benefits. When my arthritis began to spread, most noticeably affecting my hands, the children had to become more independent. My husband took over a lot of the household jobs and the children did their fair share. The reward is that now, at 18- and 21-years-old they are both responsible adults, capable of looking after themselves and skilled in all aspects of domesticity. They have also, through witnessing pain and sadness at first hand, developed caring and thoughtful natures.

With the spread of my arthritis I had to face the realisation that it was not just going to disappear and neither was it going to stand still. You do adapt to every physical change and I would say to myself each time, 'as long as I stay like this I'll be all right'. It's a way of comforting and reassuring yourself. Nevertheless, each subtle change brought fear and panic in case I might not cope. Many were the nights during the early years that I cried in bed with my husband holding me tight. I couldn't even verbalise my fears to him – all I could say was 'I feel so fed up'. I would feel guilty afterwards because

I knew he must also feel 'fed up'; it wasn't just my life that was affected, was it?

We have had ups and downs. During the first four years I tried nearly all the major drugs only to find that I was either allergic or had a poor reaction to them. Hope alternated with depression. I have to admit there were times when my joints were so painful and everything was such an effort for me that I wished I had a terminal illness. Then, I reasoned, there would eventually be an end to all the pain. Fortunately my bad spells have been interspersed with better ones when such thoughts don't surface.

Whatever my moods, I've been lucky to have the support of a very loving, caring family. The children are fortunate to have had wonderful grandparents who have eased our burden with their help and support. I feel so sorry for others with RA who don't have the family support – it must be very hard.

We don't dwell on my arthritis, in fact it is rarely mentioned at home. I suspect that both children worry that they might develop RA. They don't talk about it but I sense a fear in them if ever they have aches and pains. All I can do is reassure them that it's not likely.

The help I need is mainly with dressing and undressing, washing my hair and that kind of thing. We have a daily routine where I do what I can and then call my husband to help with the rest. We laugh a lot – that's essential! He, like me, would love it if I could wear ordinary shoes. The daily chore of lacing me into my boots is frustrating, particularly when time is short, and of course I can't get into bed until they are removed. Planning ahead is essential, as where I'm going and with whom affects my decision on what to wear. I may have to go to the toilet alone so must wear something I can fasten myself. I'm extremely lucky in having a daughter who understands the frustrations. She helps me try endless outfits till we find ones that I can manage, and spends a lot of time helping me look nice. She is sympathetic to my philosophy that if the top of me looks good then maybe people won't notice what's happening below.

Often an illness in a family can break it apart. In ours, I'm convinced rather that it has brought us closer and made us all stronger.

Coping with Pain, Work and Colleagues

I had taught at the same school for several years when I was diagnosed as having RA. Being a small staff we were friends and shared our celebrations and our problems. It was actually easier talking to them about my arthritis than to my family. Family emotions go so much deeper. You are always trying to minimise your difficulties to your family so as not to upset them further. Your colleagues on the other hand, whilst kind and sympathetic, don't spend sleepless nights worrying about you. You can often be more honest with them about how you feel.

At first I did fight against it – 'it' being the RA. I determined it would not get the better of me and got on with my job. As only my feet were affected to begin with I didn't feel too self-conscious in the classroom. I felt confident that I was still doing a good job; only my walking was slower. Whilst at home I secretly worried about the future, at school I was too busy. As anyone who has ever worked in an infant class will know, one's own worries don't get a chance to surface – children's needs are far more pressing. In that respect school freed me from my personal worries for a large part of the day.

I never felt any awkwardness with the children at school and they accepted my disabilities very easily. I was always honest. All I needed to say by way of explanation about my arthritis was, 'I've got poorly feet – they're not as good as yours.' They never made fun of the way I walked and accepted me the way I was. I always told them when I was going for a hospital appointment and they would show their sympathy by telling me, 'my grandad can't walk either', or even 'my dog's got a poorly foot.'

When my feet became very painful, at times feeling as though I had marbles in my shoes, I did become self-conscious. I hated not being able to wear ordinary shoes and looked for something more comfortable. I found I could shuffle around in school alternating between wellingtons and a pair of soft slippers. Fortunately it was winter so the wellies didn't look completely out of place! The alternative would have been to stay at home, but I was determined not to give in.

Humour seemed the best answer. I had always laughed and joked with my colleagues so it helped me to put on a brave face. If I could laugh at myself, then, I hoped, others could laugh with me and feel more comfortable; certainly the last thing I wanted was pity. Humour took a lot of the embarrassment out of situations, so whilst hating to have to wear wellingtons in school I would say to my colleagues, 'How do you like the footwear with this outfit then? Very fetching, Yes!'

Gradually my arthritis spread and things did get harder at school but whatever happened I found ways round. I was fortunate that the school was all on one level which was easier on my knees. I was also fortunate that as I taught the youngest children I nearly always had a non-teaching assistant to help. She was happy to do the jobs I found hardest: stapling, pinning up pictures and so on. I tried never to take unfair advantage of her generous nature, or of my colleagues who often came to the rescue. What was so nice was that they never made me feel bad about asking for help. In return I always tried to support them in other ways. There were often times when my disabilities could have put me at a disadvantage in school but my colleagues were always considerate. Things were always organised so that I could cope, yet I was never made to feel that I was a problem.

One of the negative ways in which arthritis affected my career was with regard to promotion. I felt confident to apply for a job at another school, got an interview but then changed my mind. The thought of how a new staff might react to my disabilities had put me off. I felt so happy and secure where I was that I decided I had more to lose by moving.

I was fortunate to work for two head teachers who gave me their utmost support. The first suffered with osteoarthritis herself, so was sympathetic and encouraging. When my shoulder worsened she would come every morning to see if I needed anything written on the blackboard. She told me never to feel obliged to give up teaching because of the arthritis. She also told me that I was worth more to her with my disabilities than some who were a hundred per cent fit. That made me realise I was still valued as a whole person and that even with disabilities I still had plenty to offer the school. When she retired I was apprehensive about how a new head would view me. I worried that she would think that I couldn't cope. I needn't have worried: she treated me the same as everyone else except that she always took a special interest in the way I managed my arthritis.

We had some very therapeutic after-school chats. To be told that I came across as a very positive person made me feel much better about myself and my condition. In a reference, she wrote that knowing me had helped her re-examine her own attitudes and understand the nature of disability in a more informed way.

My Coping Mechanisms

During my first two or three years I constantly told myself that arthritis wouldn't beat me. Besides the drugs prescribed by the rheumatologists I had tried diets and herbal remedies. I willingly tried everything and in this respect I'm sure I am no different from anyone suffering from a serious illness. With every new treatment your hopes are boosted again. Sometimes I felt better for a while but unlike the woman in the book I'd read, my relief was only short-lived. Acupuncture, reflexology and aromatherapy all relaxed me but never took the pain away. Going to church only emphasised my sadness as the minister's prayers for the sick only focused my thoughts on myself even more.

I gave up playing badminton, and found it increasingly difficult to play the piano and guitar when my wrists got bad. By now I'd had RA for about two years. At school I was coping well and loved my job. I used to say that going to school kept me sane.

Away from school I found my arthritis much harder to cope with. I hated the sideways looks I got when shopping because I hobbled as I walked. I mourned the fact that I could no longer wear fashionable shoes. I dreaded meeting people who would ask what I'd done to myself and I hated saying it was arthritis. I didn't like people's reactions, however kindly meant. 'You're so young to have it' was the commonest. I used to feel angry inside for being reminded. Saying 'arthritis' was like a password for others to tell me about their own aches and pains. It's amazing how many want to boast of their own bad shoulder, knee or whatever – just what you don't want to hear. I used to want to scream and say, 'You've no idea what it's really like' but would smile politely, my ankles stiffening all the while. Often people asked how I managed to work, sometimes in a tone that sounded as if they'd already written me off as useless. I'm afraid in the early years my emotions were extremely raw and I was very aware of other people's sensitivity or lack of it. I used to tell them that as talking was the main feature of my job – and I've never had a problem with that – I could manage very well. I would add, perhaps with sarcasm, that arthritis did not affect my brain!

It did, however, affect my confidence away from school. I began to prefer staying at home, only socialising with family and close friends. I went through a period of intense sadness and realise now that I was grieving for all I had lost. Outwardly I kept a tight rein on my emotions. I felt I couldn't share the way I was feeling with any of my family. They were upset enough by the way arthritis was affecting me physically without being burdened with my emotions too. Looking back, this was the time when we would all have benefited from counselling. I desperately needed someone to talk to about my sadness but there seemed no one available. At school I put my brave face on and immersed myself in work, but at night I would sit in the bath and cry. After several weeks of this I was crying in the bedroom one night, unaware that the children could hear me. I realised when

I heard them saying 'mum's crying' that they were upset and didn't know what to do. I remember thinking, 'How awful. They know I'm upset but they daren't ask what's wrong.' I think that's when I decided I had to take a hold on myself for all our sakes. I thought, 'It's no good moping. You can still do all sorts of things. You can still work and you've got all your family. It's not taken that away.'

I began to think more positively and I said to myself, 'Right, there is a tomorrow. Everybody is very good to you and it's time you gave them something back and showed you're determined to carry on.' Nevertheless, I do believe that time of grieving was necessary.

I threw myself into work at school, was given extra responsibilities and felt as valued as ever. I was by now not only a full-time classroom teacher but also the co-ordinator for children with special needs and curriculum leader for Art and PE. I often laughed at being responsible for PE. It seemed ironic that the most decrepit member of staff should have the responsibility for the most energetic area of the curriculum!

School work began to take up more of my time in the evenings. I didn't mind as I was involved in fewer social activities. I stopped swimming when my shoulder got bad and I found all the hassle of dressing and undressing too much. Kind friends offered to go with me but it was just too great an effort. School work stopped me dwelling on the things I could no longer do at home. Because at school I had no time to think about how I was feeling, the contrast when I was at home seemed greater. Extreme depression descended at weekends when there seemed so little that I could do. It may seem trivial to the able bodied but I longed to be able to push the vacuum cleaner round or clean the bathroom by myself. During the week I was so much more positive because I was in control, doing what I was good at.

I know my husband sometimes felt hurt by the way my moods could swing. In front of colleagues and friends I would laugh and play the clown but alone with him I was often very down and miserable, causing him to think it was his fault. The trouble is that you can put on a brave face but it's hard to keep it up all the time, and it's only those closest to you who ever really see the other side.

Some mornings I would cry with the pain and effort of getting dressed or coming downstairs, and my husband would try and persuade me to stay at home. That thought terrified me. I would plead and tell him, 'I'll be all right once I get to school.' Even the pain of driving would not stop me – I would not be beaten.

Help from Other Agencies

Four years after the arthritis began, when I was at a very low ebb, I was lucky to spend three weeks in our rheumatology hospital. I enjoyed the various treatments, particularly exercises in the hydrotherapy pool which spurred me on to swim weekly for the next three years in our local baths. The greatest benefit for me, however, was the therapeutic effect of spending time with others who had RA. I was particularly relieved to find so many others of my age-group who understood the way I felt. During two subsequent periods in the same hospital I again benefited from sharing problems and remedies with other patients. After each visit I came home with a much more positive outlook on life. The hospital stays were also valuable in offering opportunities for advice from Social Services. Life has been much easier at home since I have been provided with a special bath seat and a raised toilet seat. I was also able to try out various useful gadgets for the home in the occupational therapy department.

During my first stay in the rheumatology hospital I was visited by a nurse practitioner who did a blood test. She was involved on the research side of RA and in monitoring patients and their drugs. She asked if she could continue monitoring me during my regular visits to the rheumatology clinic and I agreed. It was one of the best decisions I ever made and I have a lot to thank her for. Seeing her regularly meant I only saw the rheumatologist if there was a problem. I liked the rheumatologist but came away feeling little had been achieved. I realise now that he was treating my physical symptoms in isolation. In my nurse practitioner I found someone who was interested not only in my physical health but in how RA affected everything in my life. She encouraged me to talk about the effect it was having on my family and my work, and helped resolve practical problems. I found I could unburden myself and for the first time I began to let go of some of my sadness. She always gave me time – time that doctors rarely have – to share my worries or achievements with her. I have laughed and cried and come away from her feeling uplifted. I firmly believe her support was crucial for my well-being and I enjoyed it for eight years. Sadly for me she moved to another hospital; but I know many patients there will benefit from her involvement.

One thing she did which is ongoing was to involve me with a Young Arthritis Care group. At first I didn't want to mix with a lot of other people with arthritis as I thought it would emphasise the fact that I was disabled. I considered myself, and still do, a normal person with a few disabilities. However, through the group I have made new friends; we have the therapeutic benefits of sharing common problems and supporting one another.

During my last years of teaching I gained help from a source discovered by my head teacher. She had enquired from the education department about getting extra help for me in school and was told about PACT – the Placement and Counselling Team affiliated to job centres who advise and provide equipment to enable those with disabilities to carry on working or return to work. After an assessment in my working environment I was provided with a swivel chair for the classroom with numerous adjustments and castors for easy movement. It was great for my painful knees and stiff neck. My class of five-year-olds thought it was great too and I could be sure that one of them would be doing a twirl on it if I wasn't using it! PACT's generosity extended to the staff room where I was provided with a magnificent high-backed chair complete with spring seat to push me out. The staff called it my 'throne'. We had some hilarious moments when, having forgotten to secure the spring lever, I would lean forward for my coffee and nearly be catapulted across the room! Later when my hands got worse I contacted PACT again. Their solution was a computer and printer to make writing easier.

More Play than Work

I've had RA for 13 years now, so should be getting used to it. Unfortunately, the nature of the disease makes it unpredictable. It's a very individual thing which is why I refer to it as 'my arthritis'. No one else's is exactly like mine. I think I've stopped fighting it as it seems to be here to stay. I don't know whether you ever totally accept it but I'm going along with it now.

After my initial worries about it ending my career I went on to teach for a further ten happy and rewarding years. Two years ago I found teaching becoming harder in all ways. I am unable to accept second best from myself and to have everything the way I wanted would have meant constantly asking for help. I decided to quit whilst on top rather than wait until I couldn't cope.

I'm glad I took that decision and retired gracefully. I realise now that although I enjoyed my work there was a lot of stress involved, much of it caused by RA. Not knowing how I would feel from day to day brought its own worries, and the physical problems of getting ready for work and getting there all added to my anxieties. Now if I have an 'off' day I can relax and take my time.

I'm enjoying the freedom to do other things I used to do. Badminton, walking, swimming, playing the piano are all tucked away in a recess of my mind. Painting, reading, pottering in the kitchen have replaced them. I've had more time to spend with my children and the rest of my family. I feel privileged that I had all those extra years and grateful to those who supported and encouraged me. I'm certain that working saved my sanity through the worst times. I wouldn't be honest if I said I never feel fed up, but time does seem to bring acceptance and most of the sadness has left me. Now I concentrate on what I can do and whilst it's the end of one era, it's the beginning of another – and who knows what's round the corner?

Chapter 2
The role of the nurse specialist in rheumatology

VALERIE ARTHUR

Introduction

In this chapter the concept of advanced nursing practice is examined before that of the nurse specialist in rheumatology. Advanced nursing must be seen in the historical context in order to understand the current controversial issues that surround it and will inevitably have implications for the future of nursing generally and more specifically for those nurses who have extended their role.

ADVANCED PRACTITIONERS MAY BE CALLED		
nurse practitioner specialist nurse	clinical nurse specialist	specialist practitioner nurse specialists
THEY MAY ENGAGE IN		
advanced practice	expanded practice	extended role

Figure 2.1: The range of titles which may be used to describe nurse specialists and their roles

As can be seen in Figure 2.1, confusion surrounds the titles and the roles of the advanced practitioner. This has always been the case and still is today. An attempt will be made in the first part of this chapter to unravel this somewhat complicated issue. There does not appear to be a universally recognised name for advanced practitioners and terms such as 'nurse practitioners', 'clinical nurse specialists', 'specialist practitioners' or more recently 'specialist nurses' and 'nurse specialists' are common titles. Further confusion arises over the terminology of 'advanced practice', 'extended role', 'expanded practice' and 'nurse-led care'. Whilst there may well be some slight differences between the generally accepted concept of these terms, for the purpose of this chapter the terms 'nurse specialist' and 'advanced practice' will be used, except where other terms are referred to from the literature. Maycock (1991) states that the confusion surrounding the role of the advanced practitioner has arisen because the posts have been set up to fulfil a medical rather than a nursing need. The titles given to nurse specialists are often lengthy and obscure, causing further perplexity not only for other nurses and health professionals but also for the general public. It appears that little thought goes into the choice of titles which exist for such nurses. Those within the profession may well understand the terminology, but does the patient know what to expect from a 'nurse practitioner', or a 'clinical nurse specialist' and does the title reflect the role? The literature suggests that titles and roles are inexorably bound together. It can be argued that as advanced practice encompasses such a wide range of functions there can be no clear-cut definition of the role or title. Roles at this level will contain core elements of advanced practice. Within specialities advanced practitioners will have responsiblity for a group of patients who have a certain medical condition, and will therefore have expert knowledge of that speciality and condition. Barker (1988) describes the confusion surrounding the specialist practitioner role as compared with that of the nurse in charge of a specialist unit. It could be argued that both these roles are seen as advanced practice. However, there is a difference between having the skill to be in charge of a specialist unit and the expertise and autonomy of a clinical nurse specialist, although in some instances it may be that both of these roles are combined. Whichever the title given to them, nurses employed within these posts should have received a training in their chosen speciality, be accountable and responsible for the management of a specific client group and be able to educate patients, relatives and nursing colleagues.

More recently, papers by Ryan (1996), and Hoover and van Ooijen (1995) describe clinical nurse specialists, advanced and specialist nurse practitioners as also being advocates, change agents, leaders and role models. In the past it may have been that these functions were understood to be integral to the role. Notter (1995) sees specialist nurses as supervising, developing and leading practice, contributing to research, teaching and supporting professional colleagues and undertaking audit.

The essential philosophy of the role of advanced practice should be that it is flexible enough to adapt to situations and patients as required. Any expansion of the role should be influenced by the necessity of improving patient care rather than filling in the gaps brought about by the reduction in junior doctors' hours (Garbett, 1996). The role of the advanced practitioner will vary depending upon the speciality, location and needs of patients and will encompass clinical, educational, managerial and research aspects.

Clinical practice Leadership	Research Advocacy	Management Role model	Education Agent of change

Figure 2.2: Components of the nurse specialist role

History of advanced practice

The nature of nursing at an advanced level originated in the United States and Canada. Nurse practitioners first appeared in the USA in the mid-1960s. They worked in rural and inner-city areas where doctors were unwilling to practise (Stillwell, 1985). Ross (1982) describes the advent of the nurse practitioner in the USA and discusses the implications for this role in Britain. Storr (1988), in a literature review, discusses how, from the early days, confusion existed not only as to the preparation, functions and responsibilities of the clinical nurse specialist but also as to their placement within the bureaucratic structure. Education to master's level was regarded as essential, and difficulty in justifying the bedside role and a suitable title for such nurses were all issues then which still pertain today. Nurse specialists remain somewhat of an enigma to management and also to themselves with regard to their position within the nursing hierarchy. Many nurse specialists have found themselves working independently with only medical colleagues for support. Nurse managers have not always fully understand the specialist role and this situation remains the case today.

Nowadays, as the number of nurse specialists increases, they form a distinct category within the nursing hierarchy and can be an effective group for the instigation, promotion and implementation of research into practice. Their essential autonomy enables them to advance practice free from many of the constraints experienced by ward-based nurses. They also form a stable group of highly motivated individuals who have chosen to remain in the clinical arena rather than climb the management career ladder.

In the UK the extended role of the nurse has been recognised since 1977 when a DHHS circular was published setting out the legal implications for nurses undertaking functions previously the responsibility of the medical profession. This increased the confusion regarding the role of advanced nursing and the debate has continued since that time. Bowling (1981), writing on the increase of nurse practitioners in the USA, asks whether the role of the nurse practitioner is really that of physician's assistant and expresses concern that nurses and doctors feel threatened by such advances in nursing practice. In the UK, Hill (1986) describes a study to evaluate a rheumatology nurse-led clinic and argues that although the criticism has been levelled at nurse practitioners – by both the medical and the nursing professions – that they provide a second-class medical service, they are in reality providing a first-class nursing service.

The advanced nurse practitioner role has developed within both the community and hospital settings. Bryan (1982) describes how in the UK the Medical Research Council arranged trials within general practice for the monitoring and screening of patients with hypertension. Nearly 200 nurses were trained to conduct the study and once it was completed they extended their roles to fill gaps in the service provided by general practitioners. Stillwell (1981) was a pioneer of nurse practitioner-led clinics in general practice. The practice nurse is now firmly established within many health centres and today such nurses specialise in health education, disease prevention, drug monitoring and the management of chronic disease. University courses now exist for practice nurses which give them the title of nurse practitioner. It would appear that this title is more commonly used by nurse specialists working within the community although the title is also used by some nurse specialists in hospital (Hill, 1986). To some extent this adoption of the title by practice nurses can be seen as a natural progression of the work of Stillwell (1984).

In the hospital setting there has been an increase of nurse-led care (Garbett, 1996) which has extended into many specialities. Most advanced practitioners have definite nurse specialist roles linked to certain conditions such as diabetes, renal disease, oncology and rheumatology. Nurse specialists are usually hospital based but they may also work in the community visiting patients in their homes, or in health centres, thus ensuring liaison between primary and secondary care. Within the hospital setting, they provide a holistic problem-solving service which supports and enhances that of their medical colleagues and ensures that patients not only receive the optimum benefit from their interventions but also continuity of care.

Education for advanced practice

Turner (1987) advocates that nurse specialists should be educated to at least first-degree level to gain a sound grounding in the behavioural sciences in order to fully realise their potential in terms of clinical practice, leadership, research, education, agents of change and role models. In the past, owing to limited opportunities, most nurse specialists gained their positions through clinical expertise and years of experience. Now, with an increase in opportunities to achieve post-registration education through the English National Board, Higher Award programme (ENB, 1991) which take into account previous experience, it is possible for nurse specialists to undertake first and master's degrees. Evans, Jackson and Shepherd (1993) describe how this model of flexible post-registration education will help to provide a research-based nursing service and thus ultimately improve health care.

The United Kingdom Central Council for Nursing, Midwifery and Health Visiting (1992) defines advanced practice as being 'a second area of professional practice' which requires 'additional skills beyond specialist practice'. One of the major additional skills is the knowledge and ability to undertake research. Education to first or master's level enables advanced practitioners to acquire this additional skill and the ability to undertake research, critically analyse the data, publish the results and institute innovations in order to increase the body of nursing knowledge. Although the ENB has established courses for the certification of specialist nursing, Turner (1987) argues that these are elementary and that the research component falls short of the level required for advanced practice. Many nurses do not see research as being relevant to practice and there is a danger of a divide between nurse researchers and general nurses (Alexander, 1989).

Specialist nurses should be able to lead by example, communicate with and involve nurses undertaking less specialised nursing. Whilst advancing the education of nurse specialists it is imperative for the profession that the vast majority of nurses are not forgotten and that the education of fellow nurses is seen as an important component of the nurse specialist role.

The advancement of nursing to the year 2000 needs to be seen in the context of integrating nursing theory, practice and research. Advanced practitioners such as nurse specialists should be in the forefront of such developments. Shaw (1993) argues that further education to master's and doctoral degree level can only improve the credibility of nursing by enabling nurses to undertake research-based practice. Consequently, the ENB framework, by offering a flexible system of study, can be considered a worthwhile mechanism to achieve this end (Bysshe, 1992).

The future: nurse specialist or junior doctor?

Advanced nursing practice may be developing in conjunction with a shortage of medical staff and the decrease in junior doctors' hours. The implications for the introduction of nurse specialist clinics are enormous, especially within those specialities dealing with chronic disease. In many rheumatology departments such clinics are already an accepted part of patient care (Hill et al., 1994).

Many procedures previously considered the domain of the doctor have become an integral part of the role of the specialist nurse (Derrick, 1989). Within rheumatology an ENB course has been designed to teach nurse specialists to perform intra-articular injections. In this case it could be argued that rather than undertaking a medical task, the nurse is providing treatment immediately instead of the patient having to wait several days, in discomfort, for a doctor to attend. This is seen as part of the holistic nursing care of the patient.

The debate about role parameters will continue to rage as more and more tasks deemed to be medical are destined to be taken on by nurses. Whether such role extension leads to advanced nursing practice is uncertain and will depend upon the task itself and the degree of responsibility it engenders. It will also depend on the motives for taking on such tasks or procedures. There is no reason why moves to extend the role should alter the essential philosophy of nursing, which is to care for patients and see to their needs. However, any adjustments to the scope of practice should abide by the principles set out in UKCC guidelines (1992). Maycock (1991) asks whether extending practice is in the best interests of patients as medical and nursing models of care are essentially different. But it could be argued that nursing is enhanced by such innovations since patients may receive immediate care. It could also be argued that unplanned and indiscriminate role expansion by nurses could lead to a situation where they will be expected to take over the tasks of junior doctors. The reason that many nurse specialist posts have been created is to ensure that patients receive information and education concerning their disease and treatment. Patients generally perceive nurses as having more time than doctors, and as being more approachable and available to answer questions (Hill, 1986). In the future, nurse specialists could find themselves almost fully occupied in undertaking 'medical' tasks, leaving them little time for the other important aspects of their role. In the rush to extend or expand nursing roles the essential value of the nurse specialist role should not be lost. Once 'medical' tasks are taken on by nurses, business managers may well see nurse specialists as a cheap alternative to junior doctors. Although the two disciplines of medicine and nursing might well overlap in certain circumstances, they are not a substitute for each other; instead they are complementary, each offering comprehensive care together with choice.

Advanced Practice in Rheumatology Nursing

The development of advanced practice in rheumatology nursing

Within the field of rheumatology the role of nurse practitioner has evolved since the mid-1970s when experienced nurses were employed in a research capacity to interview patients, and collate and analyse data which were collected for clinical and social studies undertaken by the University of Leeds (Hill, 1985). A clinical pharmacology unit was set up and these nurses were employed to make assessments and collect data for clinical trials. This discipline became known as metrology and is described by le Gallez (1981). It was found that patients who saw these nurses managed their own disease better and therefore had better outcomes. Le Gallez (1985) ascribes this to the fact that nurses were able to afford more time to answer questions, give information and educate patients and their families. State registered nurses held clinics alongside those of a rheumatologist. Patients who were prescribed specific drugs were referred to the nurses for a full explanation of the treatment, to answer any queries, for monitoring of the drug and clinical assessment of disease activity (Hill et al., 1994). These clinics arose from the patients' desire to continue in the care of a nurse once they had completed a clinical trial. Maycock (1991) describes how rheumatologists in busy out-patient clinics have been unable to meet the demand for information from patients. This has resulted in the recruitment of nurses to provide patient education and information as well as nursing care. It has been found that patients were more satisfied with the care they received from a nurse practitioner than at a normal out-patient clinic (Hill, 1986).

Two organisations which have achieved much to encourage and support rheumatology nursing are the Rheumatology Nursing

Forum and British Health Professionals in Rheumatology. The Rheumatology Nursing Forum was one of the first specialist groups within the Royal College of Nursing to publish its own standards of care (RCN, 1989). The Forum provides a network for members, organises conferences, initiates debate and sets up working parties to produce guidelines on matters relevant to rheumatology nursing. British Health Professionals in Rheumatology supports not only nurses but also enables all members of the multidisciplinary team to enlarge their body of knowledge by providing an arena for debate and information which crosses all professional boundaries.

Through the work of pioneers such as Hill, le Gallez and Maycock nurse specialists are now regarded as essential members of the multidisciplinary team in rheumatology departments throughout the country.

Specialist Nursing Care in Rheumatology

The rheumatology nurse specialist role, as with any other role in advanced practice, will be individual to the needs of the consultant and the nurse undertaking that role. However, the main aspects of the job will contain certain core elements such as clinical practice, management, education and research.

A description of the role will give insight into the highly individual nursing aspect of caring for rheumatology patients. Such patients are referred to the nurse specialist for nursing care, drug monitoring, education and counselling. The individual assessment of these patients enables the nurse specialist to plan overall nursing management and to pinpoint problems which may involve referral to other members of the multidisciplinary team (Arthur, 1994). This important aspect of the role of the nurse specialist ensures that a holistic approach is adopted and provides continuity of care for these patients. Within the speciality of rheumatology, patient education and information are seen as an integral part of holistic care. As the majority of the rheumatic diseases are chronic, this approach enables the patients to lead as normal a life as possible in spite of the vagaries of their disease. Continued research into nursing practice and also those therapies used in the care of rheumatology patients is an important aspect of the role of the nurse specialist and ensures that practice is up to date, effective and relevant.

Management of nurse-led clinics, responsibility for a patient caseload and in some instances for a department will also be important aspects of the role. Research into practice, treatments and audit of clinics and departments is essential to ensure that the best practice ensues.

In undertaking these aspects of the nurse specialist role the advanced practitioner will inevitably become a leader, role model, advocate of both patients and nurses and also an agent of change. Setting up guidelines, procedures and acting as a consultant for nursing problems within the speciality will also be an accepted part of the role.

Clinical practice

The rheumatic diseases are many and diverse. However, the majority of patients seen by the rheumatology nurse specialist will be suffering from inflammatory arthropathies such as rheumatoid arthritis, psoriatic arthritis, ankylosing spondylitis, systemic lupus erythematosus (lupus) and reactive arthritis. Therefore these patients will suffer similar symptoms whatever the underlying disease. These diseases are systemic and may affect the whole body rather than just the joints. Although the most common rheumatic disease is osteoarthritis, the nurse specialist is unlikely to see many patients suffering with this disease as they are usually managed in the general practice setting (Dargie and Proctor, 1994). However, these patients may be referred when their symptoms are poorly controlled or when they are awaiting surgery for damaged joints. Whatever the type of disease, many of the problems which patients experience are common and therefore assessment and planning form the basis of nursing care. For the purpose of this chapter diseases will be described as rheumatic diseases unless otherwise stated.

The philosophy of nursing care for rheumatology patients must be to enable them to live as normally as possible within their own capabilities, even though these capabilities may alter radically from day to day. Chronic disease can be defined as a dramatic, unforeseen and unasked for life event which presents both physical and psychological problems. As the majority of the rheumatic diseases are chronic with no known cause or cure, the nurse specialist is in a unique position as a member of the multidisciplinary team to facilitate the care of patients with these diseases. Nursing care is based on a problem-solving, holistic approach which involves education and the giving of information and advice. Referral to other members of the team not only ensures continuity of care between all disciplines but also the best possible outcome so enabling the patient to live a normal and fulfilled life.

The main problems which patients with inflammatory joint disease experience are pain, stiffness and fatigue. These problems are indirectly related to each other and also affect the patient's physical and psychological state. By assessing the patient's ability to cope with daily living activities a plan is developed which deals with all of the problems the patient may be experiencing. These will usually relate to diet, skin, mobility, self-care, body image and self-esteem as well as pain, stiffness and fatigue (see the model in Chapter 3, Table 3.3). This model is used in the Rheumatology Nursing Forum's standards of care booklet (Royal College of Nursing, 1989). Problems which arise within this group of patients tend to be common to all, although they vary in severity between individuals depending on disease activity. In order to make an assessment on which to base nursing care, it is important not only to examine the patient's joints but also to use various assessment tools. These will include asking certain questions about symptoms and restrictions to daily life. Many patients with inflammatory joint disease tend to underplay their symptoms. This may be because they have a chronic disease and live each day with pain, stiffness and fatigue to varying degrees, and their one method of coping is to try to ignore or make the best of things.

Clinical assessment of the rheumatology patient

Standard assessment procedures are recognised both nationally and internationally. They provide a valuable tool for the holistic care of rheumatology patients and they are also a useful means of evaluating outcome measures and auditing care. A baseline articular index, health and psychological status provide an initial idea of the particular problems which beset the patient (Hill, 1985). Serial assessments then provide a picture of the patient's progress and also highlight any new problems as they occur. When selecting the type of assessments to be used on a particular patient over a period of time, the nurse must bear in mind that these assessments must be sensitive to any clinical change occurring in the health status of that patient and must be relevant to the type of disease.

As with all assessments a method of storing and recording the data should be organised. Besides assisting with care plans, such data may also be used to evaluate care or to look retrospectively at outcomes. It may be advantageous to record assessments in such a way that they would be available to each member of the multidisciplinary team. It must be stressed, however, that it is essential for the same person to make the assessments and that they are performed at the same time of the day. This will safeguard against inter-observer error and any diurnal variation in the results.

Articular assessments

Assessments are made of tenderness and swelling in and around the joints. Joint tenderness may be present on movement, at rest or when digital pressure is applied. Joint swelling usually denotes a synovial effusion but can also be due to chronic synovitis. The degree of swelling may well influence the range of movement through which any particular joint can be put. When assessing the joints for swelling, joints which are enlarged due to bony deformities do not count as swollen joints. Examination of each joint gives the nurse specialist an accurate picture of those joints affected and also the degree of disability. For example, if the shoulders are painful, by asking the patient to go through a full range of movement the nurse can evaluate how that particular patient is coping with everyday activities. Questions should be asked with regard to problems patients may be having with dressing and bathing and this often encourages patients to enlarge on other complications and how their lives are affected by them. Observations can be made of other factors which can have a bearing on the plan of care such as muscle wasting, poor circulation and the state of skin. Nodules often appear on the elbows or fingers and indicate active disease. Rashes may be present when there is an intolerance to certain drugs. Vasculitic ulcers, vasculitic lesions or nail infarcts require immediate attention and referral for a medical opinion. Examination of the knee may also reveal that, where an effusion is present, a Baker's cyst may have developed. Problems can arise if the cyst ruptures and fluid tracks down inside the calf causing pain and discomfort which sometimes leads to a misdiagnosis of deep venous thrombosis (DVT).

Before starting an articular assessment, the nurse must give a full explanation of the process as pain may well be inflicted on the patient while squeezing the joints. There are several types of articular assessments (see Figure 2.3 and Figure 2.5). The *Eular Handbook of Standard Methods* (1995) of assessing disease activity in rheumatoid arthritis is a useful resource which outlines the commonly used assessment tools and has pictures and descriptions of how to undertake an articular assessment.

The Ritchie Articular Index takes a count on 53 joints (Ritchie et al., 1968). The following joints are calculated as a single unit: temporomandibular, cervical spine, sternoclavicular, acromioclavicular, metacarpophalangeal (MCP), proximal interphalangeal (PIP) and metatarsophalangeal (MTP). The shoulders, elbows, hips, knees, ankles, talocalcaneal and midtarsal joints are assessed separately (see Figure 2.3). After an explanation to the patient, the nurse puts digital pressure on the joints. The pressure that is exerted should be sufficient to whiten the examiner's nail beds (*Eular Handbook*, 1995). The patient is asked whether tenderness is felt and the

	Right	Left
Temporomandibular		
Cervical spine		
Sternoclavicular		
Acromioclavicular		
Shoulders		
Elbows		
Wrists		
MCPs		
PIPs		
Hip		
Knee		
Ankle		
Talocalcaneal		
Midtarsal		
MTPs		
Total		

Figure 2.3: Ritchie Articular Index

0 = no pain	1 = pain on pressure
2 = pain + patient winced	3 = pain + patient withdrew joint

Figure 2.4: Scoring for Ritchie Articular Index

reaction is noted. The maximum score which can be reached is 78. The joints are scored as shown in Figure 2.4.

Other indices which may be used are shown in Figure 2.5. Some indices note swollen joints only and others note both the degree of tenderness and the number of swollen joints, as can be seen in Figure 2.5. A chart is used to record the response and although different scores are used with different indices, the higher the score the greater the disease activity.

Grip strength

A dynamo sphygmomanometer can be used to measure grip strength (Figure 2.6). This is a hand-sized piece of sphygmo-manometer cuff which is attached to a dial and inflated, before assessment, to 30 mm Hg and which the patient is asked to squeeze. The scale on the dial ranges from 20–300 mm Hg. Three alternate readings are taken with each hand and the mean strength recorded for each. A note should be made of the dominant hand as this

Index	Joints	Maximum Score	Scoring
Total Tender Joint Count (as Ritchie Articular Index)	53	53	0–1
Total Swollen Joint Count (omits: temporomandibular, cervical spine, hips, talocalcaneal and midtarsal)	44	44	0–1
Thompson and Kirwan Index (omits: temporomandibular, cervical spine, sternoclavicular, shoulders, acromioclavicular, hips, talocalcaneal and midtarsal)	8	534 tenderness + swelling assessed and score weighted	0–1
American College of Rheumatology (ACR) tender joint count (as the Ritchie Articular Index but omits: cervical spine and includes the distal interphalangeal joints of the fingers and toes)	68	68	0–1
ACR swollen joint count (as ACR tender joint count but excludes the hips)	66	68	0–1

Figure 2.5: Other articular indices which may be used

reading is generally higher. In a normal hand or where there is very mild disease involvement, the reading may go off the dial beyond 300 mm Hg. However, some patients with severe disease activity can often only achieve a few points above the 30 mm Hg. Measurement of grip strength not only gives an idea of the patient's hand function but also of the degree of disease activity. Where it is significantly diminished the patient may have problems with all the functions of self-care and referral to the occupational therapist and physiotherapist will be necessary.

Visual analogue scales

Pain and stiffness can be assessed by the use of visual analogue scales, verbal rating scales or numerical rating scales. An example is given in Figure 2.7.

A visual analogue scale consists of a line of 10 centimetres; one end (0) denotes no pain and the other end (10) unbearable pain.

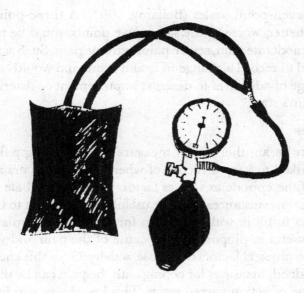

Figure 2.6: Dynamo sphygmomanometer

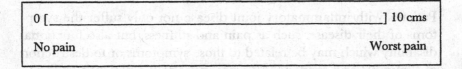

Figure 2.7: Visual analogue scale

Visual analogue scales may be drawn vertically or horizontally. Numerical rating scales are measured out from 0 to 10 against the line. The scale is explained to the patient who is then asked to place a mark on the line which represents the pain they have experienced at a given time of the day chosen by the assessor. Those with severe disease activity will score towards the higher end of the scale. This subjective assessment scale is used at each visit over a period of time and indicates how much pain the patient experiences and also whether therapy is effective. The distance from the no pain end to the patient's mark is measured in centimetres. This first recording by the patient, as with all initial measurements, is the base line, and future scores are then compared with this. Likert or verbal rating scales use adjectives to describe pain and these vary from three- to five- and seven-point scales (Bellamy, 1993). A three-point scale would use better, worse or the same. Five points would be no pain, mild pain, moderate pain, severe pain, extreme pain. Such scales can also be used to record a change in health status and would employ a similar range of adjectives to describe improvement or deterioration in the patient's state.

Pain diaries

Diaries can be another useful measure for recording pain. The patient is asked to keep a record of when the pain occurs and the duration of the episode as well as factors which exacerbate or ease the pain. In some instances it will be useful for the patient to be given a pro forma to fill in with directions for use. Such records can be extremely useful in pinpointing the cause of the pain and whether this is due to physical factors or disease activity. Once this knowledge has been gained, measures for coping with the pain can be discussed and a course of action agreed upon. This knowledge can form the basis for an ongoing assessment of the efficacy of such measures and if necessary the adoption of alternative strategies.

Health assessment questionnaires

Patients with inflammatory joint disease not only suffer the symptoms of their disease, such as pain and stiffness, but also functional disability which may be related to those symptoms or to destruction of the joints and tendons. An assessment of the patient's ability to perform everyday activities is not only useful as a measure of efficacy of treatments or interventions but is essential as a record of functional ability and quality of life. Such assessments can be made by observing how the patient undertakes certain tasks, by clinical observation or by patient self-assessment with the use of health questionnaires. These assessments enable the nurse specialist to perfect the care plan. Several validated questionnaires and indices are available to assess the rheumatology patient's functional ability.

Functional ability can be measured using the Steinbroker Index which is based on the subjective judgement of the observer whilst carefully noting the patient's functional capacity. More commonly used nowadays are the American Rheumatism Association criteria, a revised form of the Steinbroker Index. Both of these indices rate the patient's ability objectively and should be used in conjunction with a subjective assessment. The functional ability has four classifications which range from complete ability to largely or completely incapacitated (Hochberg et al., 1992).

The two most commonly used subjective questionnaires are the Stanford Health Questionnaire (HAQ) (Fries et al., 1980) and the Arthritis Impact Measurement Scales (AIMS), both of which are well validated. AIMS has been adapted for British patients (Hill et al., 1990) and asks how many times the patient was able to undertake certain activities over the previous month. HAQ has also been modified for British patients (Kirwan and Reeback, 1986) and asks patients how they manage certain activities of daily living which are divided into several categories of degrees of difficulty (see Chapter 7, Table 7.3). Both of the questionnaires are useful in deciding on the efficacy or otherwise of second-line and non-steroidal drug therapy as they can detect significant outcomes. AIMS can be completed in 20 minutes and the HAQ in eight minutes (Bellamy, 1993).

The Hospital Anxiety and Depression Scale (HAD) is a useful tool to gauge the psychological impact of inflammatory joint disease on patients. This scale was devised as a quick method to detect mood disorders of non-psychiatric patients attending hospital. It focuses on the loss of pleasureable response and has been used to suggest the need for anti-depressant therapy. It is useful for rheumatology patients as it does not include insomnia and loss of appetite, which may occur in such patients because of disease activity rather than mood changes. It is easy to complete and should take only a few minutes as a rapid response is specifically sought (Snaith and Taylor, 1985), see Chapter 5, Figure 5.1.

As with any questionnaire if patients are unable to complete the form themselves it must be remembered that the responses may not reflect accurately the patients' view. This may happen should the patient be unable to read the questionnaire because of illiteracy, poor eyesight or forgotten spectacles, or because of language difficulties. Some patients have poor hand function and for this reason are unable to fill in the questionnaire.

Physical aspects

Pain

Any exacerbation in disease activity, usually termed a 'flare', will increase the level of pain experienced by the patient with inflammatory joint disease. In order to advise and evaluate methods of pain relief, various assessment tools should be used as described earlier in this chapter. Simple analgesia such as paracetamol, co-dydramol and dihydrocodeine will normally have been prescribed for the majority of these patients. However, it is important to ascertain that such preparations are being taken regularly and at the correct dosage. The same applies for non-steroidal anti-inflammatory drugs such as Indocid (indomethacin), Naprosyn (naproxen), Brufen (ibuprofen) and Voltarol (diclofenac). These medications relieve pain as well as stiffness and swelling in the joints. Some patients are very reluctant to take medication and would prefer to use alternative means to relieve their pain. However, as with all pain control it is important to emphasise that a variety of methods can be used and that drugs can be very helpful, particularly if the pain is severe and unremitting. The nurse specialist can advise on other methods of pain relief such as hot and cold packs, rest, relaxation, joint protection, diversion and pacing of everyday activities.

When patients are in pain, any difficulty with daily activities will not only actively exacerbate their pain but will also reduce their pain threshold through the sheer effort of performing a task which is physically difficult. The Stanford Health Assessment Questionnaire (HAQ) is extremely useful for highlighting difficulties of daily living which patients commonly encounter. The answers may indicate the need for referral to the other members of the multidisciplinary team, in particular the occupational therapist who will advise on methods of joint protection including the use of splints and aids and devices such as tap turners and jar openers. Joint protection helps to prevent further damage by relieving any stress to already painful and swollen joints. Where necessary a home assessment is carried out and recommendations will be made for the provision of equipment to make life easier such as stair rails, raised toilet seats, showers and bath seats. Patients are then empowered to take control of their pain once they have the knowledge of a variety of measures which relieve or prevent pain occurring. The nurse has a unique role in assessing and enabling patients to manage their own pain.

Stiffness

Stiffness of joints and muscles, especially early in the morning or later in the day, can be a major and common problem for patients with inflammatory joint disease. There may be confusion between stiffness and pain, weakness or fatigue. It is important to decide which sensation the patient is feeling and for both the nurse and the patient to understand what is meant by stiffness (Smith Pigg, Webb Driscoll and Caniff, 1985). Joint stiffness can be described as an added sense of resistance when attempting to move a specific joint or an inability to move a joint through some part of a normal range of movement. Muscular stiffness follows excessive or unaccustomed activity and may accompany fatigue or tension. Early morning stiffness (EMS) of the joints is usually related to soft tissue swelling around the joints, particularly if the patient is undergoing a 'flare' of disease activity. EMS can last for only a few minutes or several hours and in some instances all day. The duration of EMS is a helpful guide to the degree of disease activity and indicates the amount of restriction and disability a patient undergoes before starting the daily routine. It may take hours for a patient to get up, wash and dress each morning, particularly when shoulders, wrists and hands are involved. Stiffness or 'gelling' can also occur later in the day when the patient sits down after a period of activity. Methods of relief for stiffness include the use of non-steroidal anti-inflammatory drugs, hot baths or showers, and frequent changes of position. Use of a visual analogue scale to measure the amount and severity of stiffness can assist in discussion and education about the reasons for stiffness. This helps patients to understand and use the methods of relief which are particularly suited to them and therefore to take some control of their treatment.

Fatigue

Fatigue or lack of energy is a common factor in inflammatory joint disease and is directly related to disease activity. Patients are often very concerned because they feel worn out and lethargic. Once the patients understand the relationship between disease activity and a 'flare' they often experience a profound sense of relief. They then find it easier to comply with the need for rest and relaxation when experiencing a flare, rather than trying to carry on as normal. Many patients need permission to rest as they feel guilty or upset at not being able to continue with their normal activities. As the disease activity reduces so the amount of fatigue also lessens.

Where possible other members of the family should be included in any discussions about rest and relaxation in order that they too can appreciate the need and thus help to reinforce these measures. Advice on the pacing of daily activities, for instance not completing all the ironing in one go, also enables patients to cope by reducing the strain on already inflamed joints.

Sleep disturbance due to pain often increases fatigue. Patients should be advised to take analgesia at bedtime. The use of pillows to support painful arms, shoulders and hands may also help. Some patients are provided with resting splints for wrists and legs to help relieve painful, swollen joints. Neck pain may also cause sleep disturbance and in addition to the use of analgesia the patient should be advised on how to make and use a butterfly pillow, or could be provided with a soft cervical collar. The use of pain or sleep diaries can be helpful in deciding on the cause of sleep disturbance. When the disease is particularly active patients may benefit from a period of rest in the afternoon. This will help to relax painful, tense and stiff joints, as well as muscles and tendons. In the case of a busy mother, a rest after lunch could well enable her to cope with the demanding period when children return from school. For those who go out to work, a short rest on returning home often provides the necessary respite to continue with the evening's activities.

Weight

Weight problems are common in this group of patients and a record should be kept of the patient's weight at each visit. Immobility, caused by pain, stiffness, fatigue and deformity can reduce the ability to prepare meals even if the patient is able to shop for food. Patients living on their own, particularly the elderly, may be cachexic for these reasons and also because they have difficulty in eating. Associated diseases such as Sjogren's syndrome cause a dry mouth, and some drugs such as penicillamine can cause loss of taste. Sulphasalazine and some non-steroidal anti-inflammatory drugs can cause nausea with a consequent loss of appetite.

Comfort eating, lack of exercise, steroid therapy or poor knowledge of basic healthy dietary requirements can result in obesity. Weight-bearing joints which are already inflamed or damaged by disease will be further stressed by carrying excess weight. Referral to the dietician for advice and monitoring of weight loss or gain can be helpful. The occupational therapist can provide aids and devices for the preparation and consumption of meals. For some patients it may be necessary to seek the support of Social Services for the provision of meals on wheels and a home help to assist with shopping.

Psychological aspects

Patients with chronic disease will inevitably suffer psychologically (Oberai and Kirwan, 1988). Many have to come to terms with the fact that there is no cure for their disease. When attending hospital they will see some patients who have had their disease for many years and have developed severe deformities as a result. For those who have been newly diagnosed seeing such deformities inevitably creates feelings of shock and grief. As time passes and the situation continues, maybe without any remission of disease activity, anxiety and depression can occur. Patients may also experience alterations in their lifestyle, a reduction in social activity, often loss of employment, even loss of a partner, together with severe financial difficulties. The realisation that long-term plans and expectations may never come to fruition can be devastating and cause great distress.

The nurse specialist must be aware of these feelings and have the means to assist the patient wherever possible. Sometimes it is sufficient just to provide empathy and understanding. Providing information and a means of self-help can relieve the anxiety and depression which accompanies chronic pain and stiffness (le Gallez, 1993). When patients understand exactly what is going on and how to cope with their newfound problems, they feel in control and more able to deal with the situation. In some instances the nurse specialist is unable to offer the level of counselling which severely affected patients may need, and referral to either a clinical psychologist, a psychiatric nurse specialist or a qualified counsellor is appropriate. The HAD questionnaire can be useful to determine whether the patient is psychologically depressed (see p. 110).

Alternative therapies

Unfortunately, one of the worst aspects of rheumatoid disease is that everybody knows someone who has been 'cured'. The general public tend to lump all types of arthritis together. However, arthritis is individual to each person and there is no one therapy to suit each and every patient. Patients are often urged by well-meaning sympathisers to try all sorts of treatments. Second-line drugs which induce disease suppression work by slowly building up a concentration in the body and it can take from two to four months for any benefit to occur. During this stage the nurse specialist needs to utilise her skills in order to encourage the patient to continue with therapy and manage joint pain, stiffness and discomfort by the correct use of analgesia and anti-inflammatory drugs. In addition, the patient will need support with advice about rest, relaxation and joint protection. Should the patient already be using alternative therapies there is no particular need to discourage this, providing such therapies do not lead to inadequate diet or the disuse of prescribed treatments. However, it is often worth pointing out to patients that alternative therapies can be extremely expensive and that no real proof exists as to their efficacy. But it is also worth remembering the possible placebo effect of such therapies.

Haematological and biochemical assessments

Haematological and biochemical tests are useful to detect drug toxicity as well as disease activity and efficacy. Haemoglobin (Hb), erythrocyte sedimentation rate (ESR) or plasma viscosity (PV) should be monitored. During a flare these will alter; the Hb tends to fall as the body is unable to metabolise iron properly and the ESR or PV will rise, often to dramatically high levels. A drop in neutrophil and platelet levels can reveal a reaction to drug therapy and may indicate the immediate cessation of these drugs. Non-steroidal anti-inflammatory drugs can cause peptic ulceration which results in a drop in haemoglobin. This form of anaemia is not associated with disease activity and indicates the need for further investigations, for example an endoscopy. Biochemical profiles may also reveal abnormalities due to disease activity or drug toxicity. These include raised levels of aspartate aminotransferase (AST) and alanine aminotransferase (ALT) (Alk Phos) and C-reactive protein (CRP). These chemicals are liver enzymes which can increase during disease activity. Some liver enzymes may increase without a corresponding increase in disease activity and then drug toxicity should be suspected; therapy in this instance is stopped and the test repeated. Tests may also be performed to discover levels of rheumatoid factor or of immunoglobulin levels. All second-line drug therapy requires careful and regular monitoring for which guidelines exist (BSR, 1995). These must be carefully observed for each drug. The nurse specialist should be familiar with the normal range for each haematological and biochemical test and should be aware of the possible complications of drug usage which would necessitate further laboratory examinations. Urine specimens will also be sent to the laboratory if there is an abnormality in the routine (dipstick test) clinic test. Should blood or protein be present then a mid-stream specimen of urine can be sent to the laboratory for microscopy, culture and sensitivity to rule out any possibility of a urine infection. Where protein occurs beyond +1, patients are asked to collect their urine for 24 hours and this specimen is then sent off for protein quantification. It may also be necessary to check the creatinine levels in which case a biochemical profile blood test will be necessary as well as the 24 hour urine collection.

Planning nursing care and referral to other members of the multidisciplinary team

With the variety of assessments available to the nurse specialist a clear picture of the problems experienced by patients will emerge and a plan of nursing care can be made based on the recommended solutions to these problems. However, it must be remembered that there will never be an ultimate plan as the problems which these patients experience vary from day and to day and can increase or decrease in severity. In addition to nursing care, the plan may include referral to other disciplines and care will be continued whether in the hospital clinic, ward or community.

Referrals will depend on the problem the patient is experiencing. Mention has already been made of referrals to the occupational therapist, physiotherapist and dietician. Lack of mobility can often be caused by poor footwear and the inability to purchase suitable shoes for swollen and painful feet. Referrals should be made to the orthotist (surgical fitter) for special shoes made of soft leather which are wide and deep enough to support feet which are affected by disease. Poor hand function together with restricted hip movement may result in many patients being unable to tend to their own feet. Previously simple tasks such as cutting toenails may be beyond them and referral to the chiropodist or podiatrist may be necessary.

As the rheumatic diseases are chronic, some patients may face losing their jobs and subsequent income. Therefore general advice on basic allowances such as disability and attendance allowances can be given by the nurse specialist. However, as government legislation changes frequently, more specialised and up-to-date information and help may be needed from the social worker, Citizen's Advice Bureau or Arthritis Care.

Most hospitals provide a chronic pain clinic service. In the case of severe and unremitting pain it may be necessary to refer the patient to such clinics. The specialist team consists of doctors, nurses and physiotherapists who can advise on other methods of pain relief such as the use of TENS machines, acupuncture or hypnotherapy. Patients may have a problem with body image and self-esteem. Deformed and swollen hands can cause worry and embarrassment for some patients and here counselling can often be of benefit. There may be problems of a sexual nature because of damaged joints causing pain, stiffness and the illness causing fatigue. Such difficulties with personal relationships usually require expert counselling and may be a case for referral to SPOD (The association to aid the sexual and personal relationships of people with a disability), a counsellor or clinical psychologist. However, sometimes just the sympathetic ear of the nurse will often be all that is required and advice can be given about taking relaxing warm baths and analgesia to help the situation. Where it is necessary to undertake counselling, the nurse specialist, as in all her roles, needs to be aware of any personal limitations and must be prepared to refer the patient to someone who is more experienced or appropriately qualified. Part of the nurse specialist role is having the correct information with regard to referral to other disciplines (see the section in Chapter 5, 'Sexual Relationships and Arthritis', pp. 124–32).

A nursing care plan can be made once baseline assessments have been undertaken and should include all problems and how they are to be dealt with. New problems can be added as they arise and as old problems are sorted out or change they can be altered or added to the plan. Problems will come under the headings 'physical' and 'psychological' and goals for reducing or clearing them should be set with the patient's involvement. Methods on how to achieve this should be discussed and agreed jointly with the patient. Prior to discharge from the nurse specialist's care assessments should be made to evaluate the outcomes of that episode of care.

Education

Patient information and education

Education of the patient with a rheumatic disease is vital as with all chronic diseases, and this is an essential component of the role of nurse specialist. Patient education can take several forms; it may be given as verbal information on a one-to-one basis, in group sessions using the group to stimulate questions or as written information. Various education programmes on arthritis exist and some studies suggest that such programmes are effective in changing patients' knowledge, behaviour, psychological and health status (Lorig, Konkol and Gonzalez, 1987). Research suggests that written information reinforces verbal information and should therefore be part of a planned education programme (Williams et al., 1987). Nurses as well as doctors are targeted for criticism as poor communicators by Maycock (1991) who recommends that professionals undertaking patient education should have the training and skills necessary to communicate effectively with patients (see Chapter 5).

It may be that a few words of advice and explanation are all that is needed and indeed in the early stages some patients are unable to cope with more than this at each visit. Coming to terms with a chronic disease can be a long and traumatic experience. The nurse specialist, physiotherapist, occupational therapist, pharmacist, dietician and doctor all help in educating patients. However, the nurse is often the one person in the team whom the patient sees regularly and is therefore in a unique position to instigate and continue the education and information process (Close, 1988). Patients need to understand how their bodies are affected by their disease and how their therapies should work. They are more likely to comply with treatment if they understand the reasons for it. Information should also be given about the possible side-effects of such therapies. Advice and information about how to manage their disease enables patients to make an informed choice and will affect how they eventually cope with their disease.

Written patient information

Written patient information is regarded as being essential in the management of a chronic disease. Patients themselves feel that they need leaflets not only about the management of their symptoms but more specifically about their drug therapies (Kay and Punchak, 1988). It has been shown that written information used in conjunction with verbal information increases patients' levels of knowledge (Vignos, Parker and Thompson, 1976). Ley (1982) contends that a significant degree of non-compliance is due to failure of comprehension and this aspect of written information should be regularly addressed. When compiling leaflets or any other written information account must be taken not only of readability but also of presentation, font size, durability, size and colour of the paper or the card which is used (Arthur, 1995). Dixon and Park (1990) set out guidelines for improving leaflets and put the argument forward that nurses are in a position to ensure that information is acceptable to the majority of patients.

In the field of rheumatology the Arthritis and Rheumatism Council and Arthritis Care, both charitable foundations, produce many leaflets for patients (MacFarlane et al., 1991). These cover a wide range of subjects: most of the common rheumatic diseases, drugs for arthritis and practical matters such as 'Choosing Shoes' and 'Driving with Arthritis'. Full advantage should be taken of this useful resource. However, the nurse specialist will benefit patients by producing leaflets on specific drug therapies as rheumatologists tend to have differing monitoring schedules for the second-line therapies. Although there are recognised guidelines from the British Society of Rheumatology (1995) these by no means satisfy the differing criteria which exist within different areas of the country.

Providing patients with information is an important aspect of the nurse specialist's role. The DHHS Patient's Charter (1991) states that every citizen has the right to a clear explanation of any proposed treatment. Pharmaceutical manufacturers have a legal requirement to supply patient information leaflets for all newly introduced products dispensed in their original packs as outlined in the EU directive 92/27/EEC. The emphasis in this directive is on new products and original packs. This raises the question of whether patients who obtain regular medications from hospital pharmacies, where in general original packs are not used, actually receive written information about their drugs (Furnell et al., 1994). The normal practice is that when patients receive drugs from hospital pharmacies they do not receive their drugs in an original pack. Simple instructions are written on the hospital pack and a verbal explanation is given by the pharmacist. Therefore patients may not receive a separate information leaflet.

Continuity of care

Appointments are made for follow-up or referral to other specialists and in addition liaison with the practice or community nurse is especially important to ensure that monitoring guidelines are understood and adhered to. In some instances it may be relevant for the nurse specialist to visit local general practices to assist with the setting up of arthritis clinics (Dargie and Proctor, 1994; Helliwell and O'Hara, 1995). The degree to which patients are followed up by the nurse specialist will depend on the severity of the disease activity and that patient's ability to cope. A help line is a useful resource; however, before setting up such a facility the nurse specialist must be sure that there are alternatives for manning this during periods of leave.

Research

In the past it has not been uncommon for nurses in the ward setting to act as data collectors for nurse researchers (Denyes et al., 1989). In rheumatology nursing the role of the nurse specialist developed from that of nurses employed solely to assess patients in clinical trials, as described earlier in the chapter. The discipline of advanced practice should include an element of research and thereby enable the nurse specialist to integrate theory and practice. Education to a higher level will ensure that research becomes an integral element of advanced practice and nurse specialists will be in an ideal situation to bridge the divide between researchers and practical nurses. Areas of research which should concern the nurse specialist in rheumatology are: patient education and information, nurse-led clinics, new initiatives in nursing, expanded practice such as intra-articular injections, nurse prescribing and also the psychological aspects of the disease. Research into all aspects of nursing care is essential and useful to audit and justify practice. Indeed it may well be that in the future purchasers of the service will demand that such research and audit has been undertaken and is available for them to decide whether nurse specialists provide a worthwhile service (Brocklehurst, 1995).

Clinical research studies

Clinical research studies are essential to push back therapeutic boundaries and provide patients with further therapeutic options. As the majority of the rheumatic diseases are chronic with no known cure, drug companies are continually seeking new treatments to offer patients. Many second-line drugs which are used regularly today have been the focus of such studies in the not too distant past. Specialist expertise is invaluable in helping to set up such studies by ensuring that the patient is fully informed, written patient information is comprehensible and ethical issues are addressed. Patients involved in clinical research studies may be offered a higher level of involvement with the nurse specialist, more than they would normally receive if they were being seen in a routine clinic. Visits are often fortnightly and progress to monthly intervals. This offers the nurse specialist the opportunity to use metrology skills to assess the patient, record data, evaluate progress, decide on the need for referral and ensure continuity of care. Serial clinical assessments are an essential and routine part of the evaluation of the progress of patients participating in clinical trials. Descriptions of many of these assessments have been already given in this chapter. The nurse specialist should be familiar with international guidelines (WMA, 1989) and codes for good clinical practice (Brookwood, 1996) which cover ethical considerations, patient consent, confidentiality and documentation within clinical research studies. Funding from such studies often enables departments to expand and provide patients with facilities and services which may not normally be available.

The future of the rheumatology nurse specialist

The future of the rheumatology nurse specialist will depend on the nursing profession and how nurses choose to take the role forward. Many facets of this have already been discussed earlier. It may be that patients will prefer that some procedures, previously seen as the prerogative of the medical profession, are undertaken by nurses. An experienced nurse specialist will have more knowledge and skills than a junior house officer new in post. Fund-holding general practitioners may prefer to purchase the skills of the nurse specialist rather than monitor their own patients on second-line drug therapy. This could be either in the hospital or general practice environment. Nurse-led outreach clinics and screening of patients for referral to the rheumatology consultant are already proposed within some hospital trusts. One fact is certain, that the role of nurse specialists will extend and expand further as we reach the year 2000. Nurses need to be educated to accommodate this growth of their role and the individuals who show initiative and drive will lead this advancement in nursing. Nurses will continue to be accountable for their own practice but will be in a better position to decide on their own future. By the beginning of the next century nurse specialists may well be commonplace and will provide a service based on nursing care and the holistic approach but combining some aspects of medical care.

In summary, the main issues that will influence the future of the nurse specialist will be:

(1) education to first or master's degree level;
(2) expansion of the role in conjunction with the reduction of junior doctors' hours;
(3) the ability of nurse specialists to be leaders in clinical practice;
(4) the position of nurse specialists as expert clinicians to develop nursing and influence many aspects of the current health care system.

Case Study

Patient: Mrs W. Wright
Age: 40 years
Status: Married with two children, a girl aged 10 years and a boy aged 8 years.
Disease: Rheumatoid arthritis. Disease duration of 12 months.

Mrs Wright was referred to the nurse-led clinic for the introduction and monitoring of EC sulphasalazine therapy. She had been given a leaflet about this treatment at her appointment with the consultant rheumatologist the previous week. During the 12 months that Mrs Wright had had rheumatoid arthritis her symptoms had been controlled by the use of analgesia and non-steroidal anti-inflammatory drugs. However, over the past few weeks the pain and stiffness in her joints had increased. X-rays of her hands and wrists revealed some thinning of the bones and also small erosions at the 2nd and 3rd metacarpophalangeal joints of both hands.

At the first visit, which was booked for half an hour, the nurse specialist discussed symptoms and drug therapy with Mrs Wright to discover her levels of knowledge, her worries and problems. A Ritchie articular index was performed to pin-point exactly which joints were involved and to what extent. Questions were asked about the duration of early morning stiffness, and a self-assessment health questionnaire and visual analogue scale for pain assessment were completed. Grip strengths were measured, and Mrs Wright was weighed and found to be overweight at 80 kilograms.

The main problems were:

- early morning stiffness lasting 60 minutes;
- pain in hands, shoulders, knees, and feet;
- fatigue and lack of sleep;
- decrease in mobility;
- excess weight;
- difficulties with self-care;
- worries about body image;
- decrease in self-esteem.

Use of the Ritchie articular index revealed:

- painful shoulders with restricted range of movement;
- swollen wrists, metacarpophalangeal and proximal interphalangeal joints;
- painful and swollen knees;
- painful feet with swollen metatarsophalangeal joints.

Mrs Wright filled in the Health Assessment Questionnaire herself although this was difficult with her painful hands. She was experiencing difficulties with:

- washing and dressing;
- washing her hair;
- getting into the bath;
- turning taps and opening jars;
- cooking meals and cleaning
- walking and shopping.

Plan of nursing care

The aim of the nursing care plan was to enable the patient to understand her disease and treatments in order to develop strategies and coping mechanisms for dealing with the day-to-day variations in disease activity. Once EC sulphasalazine therapy became effective Mrs Wright should be able to revert to a more normal lifestyle.

The nurse specialist helped Mrs Wright to deal with the various problems in the following ways over a period of several weeks. The plan of care inevitably varied from visit to visit in line with the flitting nature of rheumatoid arthritis. Information was given by degrees as masses of information provided in a short time is likely to cause confusion and anxiety.

Stiffness

- Mrs Wright did not like taking tablets. The nurse specialist explained how regular use of non-steroidal anti-inflammatory drugs, such as Voltarol which had been prescribed for Mrs Wright, would help decrease the stiffness in her joints. Other measures to relieve stiffness such as hot baths, showers, heat pads and changes in position were also discussed.

Pain

- The use of analgesia to gain the optimum relief from pain was explained as were other methods of relief such as heat, cold, rest, relaxation and joint protection.
- Wrist splints were provided and their use explained.

Fatigue and lack of sleep

- It was explained to Mrs Wright that disease activity affects the whole body giving symptoms of fatigue and depression. Sleep patterns and the need for periods of rest and relaxation were discussed. A leaflet on coping with a flare of arthritis was read and relevant strategies were discussed.

Decrease in mobility

- Mrs Wright was wearing shoes with high heels. Her lack of mobility was due to painful knees and feet. The nurse specialist explained that pain relief measures would help but that she would benefit by wearing shoes which supported her feet and did not place any strain on her knees. A referral was made to the orthotist to supply metatarsal pads to fit into some lace-up shoes which Mrs Wright already had.
- Mrs Wright was asked about her weight and she admitted to not being happy about this. It was explained that being overweight exacerbated the problems of inflamed knees, ankles and feet. A healthy diet was discussed and Mrs Wright asked to be referred to the dietician.

Difficulties with self-care

- Mrs Wright's problems with self-care were mainly due to her painful shoulders and hands. She preferred to take a bath rather than a shower but it was decided that a shower was the best option for the time being. As her knees were also painful and she was overweight it was difficult for her husband to help her out of the bath. A referral was made to the occupational therapist for a bath seat to help with this situation. Her husband was happy to help her with washing her hair and back and also helping her to dress. She explained that although he did this willingly she felt uncomfortable with the situation. She was reassured that this would not go on indefinitely and that she would regain her independence as her disease activity decreased.

Body image
- Mrs Wright's main concern was with wearing sensible rather than fashionable shoes. She felt that although sensible shoes would increase her mobility they did not increase her confidence in her appearance. However, she agreed to try wearing her sensible shoes whilst her feet were so painful and to keep her fashion shoes for special occasions.
- Her other concern was with her swollen hands which she felt were visible to all. The importance of rest to help reduce the swelling was emphasised and also reassurance given that as the disease activity reduced her hands would become less swollen.
- Mrs Wright has a very pretty face and hair. The nurse specialist suggested that emphasising these attributes to draw attention away from her feet and hands might help Mrs Wright to feel more confident.

Self-esteem
- Mrs Wright was not happy with herself as she felt unable to fulfil her role of wife and mother properly. Pain and stiffness caused her to get cross with the children. Her husband had to help with household chores, ironing and caring for the children as well as dressing and washing her. She was reassured that this situation was unlikely to continue indefinitely and that she would be able to take on more of her chores as her disease activity decreased. The future was discussed and Mrs Wright expressed her fear of ending up in a wheelchair. Reassurance was given that this was unlikely to happen. Emphasis was put on the need for Mrs Wright to understand the disease and therapies so that she could get the optimum benefit from treatment and cope with any exacerbations of disease activity as they arose.

To help her do this:

- Mrs Wright was asked whether she had read the leaflet about EC sulphasalazine and if she had any worries about this treatment. She did not fully understand the need for blood tests. This was discussed and reinforcement given that sulphasalazine was not effective until 10 to 12 weeks of therapy and that the Voltarol tablets should be continued. A shared care card to record blood results was given to Mrs Wright and the meaning of the results and the importance of having blood tests were discussed. The importance of taking only enteric sulphasalazine (EC) was also emphasized.
- Mrs Wright was referred to patient education classes for information and support. The groups are small and informal and patients are encouraged to participate by sharing their experiences and knowledge and by asking questions. Many patients find these sessions helpful as discussion with their peers can often bring relief when others understand what they are going through.

The following topics are covered although these may differ between hospitals:

- the rheumatology service and what to expect from it;
- the disease process, blood tests and results, X-rays;
- diet and arthritis;
- drug therapy;
- rest, relaxation and exercise;
- joint protection and aids to daily living.

Mrs Wright told the nurse specialist that she felt relieved to be able to talk to someone at such length about her disease and how it affected her and her family. It was arranged that she continue to see the nurse specialist for monitoring and referral to other team members until she was successfully and effectively established on EC sulphasalazine therapy. Regular blood tests would be taken and a visit to the consultant rheumatologist arranged before discharge to the care of the general practitioner and practice nurse. An alternative arrangement would have been for Mrs Wright to be monitored on a combined care basis. The routine monitoring would be provided by the general practitioner and practice nurse who would liaise with the consultant rheumatologist and specialist nurse when necessary.

Should the therapy not be effective Mrs Wright would remain

under the care of the consultant and nurse specialist until an effective treatment could be found. Problems would be assessed at each visit and referrals made to other disciplines as the need arose. Documentation was kept in the patient's notes. This enabled other members of the team to be aware of the nursing care plan. The nurse specialist was the one team member who saw the patient regularly and was able to ensure that continuity of care was maintained within the rheumatology team. At the last visit to the nurse specialist the assessments (Ritchie articular index, health assessment questionnaire, visual analogue scale and grip strengths) were all undertaken. Blood results (ESR and CRP) and weight and a list of referrals were also kept. These factors were to be used to evaluate the nurse specialist service and provision of patient care, and could also be used when auditing the service provided by the rheumatology team.

References

Alexander MF (1989) Nursing practitioners, researchers, teachers and managers all have the same goal. Guest editorial. Journal of Advanced Nursing 14: 991–2.

Arthur VA (1994) Nursing care of patients with rheumatoid arthritis. British Journal of Nursing 3(7): 325–31.

Arthur VA (1995) Written patient information: a review of the literature. Journal of Advanced Nursing 21: 1081–6.

Barker P (1988) A genuine art. Nursing Times 84(36): 44–5.

Bellamy N (1993) Musculoskeletal Clinical Metrology. Lancaster, UK: Kluwer.

Bowling A (1981) Should we have nurse practitioners? World Medicine June 13.

British Society for Rheumatology (BSR) (1995) Guidelines for Second Line Drug Monitoring. London: British Society for Rheumatology.

Brocklehurst N (1995) Specialists for sale. Primary Health Care 5(9): 8,10,12.

Bryan J (1982) Taking over the pressure. Nursing Mirror December 8.

Bysshe J (1992) Recent developments in the ENB Framework and higher award. British Journal of Nursing 1(13): 666–70.

Close A (1988) Patient education: a literature review. Journal of Advanced Nursing 13: 203–13.

Dargie L, Proctor J (1994) Setting up an arthritis clinic. Community Outlook (July): 14-17.

DHHS (1977) The Extended Role of the Clinical Nurse – Legal Implications and Training Requirements. HC(77)22. London: Department of Health and Social Security.

DHHS (1991) The Patient's Charter. London: Department of Health and Social Security.

Denyes MJ, O'Conner NA, Oakley D, Ferguson S (1989) Integrating nursing theory, practice and research through collaborative research. Journal of Advanced Nursing 14: 141–5.

Derrick S (1989) What are the legal implications of extended nursing roles? The Professional Nurse (April).

Dixon E, Park R (1990) Do patients understand written health information? Nursing Outlook 38(6), 278–81.

English National Board (1991) Framework for Continuing Professional Education for Nurses, Midwives and Health Visitors – Guide to Implementation. London: ENB.

Eular Handbook of Standard Methods (1995) Assessing Disease Activity in Rheumatoid Arthritis. Uppsala, Sweden: Pharmacia, Graphic Communications.

Evans B, Jackson H, Shepherd J (1993) Pathways for PREP: a consumer-orientated model. British Journal of Nursing 2(7): 375–7.

Fries JF, Spitz PW, Kraines RG, Holman HR (1980) Measurement of patient outcome in arthritis. Arthritis and Rheumatism. 23: 137–45.

Furnell M, Habing-Ridout H, Cross J, Wray L, Dodds L, Collins G (1994) Patient information leaflet. The Pharmaceutical Journal 252: 7.

Garbett R (1996) The growth of nurse-led care. Nursing Times 92(1): 29.

Helliwell PS, O'Hara M (1995) Shared care between hospital and general practice: an audit of disease-modifying drug monitoring in rheumatoid arthritis. British Journal of Rheumatology 34: 673–6.

Hill J (1985) Nursing clinics for arthritics. Nursing Times September 18: 33–4.

Hill J (1986) Patient evaluation of a rheumatology nursing clinic. Nursing Times July 2.

Hill J, Bird HA, Lawton CW, Wright V (1990) The arthritis impact measurement scales: an Anglicized version to assess the outcome of British patients with rheumatoid arthritis. British Journal of Rheumatology 29: 193–6.

Hill J, Bird HA, Harmer R, Wright V, Lawton C (1994) An evaluation of the effectiveness, safety and acceptability of a nurse practitioner in a rheumatology outpatient clinic. British Journal of Rheumatology 33: 283–8.

Hochberg MC, Chang RW, Dwosh I, Lindsey S, Pincus T, Wolfe F (1992) The American College of Rheumatology 1991 revised criteria for the classification of global functional status in rheumatoid arthritis. Arthritis and Rheumatism 35(5): 498–502.

Hoover J, van Ooijen E (1995) Back to basics. Nursing Times 91(33): 42–3.

Kay EA, Punchak SS (1988) Patient understanding of the causes and medical treatment of rheumatoid arthritis. British Journal of Rheumatology 27: 396–8.

Kirwan J, Reeback J (1986) Stanford Health Questionnaire Modified to Assess Disability in British Patients with Rheumatoid Arthritis. British Journal of Rheumatology 25: 206–9.

Le Gallez P (1981) So what's a metrologist? Nursing Times 77(45): 1927.

Le Gallez P (1985) Rheumatology health education. Nursing Mirror 160(3): 37–9.

Le Gallez P (1993) Rheumatoid arthritis: effects on the family. Nursing Standard 7(39): 30–4.

Ley P (1982) Satisfaction, compliance and communication. British Journal of Clinical Psychology 21: 241–54.

Lorig K, Konkol L, Gonzalez V (1987) Arthritis patient education: a review of the literature. Patient Education and Counseling 10: 207–52.

MacFarlane A, Gaffin J, Jones R, Seifert M (1991) General public education. Annals of Rheumatic Diseases 50: 435–8.

Maycock J (1991) Role of health professionals in patient education. Annals of Rheumatic Disease 50: 429–34.

Notter J (1995) Marketing specialist practice to managers and purchasers. British Journal of Nursing 4(22): 1330–4.

Oberai B, Kirwan J (1988) Psychological factors in patients with chronic rheumatoid arthritis. Annals of Rheumatic Diseases 47: 969–71.

Ritchie D, Boyle JA, McInnes JM, Jasani MK, Dalakos TG, Grieveson P, Watson Buchanan WC (1968) Clinical studies with an articular index for the assessment of joint tenderness in patients with rheumatoid arthritis. Quarterly Journal of Medicine, New Series 37: 393–406.

Ross F (1982) An expanded role. Community Outlook September 15: 301–2.

Royal College of Nursing (1989) Standards of Care, Rheumatic Disease Nursing. London: RCN: 1.

Ryan S (1996) Defining the role of the specialist nurse. Nursing Standard 10(17): 27–9.

Shaw MC (1993) The discipline of nursing: historical roots, current perspectives, future directions. Journal of Advanced Nursing 18: 1651–6.

Smith Pigg J, Webb Driscoll P, Caniff R (1985) Rheumatology Nursing, A Problem Oriented Approach. New York: Wiley.

Snaith RP, Taylor CM (1985) Rating scales for depression and anxiety: a current perspective. British Journal of Clinical Pharmacy 19: 175–205.

Stillwell B (1981) Role expansion for the nurse. Journal of Community Nursing 5(3):17–18.

Stillwell B (1984) The nurse in practice. Nursing Mirror 158(21): 17–19.

Stillwell B (1985) Prevention and health: the concern of nursing. Journal of Royal Society of Health 1: 31–4.

Storr G (1988) The clinical nurse specialist: from the outside looking in. Journal of Advanced Nursing 13: 265–72.

Turner C (1987) Educated for practice: the diabetes nurse specialist. Senior Nurse 7(5): 28–9.

United Kingdom Central Council for Nursing, Midwifery and Health Visiting (1992) The Scope of Professional Practice. London: UKCCNMHV.

Vignos PJ, Parker WT, Thompson HM (1976) Evaluation of a clinic education programme for patients with RA. Journal of Rheumatology 3(2): 155–65.

Williams J, Ashcroft B, Carter A, Comyn C (1987) Using printed materials effectively in health promotion. Health Education Journal 46(4): 165–7.

World Medical Assembly (1989) Declaration of Helsinki (Revised version). France: Fekney-VoltaineWMA.

Useful address:

The Association of Specialist Nurses and Advanced Practitioners (SNAP), The Nottingham Trent University, Burton Street, Nottingham, NG1 4BU, UK.

Chapter 3
The rheumatology ward and investigations

SARAH RYAN

Being admitted to a rheumatology ward can be a very daunting experience for any patient. Patients may be unsure as to the cause of their problems and be experiencing pain, depression and anxiety. Also patients are separated from both family and support networks. Welcoming patients onto the ward and familiarising them with their new temporary environment will begin to settle them and reduce anxiety. The initial perception the patients have will influence their whole stay. The nurse must be aware of the patients' feelings and acknowledge and support them at this early stage. This will enable patients to feel secure and so gain the most benefit from their inpatient stay.

Nursing can be a dynamic activity, a chance for growth, development and education provided the opportunity is taken. If it is not, then nursing will be a static procedure, rigid in its approach, dominated and structured by task with no time for individualised need. The vision for nurses caring for a patient with a rheumatological disorder must be to accept the challenge offered and utilise their skills and opportunities to engage in a therapeutic relationship with the patient, and to provide care that has meaning and relevance within the patient's frame of reference.

Throughout this chapter, the emphasis will be to examine the positive contribution that nurses can make. Practice must be centred around a philosophy of care that governs the assessment, planning, implementation and evaluation of care management within a holistic setting. There will also be focus on investigations that occur in an inpatient setting to increase understanding as to the relevance and purpose of these procedures.

The Essence of Nursing

Philosophy of care for a rheumatology ward

The philosophy of care will underpin practice and is a statement of beliefs to govern nursing actions. It is important within the ward environment that all nurses contribute to the development of a philosophy and are committed to it. This will provide ownership, leading to consistency and unity in practice. The philosophy can be divided into four main areas, but must always retain the focus on the patient (see Figure 3.1).

(1) Beliefs about the individual:
- The individual has a right to be involved in decision making and to have informed choices (e.g. exercise programmes, drug therapy, etc.).
- The individual's values, perceptions and expectations will be central to care planning (e.g. pacing activities may be viewed negatively until the benefits are experienced).
- The individual has many roles, within both the social and occupational arena, and the effect of the illness must be addressed in a holistic manner (e.g. involving family members in care planning).

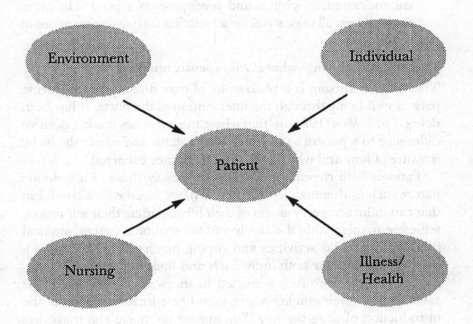

Figure 3.1: Philosophy of care

(2) Beliefs about nursing:
- The nurse will assist the patient along the continuum of adjust-ment and in the development of those skills required to obtain effective coping mechanisms (e.g. relaxation skills for pain management).
- The nurse will provide individualised care within the patient's frame of reference for both the patient and the family (e.g. advise on how to cope with a flare of the condition).
- The nurse will engage in a therapeutic relationship with the patient (e.g. spend time listening to the patient's concerns).
- The nurse will empower and educate patients about their condi-tion (e.g. when to take analgesia).

(3) Beliefs about the environment:
- The ward environment must provide an atmosphere conducive for patient involvement and be supportive in assisting the nurses in providing therapeutic care.

(4) Beliefs about illness/health:
- Health is a condition where systems of an individual are in harmony with each other. These include physiological, psychologi-cal, sociocultural, spiritual and developmental aspects. The nurse must address all these states for adaptation and well-being to occur.

Therapeutic nursing: what is therapeutic nursing?

Therapeutic nursing is a philosophy of care directed at improving patient well-being through the intervention of the nurse. It has been defined by Powell (1991) as 'that where the nurse has made a positive difference to a patient's or client's health status and where she or he is aware of how and why this positive difference occurred.'

Patients with rheumatic illnesses, especially those of a systemic nature such as rheumatoid arthritis (RA), are faced with a condition that can influence every aspect of their life including their self-image, self-esteem, role within the family and occupational system, physical functioning, social activities and coping mechanisms. It can be a bewildering time for both individuals and their family. Newly diag-nosed patients are often admitted to the ward environment for assessment of their condition and to instigate treatment such as the introduction of drug therapy. The impact the nurse can make has enormous potential; a relationship can be formed between the nurse and patients which allows the patients to express their fears and expectations within a supportive environment with a professional who has expertise and is familiar with the situation. Powell's definition includes two elements: the nurse's willingness to make a positive difference to the patient's care and the knowledge as to what the positive difference is. For a newly diagnosed patient, to be given a lot of information about the condition she or he has immediately after diagnosis may be totally inappropriate for that individual. This is why it is of the utmost importance for the nurse to reach a rapport with each individual as soon as possible so that information, support and education about the condition can be given at a time when it is appropriate for the patient and not the nurse. To provide information at a time when the patient is unreceptive will increase the potential for fear, anxiety and depression to take hold.

Therefore, if therapeutic care is to become a reality and not just rhetoric, we must ensure that the philosophy of care reflects this and that nurses are not only encouraged to practise this way, but are also provided with the mechanism and management structure to do so. If the philosophy of the rheumatology ward is to place greater emphasis on task allocation rather than individualised care, then, no matter how motivated, the nurse will not be able to practise in a therapeutic manner. There has to be a commitment from nursing management that therapeutic care is important and that resources will be available to match that commitment. Health policy, including the Department of Health's *A Vision for the Future* (1993), emphasises the importance of patients being allocated a 'named nurse' during their hospital stay. It is easy on paper to allocate a named individual, but what is more important is providing the infrastructure on both a micro- and macrolevel to ensure that the ethos behind such policies has meaning in the workplace and can be implemented. The UKCC Code of Conduct (1992) clearly emphasises that nurses should act in such a way as to safeguard the well-being and interests of the patient. If we do not seek to adopt a therapeutic role, then we are clearly not fulfilling this fundamental requirement of nursing care.

The opportunities for nurses are ever expanding in the changing face of health care. Through documents such as the UKCC Scope of Professional Practice (1992), nurses have been given a very clear mandate by their governing body to develop their knowledge and skills still further to enhance patient-focused care. Perhaps before we look to empower patients to participate in care management, we should first empower nurses so that they are able to implement the type of care that promotes adaptation and contributes to well-being.

The role of the nurse is a complex one, but the foundation from which nurses practise should be based on knowledge, thus enabling patients to adapt to their alteration in health by developing positive coping mechanisms within a partnership with a named nurse or team of nurses.

The contribution of other allied health professionals should not be forgotten here. Such is the nature of rheumatic illness that the patient will benefit from involvement with other members of the multidisciplinary team, including the physiotherapist, occupational therapist, orthotist, podiatrist, etc., but it is the nursing team that has the 24 hour contact with the patient and who will spend more time with the patient than any other health professional. This is what makes the nursing role so important and provides the opportunity for care to develop that is meaningful to the patient.

Nursing as a therapy was discussed in 1986 by McMahon, who considered four areas in which nursing can be considered to be therapeutic. These include:

(1)   the nurse–patient relationship;
(2)   conventional nursing interventions, e.g. pressure area care;
(3)   unconventional nursing interventions, e.g. massage;
(4)   patient teaching.

All of these are very appropriate to a patient with a rheumatological condition and can be practised within the rheumatology ward. Nursing must not turn away from so-called 'alternative interventions', such as massage. To a patient with fibromyalgia, massage may be the only intervention to provide relief, especially as this is a condition where medical intervention has little to offer. More research is needed in this area so that the patient can be given information as to the benefit of this and all interventions. The fundamental aspect of therapeutic nursing in the ward environment is the nurse–patient relationship.

It is only by entering into a relationship with the patient that the nurse can ascertain those areas causing greatest concern for the patient. By talking and developing an understanding of the patient as a person, it may become clear that the patient is worried about the financial implications of the illness or the ability to continue to work. If the patient is not provided with the opportunity to share this information it may not come to light. Yet the stress of financial worries could have contributed to increased pain and depression. The encounter will also enable the nurse to plan care that has relevance to the patient and arrange a visit from the disablement employment adviser.

The nurse–patient relationship

All nurses can claim to enter into a relationship with their patients, but it is the nature and substance of the relationship that is all important. Nursing has traditionally centred on physical aspects of care: feeding; caring for personal hygiene; administration of medications; recording of observations; performing aseptic procedures etc., but for patients with a chronic illness, sole concentration on physical aspects will not provide the care required to begin to assist the patient to accept the condition. It is easy to see why concentration on physical tasks predominates in some areas, as these involve little emotional commitment from the nurse and can be carried out with minimal interaction. Patients expect nurses to be competent practitioner by virtue of their occupational status, but it is their emotional style that patients equate with quality of care (Smith, 1992). If we accept that intimacy and reciprocity are the twin ingredients of a therapeutic relationship which helps to move the patient along the continuum of adjustment (Figure 3.2), then the nurse will need to involve something of themselves in the relationship.

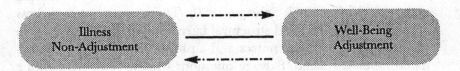

Figure 3.2: The Continuum of Adjustment

This two-way process will have benefits for both the patient and the nurse, as she or he begins to develop a knowledge base from the patient's frame of reference. Illness has meaning and significance for patients in how it impacts on their way of life. For example, a patient with an inflamed hand will not only be concerned by the visual appearance of the hand, but the limitations the synovitis may place on functional capabilities, e.g. driving, care of personal needs and work role. The continuum in Figure 3.2 is not a static entity. For example, a patient may have reached a state of well-being and adjustment but a flare of the condition, combined with non-responsiveness to drug therapy, may move him or her in the direction of non-adjustment. As a patient's condition and its impact on lifestyle alters, so will the nurse–patient relationship, with patients requiring optimum support, education and understanding when faced with a new situation or worsening of their present situation. It is at times of crisis that the patient will require an inpatient stay. To be admitted to an environment that has its roots in therapeutic care will be of great benefit to the patient. The nature of the nurse–patient relationship will influence the patient's adjustment to the situation. An approach which shows interest in obtaining the patient's perspective on care management will have real meaning for the patient.

Some patients admitted to the ward may have already achieved coping mechanisms and may not require as much support as other individuals who are struggling to grasp an understanding of their illness. The nurse will be able to act as coordinator of care options within the ward environment, engaging the services of other members of the multidisciplinary team as required, e.g. a patient with signs of clinical depression would benefit from seeing a psychologist, whereas a patient who expresses difficulty with food preparation will need to see the occupational therapist. Only by utilising the skills of motivator, supporter and coach (Benner and Wrubel, 1989) within the framework of a therapeutic relationship can the nurse begin to plan care that is individual in nature and relevant to the patient concerned.

There are critics of what has been termed a new nursing approach (Melia, 1987; Salvage, 1990). These commentators draw attention to material and structural barriers, such as a reduction in the number of qualified nurses and a philosophy of care still dominated by task. Indeed, Salvage questions whether patients desire a close relationship if their immediate concern is likely to be relief from pain and discomfort. This may be relevant to patients experiencing acute illness, but in chronic conditions it will take time and close relationships to begin to cope with aspects such as pain and stiffness that can be alleviated but not cured. This is where individual assessment is so important. A patient with RA may not perceive any benefits of developing a relationship. This must be respected as long as the patient is aware of how to renew or re-establish contact should a problem occur that is outside the patient's present domain of control. The choice must lie with the patient, but it must be informed choice. For care that is to encourage empowerment, there has to be a commitment and shared philosophy that the patient's perception, values and expectations will be part of the management plan. Without empowerment, the patient will be in a state of powerlessness, helplessness and hopelessness. Therefore, the relationship between patient and nurse can ensure that this state does not occur, or, if it does, that it is recognised and dealt with.

Aspects of Care Management

Work organisation

How a rheumatology ward decides to organise its care delivery will have a major bearing on whether or not it is possible to develop a therapeutic relationship with the patient. Work organisation should develop from the philosophy of care. In the philosophy for rheumatology nurses mentioned previously, it would not be possible to support the beliefs about the individual, nursing, environment or health if task allocation was the method of care delivery that predominated. Task allocation does still occur today and can be found in the practice of team nursing. This is not to say that team nursing cannot be a mode of implementing therapeutic care, but is a reminder that any system of care delivery can become task orientated if the nursing team does not share the same philosophy. As rheumatology nurses are advancing their practice in the ward into areas such as joint aspirations and injections, it must be hoped that nurses will not concentrate solely on technical procedures but that they will implement these procedures as part of a complete holistic care package. In fact, if nurses are competent in these skills and have already established a relationship with the patient, it will be reassuring and beneficial for the patient to have these procedures carried out by someone they can already relate to.

A nursing model

In order to apply our philosophy of care, rheumatology nurses need a model that places individuals and their related needs at its centre. The Royal College of Nursing Rheumatology Forum Model (1989) (Figure 3.3) attempts to do just that and addresses both the physical and psychological impact of illness, essential when caring for a patient with a chronic illness but often neglected in other models. An alternative model is seen in Chapter 4, Figure 4.1.

The RCN model provides a structural framework to guide the thought process when assessing and planning care. No model is inclusive but the forum model can provide the starting point for each ward to develop a model that is specific to its needs. Indeed it could be expanded on to cover the needs of the family and effects on employment, for instance.

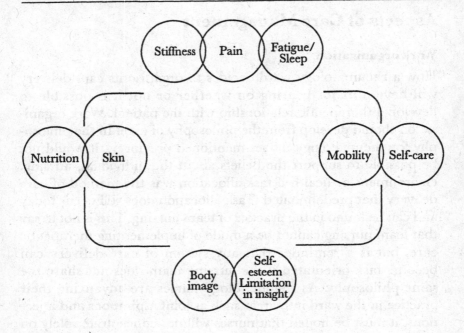

Figure 3.3: The rheumatology nursing forum problem model

Methods of Care Delivery

Task allocation

Where care organisation centres around the completion of assigned tasks and routines care delivery emphasis is on task allocation (Pearson, 1988). It advocates non-involvement, e.g. taking a patient's temperature with minimal interaction. The atmosphere is hurried, with emphasis on the importance of time. Concern is for immediate treatment rather than continuity of care. This method of care delivery is totally inappropriate when caring for patients with a chronic rheumatic condition where time must be spent exploring how the illness has impacted on a person's life so that care planning can involve the patient in an active, not a passive, role. Patient education on self-management interventions, e.g. relaxation for pain control, can only occur if the ward philosophy is committed to empowering patients.

Therapeutic nursing

Care is organised around the concerns of the patient and his or her significant others. The ward sister/manager encourages all nurses to enter into a therapeutic relationship with the patient so that care planning can match perceived needs. It necessitates nurse–patient involvement. The nurse is knowledgeable and able to identify what aspects of care provision will benefit the patient, e.g. exercises for muscle wasting. The ward sister/manager decentralises authority and enables each qualified nurse to take responsibility for the care management of an allocated number of patients. This philosophy of care can be incorporated within team nursing, primary nursing and case management.

The nursing process

Although the introduction of the nursing process has been criticised for over-concentrating on the method of delivering nursing, it has provided us with the opportunity to look at, examine and explore the nature of nursing and has been instrumental in emphasising the importance of the nurse–patient relationship. It is important that the process should not remain a static instrument, that it is dynamic in its nature and as a result it is essential to ensure that assessment, planning, implementation and evaluation of care move the patient along the continuum of adjustment.

Assessment

This is a crucial stage as it is the beginning of the interaction between patient and nurse. Time must be spent to allow a meaningful relationship to develop. It will be here that the patient's lay belief, perception of problems, aims and aspirations of the inpatient visit are obtained. It is a developmental stage whereby the patient's participation is explored and authority and power are demystified. Some rheumatology wards may find a pre-determined framework helpful to ensure that all patients' needs are considered [see 'Patient Assessment Form', pp. 64–5. An alternative method of assessment can be seen in Chapter 4, Figure 4.2]. The documentation used must encompass the philosophy and model of care. For it to be a workable tool it must have the support and be owned by all members of the nursing team involved in its use.

Planning

As the nurse–patient relationship develops, mutually realistic objectives can be set. This involves active participation by both parties and will enable continuity of care to occur during shift changes. It entails a process of helping the patient to develop a critical awareness of the root cause of any problem, plus a readiness to act on that awareness.

It includes a reinforcement of new knowledge and information and may need to include strategies to enable the patient to take control over aspects of life that can assist adjustment.

This may include advice on:

- exercise;
- joint protection;
- pacing activities;
- the condition itself;
- role of drug therapy;
- encouragement of expression of feelings and discussion with significant others.

Shared care has to be the way forward, with patients taking responsibility for their condition under the support and guidance of a nurse within a therapeutic relationship.

Implementation

This is the stage at which the patient can integrate new-found personal knowledge and skills into reality. It will be affected by the organisation of care delivery and the provision of a suitable environment. A patient with a rheumatological disorder will often benefit from an unhurried pace. This may be difficult to achieve with the erosion of specialist rheumatology wards, but is essential in whatever the clinical environment the patient is being nursed.

Evaluation

This is a crucial stage which is ongoing in nature and occurs on both a formal and an informal basis. It involves evaluating the progress in achieving the objectives or goals established at the planning stage. It is important that all goals are realistic, otherwise the patient will lose faith in the relationship and be less motivated to contribute towards further care planning. If goals have not been achieved, then a reassessment of the situation is required. This may lead to alterations in the treatment programme.

Case Study

Mrs B is a 30-year-old married woman with two young children. For the past year she has been experiencing pain and stiffness in both hands, which has prevented her working in the family's pottery business. On admission she is very frightened and depressed about her future. Investigations confirm a diagnosis of rheumatoid arthritis.

The nurse allocated to Mrs B's care welcomes her to the ward and familiarises her with the environment. Time is spent during the assessment process to ascertain Mrs B's fears and anxieties. In partnership with the nurse a care plan is formulated.

The plan involves providing Mrs B and her husband with information about the condition and allowing time to answer specific questions. This will be an ongoing process and the nurse will observe both verbal and non-verbal cues to ascertain how much information to provide at this initial stage.

The nurse begins to explore with Mrs B ways of coping with the pain and stiffness. This includes advice on the use of analgesia, relaxation and pacing activities. Mrs B is pleased to learn that she can carry out certain activities for herself, which makes her feel more in control. Arrangements are made for the occupational therapist to visit to provide information on altering work practices.

The nurse assigned to Mrs B knows her well enough to recognise that in the evenings she becomes more withdrawn. Mrs B states that she is concerned about her ability to cope with her children following discharge. The nurse arranges temporary assistance from Social Services which Mrs B greatly appreciates.

After a 10-day stay Mrs B feels better able to cope with her condition and on discharge is provided with a telephone helpline contact number. A follow-up appointment is made with the clinical nurse specialist to monitor coping strategies.

Conclusion

The nurse can make a valuable and positive contribution when caring for patients with a rheumatological disorder. Through using the skills of communication, empathy and understanding, the nurse can build a relationship with the patient. By obtaining the patient's perspective it will be possible to plan care that has meaning and relevance for the patient. The provision of a therapeutic ward environment will foster the support and education required for the patient to move towards a state of adaptation and successful management of his or her condition.

Investigations on the Ward

It is important that the nurse has knowledge of the relevance of those investigations being used to aid diagnosis, of how to monitor disease progression and of the side-effects of treatment. This will enable the nurse to explain to the patient their necessity and purpose. Routine investigations are discussed in this section (see 'Normal Laboratory Values' pp. 66–7 for a list).

Useful investigations in rheumatology include:

(1) Routine haematological investigations:

(a) haemoglobin:

The typical anaemia of RA is a normochromic normocytic anaemia (haemoglobin 10–12 gdl) and probably results from an inappropriate utilisation of iron.

A microcytic (low mean corpuscular volume MCV) hypochromic anaemia (low mean corpuscular haemoglobin MCH) may indicate gastrointestinal blood loss often attributed to the use of non-steroidal anti-inflammatory drugs.

A macrocytic anaemia can develop from vitamin B12 or folate deficiency. The use of sulphasalazine and methotrexate can also cause a folate deficiency anaemia.

Patients with musculo-skeletal rheumatism, osteoarthritis (OA) and repetitive strain injury (RSI) are likely to have a normal haemoglobin.

(b) white blood (cell) count (WBC):

The total white blood cell count should be reviewed in conjunction with a differential WBC count showing the proportion of neutrophils and lymphocytes that make up the total number of circulating WBCs.

Leukocytosis occasionally occurs in RA, but is not a typical feature. If marked, it may indicate a super-added infection (either systemic or a septic arthritis), a post-infective reactive arthritis or one of the varieties of polyarteritis.

Leucopenia can occur in systemic lupus erythematosus (SLE), and in Felty's syndrome, but the commonest cause of leucopenia in a patient with RA is marrow suppression from disease-modifying anti-rheumatic drugs (DMARDs), e.g. gold. Eosinophilia can occur following intramuscular gold.

(c) platelet count:

In musculo-skeletal rheumatism and osteoarthritis the platelet count should be within normal limits. In active RA there can be an increased count (thrombocytosis). A reduction in the number of platelets can occur in the early stages of SLE or may be a reaction to drug therapy (DMARDs) in RA.

(d) erythrocyte sedimentation rate (ESR):

If inflammation is present in the body the ESR rises. This is partly due to the changes in the red blood cells and partly to the inflammatory proteins that are present in a patient's blood. The ESR is usually raised in RA, ankylosing spondylitis, acute gout, polymyalgia rheumatica, Reiter's disease and infective arthritis. The ESR is not raised in osteoarthritis, metabolic joint diseases, repetitive strain injury or in soft tissue rheumatism e.g. fibromyalgia.

It is used in many rheumatology units as the standard test for evaluating disease activity in RA, although some areas prefer to use plasma viscosity (PV). A markedly raised ESR could also be related to myeloma (a malignant condition of the plasma cells) and requires further investigation.

(2) X-ray examination of the joints:

Although in the early stages of a condition plain radiographs may be normal, X-rays of the hands and feet may provide evidence of the onset of RA. X-ray changes can be helpful in diagnosis (see Figure 3.4). More sophisticated imaging techniques are available, such as magnetic resonance imaging (MRI) and computerised tomography (CT), for clearer definition of bony and soft tissue structures. Radioisotopes may be used diagnostically for the imaging of bone and bony lesions or for joints. They can also be used in quantity to aid assessment of inflammation. A dual-energy X-ray absorptiometry scan (DEXA) is used to measure bone density and has an important role to play in the management of osteoporosis.

Rheumatoid arthritis	Periarticular osteoporosis. Articular erosions
Osteoarthritis	Erosions of the articular cartilage, narrowing of the joint space, described as degenerative changes. Osteophytes
Ankylosing spondylitis	Irregularity, narrowing or lack of definition of the sacroiliac joints
Gout	Erosions, tophi or crystals may be seen

Figure 3.4: X-ray features

(3) Biochemical investigations:

(a) renal function: electrolytes (sodium, chloride, potassium and bicarbonate), together with urea and creatinine are usually measured. A raised creatinine level indicates renal impairment which may involve amyloidosis. The chronic renal failure of connective tissue disorders (e.g. SLE) may produce a high potassium and low bicarbonate level. The renal toxicity caused by DMARDs is most likely to be seen on dipstick testing first.

(b) acute phase reactant: C-reactive protein (CRP) is an inflammatory marker raised in the acute phase of RA and can be used to monitor disease progression and treatment effectiveness. A consistently raised CRP is associated with severe disease. In SLE the CRP remains normal and this may aid diagnosis.

(c) liver function tests: total protein, total albumin and total globulin estimates reflect hepatic function, although they can also indicate absorption and inflammation. Gamma glutamyl transpeptidase (GGT), is a more specific test of hepatic damage or alcohol abuse. Apart from lupoid hepatitis, which can mimic RA, bilirubin and AST (or ALT) are likely to be normal. Alkaline phosphatase is often raised in active RA. Medications such as sulphasalazine and methotrexate can cause abnormal liver function tests.

(d) bone metabolism: a slightly raised calcium and alkaline phosphatase level may indicate osteomalacia. In Paget's disease alkaline phosphatase is markedly raised. It is important to establish the origin of a raised alkaline phosphatase, as a similar elevation occurs in secondary neoplasms of the bone.

(e) serum uric acid: this may be raised in patients with gout or psoriatic arthritis, although a certain number of the normal population have a raised uric acid in any case. The use of uricosuric drugs such as probenecid or allopurinol will seek to maintain uric acid within normal levels.

(4) Ward urine testing:

A routine urine test should always be carried out (see Figure 3.5). If tubercule bacilli is suspected then early morning urine specimens will be required.

(5) Immunological assessment of rheumatic disease activity:

(a) rheumatoid factor: this is the most commonly requested

Proteinuria	Urinary infection, nephropathy (gold and D-penicillamine) or secondary amyloid disease. SLE - nephrotic syndrome
Haematuria	Investigate if persistent – could be an early sign of polyarteritis
Glucose	Possibility of corticosteroid-induced diabetes

Figure 3.5: Abnormal constituents of urine and their indications

immunological investigation. An IgM/IgG immunoglobulin complex occurs in 80 per cent of patients with RA of more than 12 months' duration, but in only 40–50 per cent of patients with early disease. Patients with the IgM/IgG complex are described as being rheumatoid factor positive. The rheumatoid factor is not solely diagnostic of RA as it can be found in other conditions such as liver disease and sarcoidosis. It is detected by the sheep cell agglutination (Rose Waaler) test, latex agglutination test and/or RAHA test. The Rose Waaler test is given as a titre. The higher the titre, the stronger the indication for severe disease with poor prognosis. Some patients with classic RA and radio-logical evidence of erosions test negative for the IgM/IgG rheumatoid factor. These patients are described as being rheumatoid factor negative.

(b) anti-nuclear antibody (ANA): ANA is not condition specific, as it can be raised in RA and systemic sclerosis, but it is most likely to be elevated in SLE. Of more importance in the diagnosis of SLE is the presence of anti-DNA antibodies.

(c) complement: the complement system is a complex series of proteins that play a role in the mediation of inflammation, proba-bly triggered by the immune complex function. It is therefore worthwhile to measure complement in connective tissue disorders.

(d) immunoglobulins: these can provide information when the ESR is raised for no obvious reason. In seropositive RA, serum IgM is usually raised representing rheumatoid factor in the blood. IgA, synthesised in mucous membranes, may be raised in Sjögren's syndrome. The immunoglobulin profile can show the abnormal paraprotein found in myelematosis.

(6) Histocompatability antigens (HLA):

These inherited antigens located on the sixth chromosome of the leucocyte can be useful to point towards seronegative spon-darthritic conditions. HLA B27 is the marker for this group of conditions. It is, however, worth noting that HLA B27 is present in 7 per cent of 'healthy' individuals and in 50 per cent of relatives of patients with ankylosing spondylitis, who will not necessarily get the condition. Therefore care must be taken when interpreting a positive B27 result.

(7) Antistreptolysin O titre:

The antibody to the production of streptococci antistreptolysin O (ASO) titre is raised temporarily in patients with rheumatic fever but it should be stressed that, if positive, it may simply indicate the presence of a streptococcal sore throat.

(8) Synovial fluid analysis:

Fluid should be observed under the microscope. If white cells are found the fluid should be cultured for bacterial growth. Tests on immunoglobulins may be performed. Crystals of uric acid or calcium pyrophosphate may be detected using a polarising microscope.

(9) Investigation of muscle and nerve disorders:

(a) polymyositis: if polymyositis is suspected there may be:

  • a raised level of creatinine phosphokinase (CPK) or aldelase; or
  • a raised ESR. Diagnosis is confirmed by muscle biopsy, which shows a lymphocytic infiltration throughout the muscles.

(b) electromyography and muscle biopsy: if muscle disease is suspected electromyography should be carried out. Electrodes are connected to the skin over a muscle and if a disorder is present specific electrical abnormalities are noted. If diagnosis is not clarified following this procedure then a biopsy of muscle from the limb may be taken. Routine histology can specify if polymyositis is present; however, more sophisticated histological techniques may be required if clarification between rheumatoid myopathy and neuropathic myopathy is sought.

(c) nerve conduction studies: this is performed if entrapment neuropathy is suspected. Electrodes are placed proximal and distal to the suspected entrapment on the particular nerve. The nerve is then stimulated and the time required for the nerve impulses to reach the distal recording electrode is calculated. Impaired conduction can occur in carpal tunnel syndrome.

(d) tissue biopsy: a biopsy of the skin or muscle may be necessary for the diagnosis of dermatomyositis and polymyositis respectively. Occasionally biopsy of the lymph nodes may be necessary in active RA to exclude lymphoma, as the systemic variant of rheumatoid disease with gross lymphadenopathy can mimic this condition.

Appendix 3.1 Patient Assessment Form

Name: Unit no:
Evaluation day:
Date: Time: Assessed by:
Named nurse is:
Associate nurses are:

Communication
Includes visual, hearing, speech difficulties – writing/use of the telephone owing to poor grip dexterity.

Breathing and circulation
Do you ever feel short of breath?
If so when?
Do you smoke? How many?

Eating and drinking
Do you take a special diet?
Have you any food allergies?
Have you any eating problems (indigestion, nausea, vomiting)?
Any recent weight alterations?

Washing and dressing
How well are you able to wash yourself?
How well are you able to dress yourself?
Do you take a bath or shower?

Skin condition
Have you any rashes or bruises, etc?
Have you any breaks in your skin?
Does your skin feel warm/cold/dry?
Any alteration in skin colour?
NB: Fibrosis and dryness of skin is a manifestation of connective tissue disorders.
Waterlow score is:

Eliminations
Do you have any problems passing urine?
Do you have any problems with your bowels?
How often do you open your bowels?
Do you take laxatives?
Do you take iron tablets?

Mobility
How far can you walk?
Do you use a stick, frame, etc.?

Do you have to stop walking because of pain, breathlessness, etc.?
Which joints are painful?
Have you had any joints replaced?
Do you have any neck/back problems?
How much movement have you in your arms and legs?
Do you have any sore areas from sitting, ill-fitting shoes, corns, bunions, etc.?
Do you wish to see the fitter?

Sleeping
What is your usual sleep pattern?
Do you take sleeping pills?
Do you find it difficult to get to sleep?
If so why (pain, etc.)?

Home environment
Who helps with your housework?
Do you have to look after anyone else?
Have you ever had:
Home help?   Private help?
Voluntary help?   Social worker?
District nurse?   Meals on wheels?
Would you like to see the social worker or occupational therapist?
Do you have any splints/collars, etc.?

Discharge
Do you have any particular worries about discharge that we can address now?

Education
Do you understand about your condition?
Would you like to have the Nurse Specialist see you to explain aspects of your arthritis and how it affects both home and work?
What does your family understand about your condition?

Social aspects
Are you able to work at the moment?

Psychological welfare
How do you feel in yourself (emotionally)?
Would you like someone to talk with you about the feelings that the arthritis generates in you?

Spiritual needs
Would you like to see a representative from the church?
Can we assist you with any spiritual needs?

Appendix 3.2 Normal Laboratory Values

Normal haematological values
Haemoglobin:

Men	13.5–18.0g/dl
Women	11.5–16.5 g/dl

Red cells:

Men	$4.5–6.5 \times 10^{12}/l$
Women	$3.9–5.6 \times 10^{12}/l$

Mean corpuscular volume (MCV):

Adults	76-96 fl

Mean corpuscular haemoglobin (MCH):

Adults	27-32 pg

Mean corpuscular haemoglobin concentration (MCHC):

Adults	30-35 g/dl

Reticulocytes:

Adults	0.2–2.0 %

Total leukocytes: (WBC)

Adults	$4.0–10.0 \times 10^9$

Differential leukocyte count (adults):

Neutrophils	40–75% or $2.5–7.5 \times 10^9$
Lymphocytes	20–50% or $1.5–3.0 \times 10^9$
Monocytes	2–10% or $0.2–0.8 \times 10^9$
Eosinophils	1–6% or $0.04–0.4 \times 10^9$
Basophils	1% or $0.01–0.1 \times 10^9$

Platelets:

Adults	$160-600 \times 10^9/l$

Normal biochemical values

Sodium	135-145 mmol/l
Potassium	3.6–5.0 mmol/l
Chloride	98-107 mmol/l
Bicarbonate	21-28 mmol/l
Urea	2.5–7.1 mmol/l
Creatinine	50-140 mmol/l
Total bilirubin	3-15 μmol/l
Total protein	67-82 g/l
Albumin	37-49 g/l
Globulins	24-37 g/l
Alkaline phosphatase	90–300 iu/l
Calcium	2.25–2.60 mmol/l
Phosphorus	0.8–1.3 mmol/l
Uric acid (males)	0.20–0.45 mmol/l
Uric acid (females)	0.14–0.38 mmol/l
AST	<50 iu/l
ALT	<45 iu/l

Indicators of inflammation (normal range)

ESR

Males	4-20 mm/h
Females	10-25 mm/h

CRP 0-8 mg/l
Plasma viscosity 1.50–1.72 Centipoise
Haptoglobin 0.3–2.0 g/l
Serum sulphydryl 450-600 μmol/l
Serum histidine 1.5–1.8 mg/100ml

Immunoglobulins:

IgG 128-199 iu/ml
IgA 97-181 iu/ml
IgM 60-129 iu/ml

Electrophoresis:

Albumin 36–51
Alpha 1 1.0–4.0
Alpha 2 4.0–10.0
Beta 4.0–11.0
Gamma 6.0–16.0

Complement plasma: C3 0.63–1.70 g/l
C4 0.11–0.45 g/l

Males	24–195 iu/l
Females	24–170 iu/l
CPK Male	24–195 iu/l
Females	24–170 iu/l

Gamma glutamyl transpeptide (male)   6–28 units/l
Gamma glutamyl transpeptide (female)   4–18 units/l

References

Benner P, Wrubel J (1989) The Primacy of Caring. Stress and Coping in Health and Illness. Wokingham: Addison-Wesley.

Department of Health (1993) A Vision for the Future. London: NHS Management Executive.

McMahon RA (1986) Nursing as therapy. Professional Nurse 1(10): 270–2.

Melia K (1987) Learning and Working. The Occupational Socialisation of Nurses. London: Tavistock.

Pearson A (1988) Primary Nursing – Nursing in the Burford and Oxford Nursing Development Units. London: Chapman & Hall.

Powell J (1991) Reflection and the evaluation of experience: prerequisite for therapeutic practice. In McMahon R, Pearson, A (Eds) Nursing as Therapy. London: Chapman & Hall.

Royal College of Nursing (1989) Standards of Care. Rheumatic Disease Nursing. London: RCN.

Salvage J (1990) The theory and practice of the 'new nursing'. Nursing Times 86(4): 42–5.

Smith P (1992) The Emotional Labour of Nursing. London: Macmillan.

UKCC (1992) The Code of Professional Conduct. London: UKCC.

UKCC (1992) The Scope of Professional Practice. London: UKCC.

Chapter 4
Rheumatology:
care in the
community

CHRISTINE WHITE

Introduction

Care in the community means the help and support that people need to live as independently as possible in their own homes or in homely settings within the community. The network of services providing community-based care includes the health service, social services and the independent sector who run private residential homes. Most people in need of care receive this at home and the carers are usually relatives and friends.

A large majority of patients with musculoskeletal disorders receive medical care from their general practitioner (GP), with only 4 per cent of patients being referred to a consultant rheumatologist (Symonds and Bankhead, 1994) and an even smaller percentage requiring hospital admission. The major burden of rheumatological care is therefore in the community.

A number of factors influence the provision of community care; these include government legislation and more specifically coordination, communication and cooperation between the local services. Patient management should therefore be carefully planned and aimed to include team delivery of care, with the patient and carer in partnership. Effective team care requires the skills of social workers, nurses and other members of the health and social services. Clarification of responsibilities is essential and joint initiatives should ensure a seamless delivery of service. Shared care protocols need to be clearly identified and easy access to the hospital service for information and advice should be provided.

The Prevalence of Rheumatic Disease in the Community

Musculoskeletal disorders is the term used to describe those diseases affecting joints, bones, soft tissue and muscles and includes 200 different conditions. Although a large number of these are confined to the musculoskeletal system, some also affect other organs and systems and this requires complex management (BSR,1995a). Musculoskeletal disorders are the principal cause of severe physical disability in the United Kingdom affecting nearly 8 million people. (BLAR, 1994).

The severity of these conditions ranges from mild and self-limiting to life-threatening. Evidence suggests that early treatment to suppress inflammation significantly slows disease progression and reduces joint damage and deformity (Donnelly, Scot and Emery, 1992). Treatments can thereby improve quality of life and minimise functional consequences. Many patients can be managed in the primary care setting whereas other patients will benefit from the diagnostic expertise and management of a specialist hospital unit, including education, medication and investigative techniques (BLAR, 1994).

Musculoskeletal disorders affect all age-groups but the prevalence rises with age and as the number of elderly people in the community increases so will the number of people exhibiting musculoskeletal problems (Bradley, 1991). This age trend is expected to continue. At present 'arthritis and rheumatism' are the most frequent and persistent conditions in Britain, with the rate of 80 per 1000 adult females and 40 per 1000 adult males affected (HMSO, 1989a).

Community studies have shown that a number of patients with potentially treatable musculoskeletal disease have never been referred for evaluation. This is most noticeable for non-inflammatory forms of arthritis, with less than half of those severely disabled referred for evaluation (Foster, Pyle and Walker, 1991).

Rheumatoid arthritis

Rheumatoid arthritis is the most common cause of treatable disability which can lead to morbidity and mortality comparable to those caused by malignancy (Emery, 1993). The annual incidence of rheumatoid arthritis is estimated at 36 per 100 000 for women and 14 per 100 000 for men with a female:male ratio of 3:1 in younger patients. In the elderly the incidence is similar for men and women (Symonds and Bankhead, 1994). Juvenile chronic arthritis, which affects patients under 16 years of age, was estimated to affect 11 per 100 000 in 1989–91 with 30 per cent having severe functional impairment (Scott et al., 1987).

Osteoarthritis

This is also a very common form of musculoskeletal disease causing disability but it is difficult to estimate the incidence of osteoarthritis as the joint pain and diagnostic features are insidious. However, the prevalence of osteoarthritis is higher in females than males at all ages and rises with age, with 60 per cent of those aged 65 years having moderate to severe osteoarthritis in at least one joint (Symonds and Bankhead, 1994). Risk factors include obesity and occupations involving lifting and bending. The most disabling features of osteoarthritis occur where either the knee or the hip are involved, as this impairs walking function as well as causing pain.

Back pain

Another common problem is back pain which should be described as a symptom rather than a disease and may be the result of numerous different factors. The majority of back pain cases settle within six weeks but recurrence of back pain is common and one episode is a strong predictor of future problems (Liang and Komaroff, 1982). Back pain is more common in males aged between 25 and 44 years, but more common in women at all other ages. Walsh et al. (1992) showed that back pain in men approaches 70 per cent by the age of 60.

Osteoporosis

Osteoporosis is a growing problem due in part to the relative increase in the numbers of the elderly and there is now an increasing prevalence in men as well as women. Osteoporosis is associated with an increase in all types of fractures. In the UK it has been estimated that 60 000 hip fractures, 50 000 distal forearm fractures and 40 000 vertebral fractures occur each year in post-menopausal women (Cooper, 1993). There is now evidence available to show that osteoporotic fractures may lead to substantial disability and death (Royal College of Physicians, 1989), the latter due to perioperative problems such as bronchopneumonia, pulmonary emboli, etc.

Systemic lupus erythematosus

It has been estimated that about three in 10 000 people in British cities have systemic lupus erythematosus (Johnson et al., 1995). It is thought to be nine times more common in women than men. These figures are thought to be an underestimate as many mild cases may be undiagnosed (Johnson et al., 1996).

Scleroderma

Scleroderma is one of the most uncommon of the rheumatic diseases.

The overall incidence is estimated at around one per million males and six per million females (Symonds and Bankhead, 1994).

Ethnic differences in disease

There are marked differences in the way that rheumatological conditions affect varied ethnic groups. For instance, the prevalence of rheumatoid arthritis is similar across European urban populations but it appears less common in rural African communities. Similarly a milder and less progressive form of rheumatoid arthritis appears in the Asian population (Nichol and Woodrow, 1981).

Osteoarthritis has a worldwide distribution but affected joints vary in different cultural groups. However, compared with Europeans there is an increased knee involvement and a decreased incidence of hip involvement in both the Indian and African populations. The incidence of ankylosing spondylitis is four times higher in Caucasian subjects than in Africans or black Americans (Mukhopadhaya and Barooah, 1967; Ebong and Lawson, 1978).

Studies have shown that systemic lupus erythematosus is between three to five times more prevalent in the black Afro-Caribbean population and twice as prevalent in the Asian population compared with Caucasians (Johnson et al., 1996).

Osteoporosis is less common in the Afro-Caribbean populations who have been shown to have a greater bone mass (Morrison et al., 1994). Vitamin D-deficient osteomalacia and rickets are common in the Asian population, with up to 30 per cent of Indian and Pakistani immigrants showing some evidence of these conditions, which may present with proximal myopathy and bone pain (Maggi et al., 1991; Linton and Situnayake, 1993).

The Cost of Disability to the Individual and to Society

Chronic and disabling diseases such as rheumatoid arthritis and osteoarthritis have the greatest burden in the terms of cost. Rheumatological disorders increase the cost of personal care along with more expensive items of clothing and footwear that are designed for the disabled. The extra heating and lighting required and alterations in diet to cope with difficulties of food preparation add to the family budget. Adaptations and appliances to aid independent living are also very expensive. Travelling costs increase with the use of taxis and ambulances which are frequently needed because of disability. There is also the cost of loss of earnings related to the disability and often a personal cost because relationships also breakdown as a result of disability. Patients often seek alternative therapies when conventional therapies cannot offer a cure or even alleviate distress, and the costs can be substantial during the course of an illness. The cost of pain and the distress resulting both to the patient and the family represent a cost which cannot be counted in monetary terms (Silman, 1995).

Health-care provision to treat an individual can be expensive and includes the cost of drugs, appliances such as splints, and investigations including X-rays and blood tests. More sophisticated tests such as MRI scans and new therapies lead to a massive increase in the cost of care. Inpatient care is expensive and includes hotel services, in addition to medical, nursing and therapy staff costs, along with the cost of investigation, treatments and possible joint replacements. Capital expenditure such as ancillary staff, equipment and running costs must also be included. Provision of social care and support, including social welfare payments and adaptations to enable independent living, increases the considerable impact of cost caused by rheumatological disorders.

Prevention

Most acute and chronic musculoskeletal disorders are idiopathic but some may be affected by factors that are amenable to change, for example, gout in association with high alcohol intake or inappropriate diuretic therapy, accelerated osteoarthritis in obesity and work-related disorders such as repetitive strain disorders. Undoubtedly osteoporosis is the most important disorder in which prevention has a major role. The impact in terms of mortality, morbidity and cost is well recognised. Convincing evidence exists that therapy can delay or prevent osteoporosis and treatment of patients who have one or more vertebral fractures can significantly reduce further fractures. Back problems affect 80 per cent of the population at any one time and education with regard to posture, lifting and the sensible use of body mechanics can significantly reduce the incidence of back pain. The introduction of no-lifting policies together with teaching good lifting techniques can also significantly reduce the number of back problems. Work-related problems can often be solved by the use of appropriate equipment, seating or good posture. Anxiety and depression can also intensify rheumatological problems and appropriate relaxation and stress relief can significantly reduce the effects of many related conditions. Exercise has also proved to be beneficial in maintaining muscle tone, reducing pain and managing many rheumatological conditions.

The primary care team has an important role to play here. Much can be done for patients with rheumatological conditions by early recognition of the disease, followed by appropriate GP referral, treatment and management. All are crucial factors affecting the outcome of the disease.

The use of disease modifying drugs (DMARDS) can significantly reduce the incidence of severe deformity and joint destruction. The side-effects of the drugs should be balanced against the effects of untreated disease, which can be costly in terms of health and social care as well as personal cost of disability. Maintaining patients on disease-modifying drugs is also costly in terms of drug monitoring combined with frequent visits to health professionals.

Government Legislation

The Chronically Sick and Disabled Persons Act

The Chronically Sick and Disabled Persons Act (HMSO,1970) (section 2) requires the social services department to arrange various services which it considers a disabled person may need.

The Government White Paper

The government White Paper *Working for Patients* (HMSO, 1989b) was aimed at drastically altering the basic concepts of Britain's health care provisions. The paper was aimed at increasing accountability and encouraging initiatives to respond to local needs. Central management for the National Health Service (NHS) aimed to fund each district according to its population and hospitals were to become self-governing NHS Trusts. GPs were also given their own practice and drug budgets which were to be managed locally.

Charges for drugs

The Charges for Drugs and Appliances Regulation (HMSO,1989c) and subsequent amendments allow exemption for some sufferers of chronic disease but rheumatology patients, who are often crippled and on numerous drugs to enable them to function, presently receive no such exemption, unless they are on a low income.

The new GP contracts

In 1990 the government imposed new contracts on general practitioners (GPs) requiring them to provide a range of screening and health promotion services, and these have subsequently been amended. Apart from services already offered to patients, the new contracts required GPs to be responsible for:

- adult health checks;
- child health surveillance;
- health promotion clinics;
- minor surgery.

Fees or target payments can be claimed for these services (HMSO, 1989c)

Community Care Act and the Health of the Nation

In 1989 the NHS and Community Care Act was introduced and in 1992 the *Health of the Nation* White Paper was published, and the effects have clearly benefited some patient groups. The framework set up by the NHS and Community Care Act (1989d) requires that the assessment of the health needs of the community should be met by planning and purchasing appropriate services. Thus, since April 1993, it has become the responsibility of the local authority social services department to purchase social care and thereby, it is hoped, reflect the needs of local patients, and to use care management appropriately to achieve effective care. Community needs assessment has been defined as 'a description of those factors which must be addressed in order to improve the health of the population' (Harvey, 1994). The social services department has the responsibility for social care provision and the health authorities bear responsibility for health care provision

The Patient's Charter

In 1992 patients acquired new rights as consumers through that part of the Citizen's Charter relating to the NHS. The Patient's Charter was aimed at putting the patient first and setting standards which patients might expect to receive (DHSS, 1991).

Residential care fees

New arrangements came into force in April 1993 for the payment of residential care fees. People requiring residential care are now means-tested by the local social services department who decide how much individuals can afford to pay towards their own residential care cost.

The Carers Recognition and Services Act

From 1 April 1996 the Carers Recognition and Services Act, otherwise known as the Carers Act (HMSO, 1995), recognised the rights of carers, and gives them a right to separate assessment of their ability to provide and continue to provide care. Carers are people who look after and support elderly and disabled relatives and friends and they have the right to ask for an assessment and to have their requirements considered.

GP fundholding

Fundholding practices receive funds from the Family Health Services Authority (FHSA) to cover the cost of running a practice including staff, premises and equipment. A drug budget is also set to indicate the limits of prescribing. Purchasing authorities set budgets for purchasing inpatient and outpatient services, as well as district nursing and health visiting (HMSO, 1990a).

The Effects of Government Legislation

The government's health focus has been based on mortality statistics. Few patients suffering from rheumatic conditions die rapidly from their condition and as a result the rheumatic diseases receive no emphasis in the government's scheme. It appears therefore that the health care needs of a large proportion of the population have been discounted.

Cerebro- and cardiovascular disease is the major cause of death and disability in the UK, thus the *Health of the Nation* (HMSO, 1992) targeted this as the principal area for promoting preventive health measures. Asthma and diabetes were also highlighted. Major developments and improvements in the provision of health needs in these areas have resulted in specialist clinics in general practice for patient education and also screening clinics, e.g. for hypertension. As it is mainly practice nurses who run such screening clinics their skills have had to increase and this clearly benefits affected patients. Because the *Health of the Nation* does not specifically mention the rheumatological conditions, no stimulus exists for practices to improve rheumatological care. Despite the concentration in the *Health of the Nation* manifesto on coronary heart disease, stroke, asthma and diabetes, and notwithstanding the intention to ensure that health promotion is appropriately and adequately resourced, the legislation can also allow other priority needs to be addressed. The previously quoted statistics show that rheumatology patients need to become a priority group.

The Effects of the Community Care Act on Rheumatology Patients

This act has significantly changed the concept of community care. A survey was carried out by the British League Against Rheumatism (BLAR, 1994) to ascertain whether or not the advent of the NHS and Community Care Act (HMSO,1989d) had brought about improvements in community care and healthcare facilities for those with physical disability resulting from arthritis. The BLAR (1994) survey, carried out following implementation of the Community Care Act (HMSO 1989d), showed that no significant improvements had occurred compared with a survey carried out prior to the implementation of the act. Access to useful support services such as physiotherapy had also not improved. The BLAR 1994 survey also showed no apparent improvement in the provision of home adaptations designed to facilitate independent living. Thus, despite the fact that physical disability in the study group had been shown to have increased, there has been no increase in the level of support available. Clearly these findings raise doubts about the effectiveness of the NHS and Community Care Act (HMSO, 1989d) in reforming service provision to the individual with arthritis-related disability.

Included in the management of the rheumatic diseases is the aim to minimise pain and stiffness, and to maximise physical function and so improve quality of life. Even the absence of deterioration constitutes success because the natural history of most of the arthritic diseases is progressive deformity and disability. Most are age related and therefore the burden of the disease will increase as the number of old people in the UK grows. These issues need to be addressed by the government in its directives if it is really concerned about the health of the nation.

Primary health care

Primary health care refers to care within the community including health promotion, compared with secondary care provided by hospitals and specialist services.

The practice team

A practice team incorporates the doctors, practice nurse(s), practice manager and receptionist(s). Larger practices may employ or facilitate other professional staff including dietician, physiotherapist, counsellors and chiropodist, increasing the range of services for patients.

Shared Care

The workload of general practitioners (GPs) has been shown to include between 15 per cent and 20 per cent of consultations for musculoskeletal symptoms and this trend is expected to increase. Hospital-based rheumatologists see only a minority of affected people as diagnosis of most minor rheumatological conditions is well within the scope of the general practitioner. However, some musculoskeletal disorders include complex multi-system life-threatening complications which need to be recognised and treated early. Furthermore, management of many established diseases can be complex and difficult, and requires considerable knowledge, skills and experience (Dieppe, 1994). Rheumatologists have diagnostic experience and access to special investigations as well as to the multidisciplinary team, so ensuring effective management. For instance, prevention of disability and early mortality in rheumatoid arthritis patients depends on early recognition and appropriate treatment. The GP therefore has a key role in early recognition followed by immediate referral. Shared care is thus where the actual responsibility for patient care is split between the hospital-based specialist and his or her team, and the community-based team led by the GP.

Shared care in rheumatology should aim at reducing the number of hospital visits and improving patient care. Once patients are established on disease modifying anti-rheumatic drugs (DMARDS), shared management between hospital and primary care is the most appropriate arrangement with open access to hospital services as needs arise. Shared care in rheumatology usually means shared drug-monitoring responsibility. Ready access for emergencies would seem more appropriate than regular attendances when active problems do not exist. In addition, open access to a specialist rheumatology nurse via a telephone help-line will facilitate this process. Shared care is dependent on cooperation, communication and coordination of services and requires provision of clear protocols, which should be produced by the local rheumatology department. Clarification of responsibilities is needed to avoid disputes about responsibilities of care.

The practice nurse is in the ideal position to provide routine information and advice for patients in the community, especially for those who have never seen a consultant rheumatologist and therefore do not have the benefit of education from the hospital-based multidisciplinary team. There should be an educational package that is formulated by the hospital-based rheumatology team, which should include the GP and other health professionals.

Shared care monitoring

Disease-modifying drugs have potentially dangerous side-effects which require safe and effective monitoring. Monitoring reflects the safety precautions for each drug and good professional practice and includes the national guidelines of the British Society for Rheumatology (BSR, 1995b). General guidelines on monitoring are given in this chapter but for more specific guidelines and advice on abnormal results and side-effects see Chapter 6.

Provision of patient information about disease-modifying drugs

Patients should be informed about the benefits and the side-effects of the relevant drugs. This information should be provided by the prescribing department but in addition written information should always be given to reinforce verbal information. The importance of regular monitoring should be stressed and the frequency of the tests explained. A monitoring booklet should be supplied in which the monitoring person should record the results and this should be carried by the patient and shown to the prescribing doctor as well as the hospital consultant. The GP should also be provided with information about the drug, its side-effects and the monitoring protocol. See Chapter 5 on patient education.

Monitoring of patients on disease-modifying drugs

Patients may be monitored in specialist monitoring clinics which are usually hospital based or at their local GP's surgery. It is important that patients know who is responsible for their monitoring. Generalist care is provided at the primary care level and this should be complemented by easy access to the hospital service. A specialist nurse in rheumatology is usually the link person employed in most rheumatology departments and should be easily accessible via a telephone help-line to support and advise the practice nurse or GP.

Maintenance of therapy

The range of disease-modifying drugs is small and every effort should be made to maintain patients on therapy. The decision to stop a disease-modifying drug should be taken with care and requires consultation with the appropriate rheumatology department.

Responsibility of the practice nurse in relation to monitoring

The practice or district nurse is usually responsible for the monitoring of DMARDs in the community and it is important that he or she is aware of the relevant observations and tests and the action to take. The practice nurse should have the skills and expertise to provide each patient with appropriate education and support with regard to the disease and its treatment. Adequate literature should be available within the surgery; this is provided by the charitable organisations Arthritis and Rheumatism Council and Arthritis Care free of charge.

Requirements of a monitoring visit

Monitoring of patients on disease-modifying drugs not only ensures patient safety but is also a way of maintaining contact with the patient for support and early identification of complications or deterioration of the disease. Ideally, a monitoring visit should also include general assessment and education of the patient, with early detection of problems and appropriate intervention. However, in primary care monitoring and general health assessments only are made. Education and counselling is left to the nurse specialist and other hospital-based professionals.

General guidelines for monitoring

At each visit the nurse should:

- inspect the skin for rashes and ask if any pruritis has been experienced;
- ask the patient if he or she has developed any mouth ulcers, sore throat or loss of taste;
- inspect the skin for bruising;
- enquire whether the patient has experienced any undue bleeding such as epistaxis or bleeding gums;
- ask if the patient has experienced any influenza-like symptoms or noticed anything unusual about his or her health;
- ask about any breathlessness or persistent cough;
- test the urine to ensure it is free of protein and blood if patients are having gold or penicillamine;
- ascertain whether bloods have been taken according to the relevant monitoring requirements;
- ask how the patient has been since the previous visit and whether there is any increase in disease activity, hot painful joints, increased morning stiffness or any new problem;

- ensure that recent results are available and have been checked against the previous results by the nurse or prescribing doctor *before* any further medication is given;
- record dose of drug and the most recent results in the monitoring booklet and note any adverse reactions;
- inform the local doctor or contact the rheumatology department should any problems or queries arise from the visit.

Adverse reactions

Reactions usually occur early after starting a new drug but may occur at any time during the course of the treatment. The following are general guidelines and local protocols should be adhered to as well as advice on individual drug administration.

Gastrointestinal tract

Gastrointestinal upsets occur with most of the disease-modifying drugs and can also occur more frequently with non-steroidal anti-inflammatory medication and steroids. Upper gastrointestinal upsets: nausea, vomiting, anorexia, dyspepsia and reversible taste disturbance can occur with any drug.

Action:
- Ensure that steroids and non-steroidal anti-inflammatory drugs are taken with food.
- If on MTX may require folic acid adding to the regimen.
- May require anti-emetic therapy or a reduction in dose especially if taking sulphasalazine or D-penicillimine.
- Stop if severe.
- Review.
- If persistent, patient may need upper gastrointestinal tract endoscopy to exclude ulceration and gastric bleed.

Lower gastrointestinal tract: abdominal pain and diarrhoea. May be due to auranofin (oral gold), methotrexate or occasionally intramuscular gold. Also, check for constipation which may be due to certain analgesics.

Action:
- Reduce dosage and encourage more fibre in the diet or introduce a bulking agent.
- Stop if severe.
- Review.

Skin manifestations

Skin changes may be due to a variety of causes such as a complication of the disease, e.g. vasculitis, leg ulcers and allergies, or steroid therapy resulting in skin thinning.

Rash: may occur with any medication. Can vary from urticaria or eczematous pruritis to severe exfoliative dermatitis.

Action:
- Ensure that there is no other cause for the skin rash.
- If the rash is severe, persistent or generalised stop the drug and inform the rheumatology department. A dermatology referral may ensue.

Itching
Action: If the itching is:
- troublesome – reduce the dosage and review in three weeks.
- unbearable – i.e. patient cannot sleep, stop the medication until the itching is resolved. Review in three weeks. If the rash has cleared recommence medication at a lower dose. If the rash persists the drug should be stopped altogether and the rheumatology department contacted. A dermatology referral may ensue.
- Always ask the patient to return if the condition becomes worse.

Mucous membranes: stomatitis and mouth ulcers can develop in some patients and may be due to a reaction to the medication, vasculitis or lupus.

Action:
- Check white cell count.
- If mouth is sore but there is no visible ulceration suggest mouthwashes.
- Ensure that dentures are fitting correctly.
- Review.
- For one or two minor ulcers in isolation suggest Bonjela or hydrocortisone lozenges.
- Cyclosporin is known to cause gum hyperplasia.
- Review.
- If leucopenic or with an acute and severe crop of mouth ulcers check for signs of vasculitis, stop the drug and inform the rheumatology department.

Alopecia or hair thinning: can occur whilst taking cytotoxic drugs, i.e. cyclophosphamide or methotrexate.

Action:
- Reduce dose.
- Can wear a wig if severe.

Hair growth. Can occur while taking cyclosporin.

Action:
- Stop drug, or
- bleach facial hair, shave.
- Electrolysis depending on the site.
- If troublesome or severe, stop and inform the rheumatology department.

Urinary manifestations

Urinary abnormalities may be due to:
- the disease itself and its complications, e.g. amyloidosis or vasculitis;
- gold or penicillamine and occasionally sulphasalazine or methotrexate.

Asymptomatic urinary tract infections are common in RA patients.

Proteinureia

Action:
- If a trace or + in isolation, ignore.
- If urine shows ++ send MSU. Establish whether the patient has any recognised signs of infection, i.e. burning or frequency of micturition, incomplete feeling of voiding, offensive smell or concentrated urine, or vaginal discharge.
- If MSU reveals no infection but ++ of protein arrange a 24-hour urine collection.
- If +++ of protein collect a 24-hour urine. Discontinue drug, usually penicillamine or gold, until the result of the 24-hour protein is known.
- If the 24-hour urine shows more than 500 mg protein stop the treatment and contact the rheumatology department.

Muscle problems

If the patient notices weakness, ptosis, double vision or speech difficulties this raises the possibility of an associated myositis (inflammation of a muscle) or drug-induced myasthenia gravis (disorder of the neuromuscular junction due to penicillamine). **Inform the doctor immediately**.

Headaches

May occur with any DMARD but particularly sulphasalazine and methotrexate. NSAIDs can also cause headaches.

Action:
- If mild, decrease the dose and increase again when headaches have stopped.
- If severe stop the drug. It may be possible to reintroduce gradually later when headaches have stopped. With NSAIDs stop the drug and do not reintroduce; find an alternative NSAID instead.

Chest symptoms

Breathlessness with or without a cough may be due to pneumonitis or fibrosis in rheumatoid arthritis (RA) patients taking methotrexate or intramuscular gold. Fibrosis can occur in RA without the complication of methotrexate.

Although acute methotrexate pnuemonitis is rare it can be life-threatening if ignored and should be considered if the patient has a dry cough or has experienced recent onset of breathlessness.

Action:
- Stop the drug.
- Collect a sputum specimen in the event of a productive cough.
- Inform the doctor so that he or she can listen to the chest and arrange X-ray and lung function tests if required.
- Contact the rheumatology department if chest symptoms are unresolving or troublesome.

Pharyngitis

Pharyngitis may be suggestive of leucopenia.

Action:
- Repeat full blood count and await result.
- If leucopenic refer to rheumatology department.

(Adapted from guidelines produced by the Department of Rheumatology, Cannock Community Hospital.)

Outreach Clinics

The emphasis on community-based care includes the provision of outreach clinics in some locations. The consultant rheumatologist may thus provide clinics in general practice health centres. Such clinics help to provide expertise in the community and are more convenient for many patients who previously had to travel long distances, and found difficulties with transport or parking when they attended large hospital centres. This is particularly attractive in rural areas although patients may still have to visit a hospital for diagnostic testing. Specialist nurses also provide specialist support regarding disease management and monitoring in the health centre setting.

Discharge Planning of Rheumatology Patients

The planning of services to enable patients to cope at home should begin as soon as they are admitted and should ensure a multi-agency approach. It should include all relevant parties to facilitate the safe and seamless return of the patient to the community. This process should include identification of 'at risk' patients who in relation to diagnosis, disability follow-up care, social support and home circumstances require involvement of members of the multidisciplinary team or multi-agency assessment (Elliot, 1995).

The process of discharge planning has been described as having four phases and this applies to rheumatology patients. These include:

- patient assessment;
- development of discharge planning;
- provision of services including patient education and service referrals;
- follow-up/evaluation.

Patient assessment

The named nurse or associate nurse should ensure that the patient and the carer are involved with the appropriate members of the multidisciplinary team in discussing all aspects of continued care. The complex health needs of rheumatology patients require involvement of the multidisciplinary team, which includes the consultant rheumatologist, specialist nurse, physiotherapist and occupational therapist, chiropodist and appliance officer.

An integral part of the first phase should include assessment of how carers and health professionals have been involved before admission. Patients are often discharged in a matter of days and therefore assessment and discharge planning should begin at the time of admission (Elliot, 1995).

Complete assessment of the rheumatology patient needs to be based on three main areas:

- disease management and knowledge;

- self-care abilities;
- environment and social factors.

The components of these three areas are identified in the model of management for rheumatology patients in Figure 4.1 and this can be used as a framework to identify patients' individual needs (White, 1996). An alternative model is described in Chapter 3.

Disease management and knowledge about the disease process enable patients to take control and participate in the management of their care and should form the basis of management for rheumatology patients.

The patient's self-care abilities are often limited and can be affected in either a positive or negative way by the disease activity, disability, time of day and provision of aids and appliances.

Environment and social factors can also affect disease control and management. Adjustments and necessary changes such as a stair lift, shower, hand rails and tap turners can significantly improve quality of life.

Social needs assessment

Rheumatology patients often have many roles including caring for a family and/or being the wage earner contributing to the family budget. Patients are often carers themselves, with elderly parents or relatives they are expected to care for despite their own difficulties. It is therefore important to identify those giving support as well as those requiring support. The social needs assessment in Figure 4.2 clearly identifies the client and their role(s) and also significant others, and allows for clear documentation of those giving support and those requiring support. Professional input is also easily documented and a summary of needs can then be identified.

Multidisciplinary assessment

All patients require an assessment by the appropriate health care professionals and a care plan to be formulated which can be carried through into the community. Specialist nurses who have greater knowledge of rheumatological conditions as well as a close working relationship with the consultant rheumatologist, physiotherapist, occupational therapist and social worker are ideally situated to identify the continuing health care needs. In conjunction with other health professionals they can commence care plans that include consultation with the patient and focus on rehabilitation and recovery. The information should always be reported back to the primary nurse.

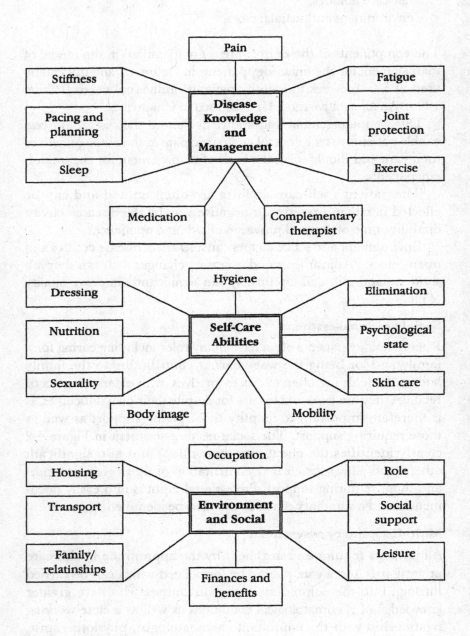

Figure 4.1: Model of management for rheumatology patients
Source: C.E. White, unpublished dissertation (1996).

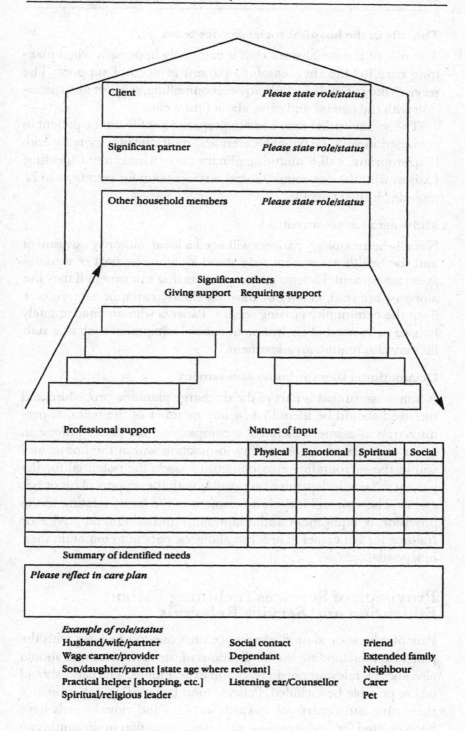

Figure 4.2: Social needs assessment
Source: C.E. White, unpublished dissertation (1996).

The role of the hospital social service team

The role of the social work staff is extremely important when planning care for the rheumatology patient in need of support. The services they provide include advice, counselling, support and discussion with the patient and carer about future care.

The social worker may need to prepare a profile on the patient in conjunction with the patient, carers and multidisciplinary team and, if appropriate, call a multidisciplinary care management meeting. Liaison with the community social services team for resources to be provided is then possible.

Multi-agent assessment

Not all rheumatology patients will need a local authority assessment and the health assessment may stand alone or be part of a multi-agent assessment. Patients may require further assessment if they live alone or are frail, elderly or have an elderly carer, or require care from the community nursing service. Patients who are inadequately housed or in need of environment control equipment such as a stair lift may also require an assessment.

Occupational therapy home assessment

A home assessment is part of the discharge planning procedure and the need should be identified by any member of the team. A pre-discharge assessment includes accompanying the patient home in order to assess his or her ability to function within the home, and within the surrounding environment to assess the potential for the patient to be as independent as possible with the support of his or her carers. The visit will include assessment of the home relating to the provision of equipment and adaptations and additional advice or training for the carers in order to allow the patient to maintain their independence.

Provision of Services Including Patient Education and Service Referrals

Patient education should commence on a one-to-one basis with the patient understanding the implications of the condition, and should also address relevant needs, fears and expectations. The carer should where possible be included. Patients must believe they can influence their care and contribute towards it. Once individual needs have been catered for, inclusion in a structured education programme can follow. Patient and carer education sessions are usually run on an outpatient basis and include the multidisciplinary team (Ryan, 1995). The identification of the need for service provision should be identified from the assessment and care plan in Figure 4.2 and can subsequently be arranged with the relevant health professional.

Follow-up and Evaluation

The follow-up arrangements should be dependent on the assessment. Specialist rheumatology nurses usually run their own clinics and are able to assess the needs of the patient and refer for further therapy assessments and treatment as required. It is thought to be more appropriate if patients are seen on the occasion of a flare. Also, if circumstances allow, it is more convenient to allow a system of open access where patients can refer themselves if the need arises. The long wait for outpatient appointments to see a consultant caused by the extremely high workload of most rheumatologists is balanced by open access to the nurse who can consult with the medical team as appropriate. Physiotherapy and occupational therapy assessments are organised as appropriate. The rheumatology team can refer to other team members whenever the need arises. Evaluation should occur as part of the review procedure and any changes required can be arranged with the appropriate member of the multidisciplinary team.

Rheumatology Outpatients

Many rheumatology patients are only seen on an outpatient basis as every effort is made to avoid hospital admission where possible. Many outpatients are severely disabled and need to be exposed to the same assessment and referral procedure. Every effort should be made to ensure that the assessment of all aspects of the rheumatology model of management in Figure 4.1 are carried out. The outpatient should have access to the same multidisciplinary team and education session. Carers of outpatients also need to be considered.

Community Assessment and Care Planning

Patients have an entitlement to expect that an assessment of community care needs will be carried out to a high standard. This includes listening to and taking account of patients' needs, and their views on how those needs can best be met. This should include the opportunity for patients to have a relative, friend or other person present to support them or speak on their behalf. Coordinating the involvement of different agencies to provide the most comprehensive assessment with the minimum of inconvenience to the person concerned should then follow. Accurate information about the different services that might be available and information about any charges patients may have to pay should be provided (DHSS, 1994).

Community care plan

Following the assessment patients have an entitlement to expect a care plan in writing which is shared with multi-agency users and carers. The plan should state what services are to be provided, by whom and when. Contact numbers should be given for problems, especially outside working hours.

The community assessment is available to anyone regardless of whether it is arranged during an inpatient stay or as an outpatient. Patients or carers may self-refer.

Support available for patients in the community

Services and support should be made available depending on particular needs to enable persons disabled with rheumatological conditions to live in their own homes and maintain maximum independence. The following are some of the services that should be made available.

- home care or home help; someone who can assist with more personal tasks such as dressing;
- meals on wheels;
- sitting services or respite care;
- aids and equipment to cope with everyday tasks;
- counselling;
- occupational therapy;
- physiotherapy;
- chiropody;
- rehabilitation services for people with a visual impairment including mobility training;
- appliance officer;
- temporary or permanent accommodation in a nursing or residential home;
- help with holidays;
- help with transport;
- help with installing a telephone and special equipment to help with its use.

It is worth noting that many services will be means tested.

The Needs of the Carer

Carers are people who look after relatives or friends who, because of disability, illness or the effects of old age, cannot manage at home without help. A carer is someone who provides a substantial amount of care on a regular basis, may not be the only carer and does not need to live with the person being cared for.

Historically the carer has not been considered when planning care. However, carers have rights too and they should always be taken into account when planning care. Carers need to recognise themselves as carers, and to be recognised and valued for the work which they do. They need support, and access to services at the appropriate time, as well as accurate information and advice. Most community care is provided by family, friends and relatives who also have needs of their own and may themselves be old or disabled (HMSO, 1995).

Special Needs of Carers of Persons with Rheumatological Conditions

The needs of the carers are often ignored and yet our patients are frequently very dependent on them for many aspects of care. Carers of patients with rheumatological disease require an understanding of the disease process, the effects of the disease and the differences in mobility, stiffness and fatigue which affect the sufferer's ability to cope with everyday tasks. It is important that carers understand the changing nature of the condition which means that the sufferer varies according to the time of day, previous activity or inactivity. Learning pain management techniques often helps the carer to ease the suffering of the patient and this in turn helps to give a feeling of being in control. It is important to include carers in education programmes and to offer support and counselling should they require it. The needs of the carer are as important as those of the patient if the partnership is going to be successful.

Where necessary carers should be taught lifting and transferring by a trained therapist and adequate provision of equipment should be made to help with moving the severely disabled rheumatoid patient.

Carer assessment

All carers now have the right to an assessment which should offer a private interview or a joint assessment with the patient if this is the request of the carer. If a person in need of care is being assessed under the NHS and Community Care Act (1989d) the carer also has the right to ask for a separate assessment and should be informed of this right. If the person needing care has already had an assessment and circumstances change he or she may have a reassessment and at this point a carer may also ask for an assessment. The carer does not have to pay for the service; the person in need of care will be assessed to pay for the service.

Support Groups and Voluntary Organisations

There are numerous voluntary organisations that provide support for rheumatology patients, including Arthritis Care and the Arthritis and Rheumatism Council, and these are listed at the end of the chapter. Local support groups are also run in many areas and libraries, carer groups, rheumatology specialist nurses, national organisations and local GPs' surgeries may have information about the location and frequency of group meetings.

Conclusion

Much needs to be done to improve care within the community. Financial restraints prevent the provision of adequately resourced services within the community. Courses are now being set up to provide training for nurses in rheumatology care and time and money needs to be available so that community-based rheumatology can match the care provided for patients with some other health problems. Improved resources, better training and facilities could significantly reduce the suffering caused by pain and disability. Community rheumatology should expand and develop if we are to cater for the health needs of the majority and reduce the financial burden of long-term care.

Useful addresses including support groups and national organisations

The Arthritis and Rheumatism Council (ARC)
Copeman House
St Mary's Court
St Mary's Gate
Chesterfield
Derbyshire S41 7TD
Tel: 01246 558 033
Fax: 01246 558 007

Arthritis Care (AC)
18 Stephenson Way
London NW1 2 HD
Tel: 0171 916 1500
Helpline, Tel: 0800 289170

The British Council of Organisations of Disabled People
(BCODP)
Litchurch Plaza
Litchurch Lane
Derby DE24 8AA
Tel: 01332 295551

The British Sjögren's Syndrome Association
20 Kingston Way, Nailsea,
Bristol, BS19 2RA
Tel: 01275 854215

Carers National Association
Ruth Pitter House
20–25 Glasshouse Yard
London EC1A 4JS
Tel: 0171-490 8818
Carers line, Tel: 0171 490 8898
Fax: 0171 490 8824

Disabled Living Foundation
380–384 Harrow Road
London W14 3NS
Tel: 0171 289 6111

The Ehlers-Danlos Support Group
Valerie Burrows Founder/Organiser
1 Chandlers Close
Richmond
N Yorks DL10 5QQ
Tel: 01748 823867

Fibromyalgia Support Group
PO Box 206
Stourbridge
DY9 8YL
Tel: 01384 820052
Fax: 01384 869467

Lupus UK
Queens Court
1 Eastern Road
Romford
Essex RM1 3NH
Tel: 01708 731251
Fax: 01708 731252

The National Ankylosing Spondylitis Society
3 Grovenor Crescent
London SW1X 7ER
Tel: 0171 235 9585

National Back Pain Association
16 Elm Tree Road
Teddington
Middlesex TW11 8ST
Tel: 0181 977 5474
Fax: 0181 943 5318

National Association for the Relief of Paget's Disease
1 Church Road
Eccles
Manchester M30 0DL
Tel: 0161 707 9225

The Raynaud's and Scleroderma Association
112 Crewe Road,
Alsager
Cheshire ST7 2JA
Tel: 01270 872776
Fax: 01270 883556

Psoriatic Arthropathy Alliance
PO Box 111
St Albans
Herts AL2 3JQ
Tel/Fax: 01923 672837

The National Association to Aid the Sexual and Personal
Relationships of People with Disability (SPOD)
286 Camden Road
London NW7 0BJ

The National Osteoporosis Society
PO Box 10
Radstock
Bath BA3 3YB
Tel: 01761 471771
Fax: 01761 471104
Helpline, tel: 01761 472721

References

BLAR (1994) Disability and Arthritis, report of a survey. London: British League
    Against Rheumatism, 41 Eagle Street, London, WC IR 4AR.
Bradley EM (1991) Population projection and the effects of rheumatology. Annals
    of the Rheumatic Diseases 50:3–6.
BSR (1995a) Musculoskeletal Disorders: Providing for the Patient's Needs. A Basis
    for Planning a Rheumatology Service. London: British Society of
    Rheumatology.
BSR (1995b) Guidelines for Second Line Drug Monitoring. London: British
    Society for Rheumatology.
Cooper C (1993) Epidemiology and public health impact of osteoporosis. Baillière's
    Clinical Rheumatology 23: 8–12.
DHSS (1991) Patient's Charter Raising the Standard HPCI 51-1003 10/91 C5,00.
    London: Department of Health and Social Security.
DHSS (1994) A Framework for Local Community Care Charters in England,
    F16/003 1P 100K. London: Department of Health and Social Security.
Dieppe P (1994) Referral guidelines for GPs. Arthritis and Rheumatism Council for
    Research Chesterfield Series 3 Practical Problems January. Collected Reports
    on Rheumatic Diseases 31–4.

Donnelly S, Scott DL, Emery P (1992) The long term outcome and justification for early treatment. Clinical Rheumatology 6(2): 251–60.

Ebong WW, Lawson EAL (1978) Pattern of osteoarthritis of the hip in Nigerians. East African Medical Journal 55:81–4.

Elliot M (1995) Care management in the community: a case study. Nursing Times 91(48): 34–5.

Emery P (1993) Early rheumatoid arthritis. Rheumatology in Practice, 1(1): 10-12.

Foster HE, Pyle C, Walker DJ (1991)The provision of medical and community services to people with severe arthritis; an audit. British Journal of Rheumatology 27: 54–61.

Harvey J (1994) Assessment of Population needs. Paper presented to the RCN Public Health Conference, London, July (unpublished).

HMSO (1970) Chronically Sick and Disabled Persons Act. London: HMSO.

HMSO (1989) The NHS and Community Care Act. London: HMSO.

HMSO (1989b) Working for Patients. London: Department of Health/HMSO.

HMSO (1989c) NHS (Charges for Drugs and Appliances) Regulations. London: HMSO.

HMSO (1990a) The NHS (Fund Holding Practices) (The Application and Recognition) Regulations. London: HMSO.

HMSO (1992) The Health of the Nation, Government White Paper. London: HMSO.

HMSO (1995) Carers (Recognition and Services) Act. London: HMSO.

Johnson AE, Gordon C, Palmer RG, Bacon PA (1995)The prevalence and incidence of systemic lupus erythematosus. Relationship to ethnicity and country of birth. Arthritis and Rheumatism 38: 551–8.

Johnson AE, Gordon C, Hobbs FDR, Bacon PA (1996) Undiagnosed systemic lupus erythematosus in the community. Lancet 347: 367–9.

Liang M, Komaroff AL (1982) Roentgenograms in primary care patients with acute lower back pain: cost-effective analysis. Arthritis and Rheumatism 142: 1108–112.

Linton S, Situnayake D (1993–95) Multi-ethnic rheumatology. Rheumatology in Practice, 1(5): 8–10 Vol 1 Part 4. Hayward Medical Communication.

Maggi S, Kelsey JL, Litvak J, Heysey SP (1991) Incidence of hip fractures in the elderly: a cross-sectional analysis. Osteoporosis Int Vol 1 Part 4: 232–241.

Morrison NA, Qi JC, Tokita A, Kelly PJ, Croft L, Nguyen TV, Sambook PN, Tisman JA (1994) Prediction in bone density from vitamin D alleles. Nature 376 (January): 284–7.

Mukhopadhaya B, Barooah B (1967) Osteoarthritis of the hip in Indians: anatomical and clinical study. Indian Journal of Orthopaedics 1: 55–63.

Nichol FE, Woodrow JC (1981) HLA-DR antigens in Indian patients with rheumatoid arthritis. Lancet i: 220–1.

OPCS (1989) General Household Survey. London: HMSO.

Royal College of Physicians (1989) Fractured neck of femur, prevention and management. Summary and recommendations of a report on the Royal College of Physicians. Journal of the Royal College of Physicians of London 23: 8–12.

Ryan S (1995) Sharing care in an outpatients' clinic. Nursing Standard 10: 23–5.

Scott DL, Symonds DPM, Coulton BL, Popert AJ (1987) Long term outcome of treating rheumatoid arthritis: results after 20 years. Lancet i: 1108–1111.

Silman A (1995) Rheumatoid arthritis: the health economic burden. Rheumatology in Practice 2(4): 16–19.

Symonds DPM, Barrett EM, Bankhead C, Chadkravarty K, Scott DGI, Silman AJ (1994) The incidence of rheumatoid arthritis in the United Kingdom: results from the Norfolk Arthritis Register. British Journal of Rheumatology 33: 735–39.

Symonds D, Bankhead C (1994) Health care needs assessment for musculoskeletal disease: the first step – estimating the number of incidents and prevalent cases. ARC Arthritis and Rheumatism, Chesterfield.

Walsh K, Cruddas M, Coggan D, Low (1992) Back pain in eight areas of Britain. Journal of Epidemiology and Community Health 46: 227–30.

White CE (1996) Model of management for rheumatology patients and social needs assessment form. Unpublished dissertation.

Chapter 5
Patient education and self-management

PATRICIA LE GALLEZ

A physical disability handicaps not only the person in whom it occurs, but frequently those who enter social relationships with them. (Hilbourne, 1973)

Introduction

In rheumatology, patient education (PE) emerged, at least in this country, in the early 1980s. Prior to this patients had received little information. The reason for this attitude was that as there was no known cure or control, there was little point in education, and as a result patients were simply told to 'Go home, and learn to live with it.' The consequence of this attitude was that patients were offered virtually no support, or means of communication, just a brief summary of the disease with little opportunity for questions. The result can still be seen in our clinics today: patients who, many years after diagnosis, still remain ignorant of most facts which relate to their illness and are overwhelming in their praise following just a few minutes spent explaining some minor detail of their drug therapy or treatment to them. The diabetic or asthmatic patient has long been the recipient of excellent PE. The reason for this is clear; these illnesses are life-threatening and failure to inform the patient about his or her condition and treatment would result in the patient's death.

In rheumatology task nursing was the accepted method of nursing care, and this, because of its philosophy, left little opportunity for the nurse or the patient to develop a unique relationship which would allow for the sharing of information, or for giving psychological support. Indeed, had the nurse presumed to spend time actually talking, and as importantly, listening to the patient, she would have been accused of wasting time, time which could have been spent on yet a further task even if that task involved straightening the beds or tidying a cupboard. All were deemed more important than actually communicating with the patient.

We now live in a more enlightened society, one in which social attitudes have been turned upside down. If we fail to inform the patient adequately with regard to the disease or drug therapy, or just as importantly the outcome of surgical intervention, then litigation may well be threatened. In addition, with the advent of Trust Hospitals, GP fundholders and purchaser power, the role of the doctor has also changed considerably and he or she is no longer considered the sole conveyer of information to the patient as was the case in the recent past. Because of this change in attitude, each discipline within the health field has a role to play in passing information to the patient, and to the relatives, so enabling the individual to regain control of the future. Fortunately, rheumatic patients rarely die of their disease, though it is now known that they do have a reduced life expectancy (Scott et al., 1987). Even so, their lives will be changed dramatically by a cruel and debilitating illness. Although this illness may not cause their death to be imminent, it may well deny them the freedom of mobility, which to many people is the very essence of life. How can such patients be helped? Our aim must be to do everything possible to alleviate the mental and physical anguish, to assist each person to develop independence, to come to terms with their individual problems, and to live as pain free and as mobile an existence as is possible.

At the introduction of PE many years ago the term 'education' was considered appropriate. Now, some say it is condescending to the patient to refer to the giving of information in this way and the term should therefore be avoided. Whilst I have a certain sympathy with this assumption, finding a substitute is not easy. Though 'information' appears to be a reasonable option I have nonetheless decided to continue to refer to the subject as education, because, quite frankly, when writing about it, it is easier to do so.

Patient Education and Self-management

Basic nursing requirements

For the nurse to provide the patient with the best possible help via education and information, they will need to know the disease they are dealing with. They must be fully informed in every aspect of care which lies within their province. Though they will not be expected to know everything about joint protection, which is the role of the occupational therapist (OT) or about a daily exercise programme which is a function of the physiotherapist (PT), they will be expected to have sufficient knowledge to enable them to give useful information to the patient, certainly sufficient for them to reinforce what has been taught by the OT or the PT, or the orthotist or the dietitian. Of course the same applies to the disease process, drug therapy, disease outcome, sexual and social aspects, psychological impact, resources and so on. To try to inform someone else when one is oneself ignorant, apart from being foolish and unprofessional, is also dangerous.

Why educate the patient?

Patient education is a caring, constructive method of disease control. As we have no other 'control' to offer patients, drug therapy being a holding device and not a control, surely, giving the patients information which empowers them to make informed decisions is a giant step along the way?

Even so, before answering this question in any depth, let us consider the consequences of a chronic and, in some instances, a disabling illness for both patients and their families. Patients with a rheumatological problem, whether mild or severe, will be affected emotionally, physically, psychologically, sexually and financially. Repercussions will follow which will themselves influence the patients' relationship with their partners, families, friends and colleagues at work. As a result of these changes the following may well take place.

A change in lifestyle: The patient will live at a much slower pace, may have to stop work (Reisine and Grady, 1989), or worse still, unwillingly lose his or her job (Meenan et al., 1981). A housewife may find she can no longer accomplish her housework. As a result, she may find she can no longer care adequately for her family. Recreation, as the patient knew it, may now be a thing of the past.

Because of these alterations in lifestyle the patient's quality of life will be diminished: The patient may experience a loss of income, and no longer enjoy the pleasures of holidays (le Gallez, 1993). Children in the family may develop behavioural difficulties. In more extreme cases the patient may be confined to the home. Divorce or separation may ensue (Hawley et al., 1991).

The systemic illnesses result in fluctuations of the disease with exacerbations, followed by remissions: The consequences of such fluctuations produce uncertainty (Wiener, 1975). It then becomes impossible to plan ahead, whether it is a day, a week, a month or a year. The uncertainty is all-encompassing, and can take control of the patient's life.

Because we lack a cure, we can offer only limited control of the disease: As a result there is a deep fear as to what the future holds. This fear is experienced in particular by someone who is newly diagnosed (see Chapter 1).

Though the normal lifespan may be shortened as a result of the disease, the patient should live for many years: In order to retain a semblance of normality patients will now be subjected to a life time of drug therapy, coupled with various form of painful treatment and possibly multiple orthopaedic surgery. Many will constantly be faced with the dilemma of treatment versus side-effects.

Pain will dominate the patient's life: It is because of this particular symptom that, in all probability, you will find yourself face to face with a patient seeking your help and support. What better way is there to provide for the individual's needs than to supply the relevant information, so empowering the patient to make informed decisions with regard to the illness. In this situation the nurse will not only require educational skills; counselling skills will also be called upon. Education and counselling are quite distinct from each other in their method of approach and yet the outcome is much the same. When dealing with a patient with a rheumatic condition the nurse will be called upon, time and time again, to provide both these skills. It will be up to each nurse to decide the most appropriate path to take with regard to each individual patient, at any one moment in time.

Who should act as educator?

Clearly, I am advocating nurses as an obvious choice, though they are by no means the only one. Every discipline involved in the care of the patient will wish to offer information and rightly so. The problem arises when an individual discipline interested in PE then puts together a package in total isolation. In this instance, the opportunity for a team approach is lost and in rheumatology this would be an unworkable scenario as we need to work together to give the same message, if we are to achieve optimum care for the patient. Therefore, those professionals involved in caring for the patient with a rheumatic problem should work together to provide an educational package that covers all aspects of care.

Traditionally, the doctor alone would have provided the patient with such information as he or she thought fit, but does the modern doctor wish to spend time educating the patient in detail? In most instances the answer would be no! At least, not in great depth. Not because doctors are unsympathetic to PE but simply because they are trained to diagnose, and therefore a large proportion of their time is already committed, and they have little time to spare. Doctors are usually seen working in busy outpatient clinics or wards, and working under great pressure. The degree to which they are able to offer education is severely limited and therefore they move on to the next patient, giving the minimum information as they go. This is an acceptable situation provided the doctor is fully aware of the needs of the patient and the family and makes certain someone else is employed to carry out the task instead. In rheumatology we now have nurse specialists (see Chapter 2), nurses who have vast experience in the speciality and whose main concern is education and counselling of both patients and their families, whether as inpatients or outpatients.

The patient as educator

As the central figure in any education programme is the patient, perhaps the best person to pass information on to a patient is a fellow patient? Certainly, in America, this method of informing the patient has existed for many years (Lorig et al., 1986). Sessions involving a group of people with different forms of arthritis, and lasting approximately two hours, are held on a regular basis, usually for six consecutive weeks. The whole programme is taught and run by people (trainers) who have some form of arthritis. A major component of these sessions is for 'contracts' to be forged between the group and the patient and which the patient aims to meet by the next meeting. An example could be agreeing to exercise three times a week, instead of only once or not at all. The research carried out leads us to believe that this method of education is a useful adjunct to the more formal teaching programme to be discussed later (Lorig et al., 1985; Cohen et al., 1986). In this country, Arthritis Care is in the throes of a research programme which is attempting to emulate the American findings. The programme is based on that designed by Kate Lorig and described above. The trainees (teachers) must first go through a training programme before they are allowed to act as trainers themselves. It will be some two years before we know the outcome of the programme in this country, though unpublished results look promising so far.

Anxieties about such topics as the disease process, drug therapy and exercise programmes being taught by laypersons, even though they are patients themselves, are resolved by the group using the Lorig and Fries (1980–95) manual as a guide, with instructions not to deviate from its content.

In addition to these group sessions, arrangements can also be made for an individual patient to counsel a fellow patient in a one-to-one situation. This can provide much useful support in respect of the emotional and psychological impact, and also they can each share their experiences of coping with the disease. There can be no one better experienced to do this. However, a word of caution. The patient who is to counsel needs to be selected with great care otherwise the result may prove to be unsatisfactory.

Formal education sessions and how to approach them

Formal sessions can be arranged for inpatients or outpatients; they can also be one-to-one or group sessions. Either session can include members of the patient's family. Indeed, this should be encouraged wherever possible. Even young children can be included in a session providing they are not overwhelmed. Children who accompany their parent to hospital provide an excellent opportunity for the nurse to explain Mum's or Dad's problems to them in a very simple way. It is also an ideal opening for the nurse to appeal to children to help if they can, particularly in the following ways. The nurse might suggest keeping their room tidy, or offering to set or clear the table without having to be asked, and when Mum or Dad is having a bad day, remembering to give them a gentle cuddle and ask if they can do anything for them. Children will usually listen when spoken to by someone other than the family. And of course Mum or Dad can always remind them of what the nurse said, should they forget!

If older children attend with their parent the opportunity should be grasped to discover the children's views on whether or not they are concerned in case they too might develop the illness. Sadly, it has been shown (le Gallez, 1993) that children do worry about developing the illness themselves and have often been misinformed into thinking their parent's illness is hereditary. These fears must be quickly allayed by the nurse (Spector, 1996). Of course, ward staff have a much better chance of meeting the children whatever their age, as they will usually be visiting their parents on the ward. After obtaining permission from the parent the nurse could take the children to one side, preferably into a private room, to offer them the opportunity for discussion, if they should wish, either at that time or on another occasion. Sometimes simply suggesting to the parent that they approach the children with the same offer also works.

Group sessions

If the idea of group sessions appeals, you will first need to consider patient numbers. If you have access to large numbers of patients, whether inpatients or outpatients, you may well achieve a good response. If you have only a few inpatient beds, perhaps only between 4 and 8, then it will be difficult realistically to educate inpatients in a group. The chances are your group of inpatients will be suffering from a variety of rheumatic problems making group education difficult as the accumulated problems will be diverse. Here, a one-to-one educational approach should be considered. A good supply of educational videos can be a tremendous asset, though it is imperative that patients are never left to watch such videos without professional supervision or they may misinterpret information which could result in extreme distress. If a well-informed member of staff is available to answer questions while the patient is viewing, much can be gained from well-documented educational videos.

If group sessions are to be seriously contemplated then the implementation will require organisation and cooperation from all disciplines involved. Generally speaking, sessions are best broken down into specific illnesses. What is more, because time is at a premium for all the professionals concerned, most classes concentrate on rheumatoid arthritis with the less common systemic illnesses dealt with on a one-to-one basis. Education on the non-inflammatory disease osteoarthritis is rarely offered to patients in group sessions. These patients are usually given information and advice, on a one-to-one basis, by whomever they see in the clinic situation. Patients with ankylosing spondylitis (AS) are usually the concern of the physiotherapist (PT). The PT will organise group sessions as outpatients or, if they are lucky enough to have adequate resources, groups of inpatients are admitted for two weeks for intensive physiotherapy and hydrotherapy, which includes education. This is because it is in the best interests of AS patients to adhere to a daily exercise programme if they are to remain upright and mobile.

The above description of separating out different diseases into groups is in direct contrast with the patient-taught classes previously mentioned, both here and in USA. These classes will include, at any one time, any arthritic condition, from the more serious inflammatory illnesses to the less seriously ill with fibromyalgia, or low back pain. This method of education, at least from a professional point of view, can make the task of successfully informing such a diverse group of people somewhat difficult. Because of this, for educational purposes, professionals will in the main tend to separate groups into diseases.

Once a decision is taken to hold group sessions, whether for in- or outpatients, a committee consisting of the disciplines involved should be formed. If getting everyone together proves impossible because of other commitments and pressure of work, then someone in the team could take the initiative and act as coordinator. He or she could put together an outline of the intended classes and distribute this to all who have expressed an interest in being involved. This would allow those interested to comment on the content of the proposal and at the same time they would have the opportunity to commit them- selves to the programme, or not. Once committed it is vital they see through their part in the programme. Should they be taken ill they must organise a suitable substitute. As a last resort, if a session is organised and patients are arriving and the educator cannot be present then a video, run by a substitute professional, can be shown instead. Occasionally, group sessions can include patients with other rheumatological problems though only in certain of the classes – in relaxation for example, as this is a very useful skill for all to learn, or a class on 'improving your posture' would also be suitable for all.

One-to-one sessions

In many ways, this is perhaps the most satisfactory way to educate and inform a patient. It is more relaxing for the patient, and the privacy helps to develop an atmosphere of trust between patient and professional. It is of course nurses above all other professionals who usually have the time and the opportunity, because of the 24-hour cover, to offer one-to-one sessions, or because they are employed specifically for this role, as with the nurse specialists (see Chapter 2). To reiterate the previous advice, in order to offer education the nurse must be proficient in the chosen speciality. However, if your specialist knowledge is limited, then you can, at the very least, offer to listen to the patient's anxieties with the express aim of finding someone more knowledgeable to answer the questions or provide solutions to the problems. It is also an excellent opportunity for improving your own skills and gaining experience. When contemplating one-to-one education, always find a private room, even if it is a closet – this is imperative. The alternative is an open ward and the patient trying to express personal worries and anxieties while the other patients listen to every word and this is not a good idea. Even though space is at a premium in all hospitals, the setting aside of a small private room specifically for this purpose should be a priority.

Drop-in centres are springing up in many specialities. They are not strictly venues for education, for the atmosphere is usually geared towards offering support together with a social component. Informal advice may be offered, or contacts made which lead to a formal education group. A further consideration must also be taken into account. Whilst the general idea of drop-in centres is excellent, they are very demanding as the staff usually help to run these centres in their own time in conjunction with interested patients. Unlike a planned education programme, drop-in centres, once established, must fulfil their obligation each week or month, indefinitely. For drop-in centres to work successfully they require a dedication and commitment from staff perhaps beyond the call of duty.

Planning outpatient group sessions

Having decided to go ahead with outpatient group sessions, the following should be taken into account. Much of what is about to be suggested will apply to inpatient sessions also.

The building should be situated in an area which has car parking suitable for people with a disability, plus convenient public transport. The area around the building should be well lit if sessions are held in the late afternoon or evening. Suitable access is vital for those with walking difficulties or in wheelchairs. Accordingly, ramps must be provided. Wooden ramps are obtainable to fit over steps and can be a worthwhile investment.

Rooms: Once inside the building lifts to different levels will be essential if steps are the only other means of approach. The rooms themselves should also have easy access, with doors that are manageable, hence not too heavy, and handles not too difficult for someone with hand problems to open. The width of the door should accommodate a wheelchair easily. Lighting should be adequate. The room should not be too hot or too cold. The room itself should be situated away from distracting noise. Seating should be varied so as to accommodate different needs. There should be sufficient space for people to get up and move around.

Essential extras: Electricity points need checking beforehand if slides or videos are to be shown. Curtains at the windows will be required in this case. You may need to provide a hot drink, so make certain you have a kettle plus everything else necessary.

Toilets: These must be provided and they must have easy access for those who are disabled.

Transport: If people do not have their own transport and public transport is out of the question, try and arrange for others to provide a pick-up service; many voluntary bodies will do this willingly. At the end of a session ALWAYS make sure everyone has a lift home.

Before the meeting: Always remind those attending to bring their glasses, hearing aid and spare batteries; pens or pencils too, if they are required.

In addition to holding formal and informal groups the nurse specialist should be particularly vigilant and consider intervention at the following times, all of which demonstrate a critical period in the day-to-day life of a patient:

(1) When the patient is first *diagnosed.*
(2) During or following the *first serious flare.*
(3) When the patient is *considering stopping work.*
(4) When the patient is *deciding whether or not to have children.*
(5) At times of *emotional upheaval,* for example, difficulties with children, financial difficulties, death in the family.
(6) At times of *marital stress,* particularly divorce or separation.

What to teach

Many papers have been written which describe patient education programmes, and their benefits (Bellman, 1994; Close, 1988, 1992; Hilton, 1992; Lindroth et al., 1989; Lorig, Konkol and Gonzales,1987; Lorish et al.,1985). Also, Hill et al. (1991) suggest a means of evaluation by use of the Patient Knowledge Questionnaire. This chapter therefore gives a brief description of those areas which should be covered, whether on a one-to-one basis or in a group session.

The patient should be referred for education and counselling as soon as a diagnosis has been made. In this way success in helping the patient adapt successfully to the illness is likely to succeed. This is not to say that the patients who has been diagnosed for many years will not benefit from education, for of course they will.

The following are some of the major problems encountered and common to most rheumatic diseases.

(1) an altered emotional state;
(2) lack of medical knowledge pertinent to the disease;
(3) understanding and accepting complicated drug therapy;
(4) mastering pain control;
(5) coping effectively with everyday tasks, both at home and at work;
(6) maintaining good mobility and preventing joint deformity;
(7) identifying and surviving a flare;
(8) resolving reduced social isolation;
(9) adjusting to an altered sexual lifestyle;

(10) coping with concomitant illnesses as a result of medication or the initial disease;

(11) eating sensibly so as to maintain a balanced diet and a healthy weight.

The following suggestions will enable the health professional caring for the rheumatic patient to provide a concise educational programme. Subsequently such diverse problems as those experienced by patients suffering from OA or AS can be met from this programme as, indeed, can those problems associated with more serious systemic diseases, for example systemic lupus erythematosus (SLE) or RA.

Content of an educational programme

(1) Altered emotional state

Intervention - counselling: The emotional state may be characterised by acute anxiety or by an expression of self-denial; rarely do patients accept the diagnosis without some emotional trauma. At this stage the nurse must assess the patient and decide how much information to give. It is possible that appropriate counselling must first be considered and a positive response obtained before any education can be given. Ideally, this would be the recommended approach. Unhappily, the patient with a rheumatic condition is likely to be suffering severe pain and will therefore require instant therapy, in which case certain information has to be given in order for the patient to start treatment.

Providing the nurse has a sound understanding of the disease process and is aware of the problems which may result, whether they be physical or psychological, social or sexual, she will be in the ideal position to provide the basic guidance and care. Whilst more hospitals are now employing clinical psychologists as team members they are still in very short supply and those that do exist have very long waiting lists. Because of this situation it is generally the nurse who cares for the majority of distressed patients. With the help and support of the family, the patient generally pulls through and eventually adapts to the illness, though this may take as long as five years (Manne and Zautra, 1992). Those few patients who cannot come to terms with the problems can, in addition to seeing the nurse, be referred to the clinical psychologist. Patients who live alone for whatever reason, and regardless of their gender, appear to have more difficulty coping and adapting to the illness, and this is quite understandable. When ill, we rely on others to help pull us through, and if companionship is lacking it may well take longer to adjust to the constraints of the illness. This is an important point of which to be aware. Such patients often make heavy demands on the nurse specialist in particular.

A subjective assessment can be made by listening to the patient describe how the illness started and how it is progressing and also the extent to which the patient's life has now been altered because of it. Some patients will be both receptive and talkative; others will be in a state of mental shock and incapable of understanding or retaining anything said to them. In the latter case the situation will need to be approached with great sensitivity, and at this juncture education may well consist only of basic information on the drugs prescribed and how to cope with pain. Meanwhile, encouragement and support for the patient and the family will be supplied by all the hospital staff as the patient comes into contact with them.

A more objective assessment of the patient's mood could be obtained at this point using the Hospital Anxiety and Depression Scale (HAD) (Zigmound and Snaith, 1983, Figure 5.1) (see Chapter 2). If the score suggests depression and/or anxiety is present then you will need to act accordingly. Either antidepressants can be prescribed on a short- or long-term basis, or referral to a clinical psychologist may be appropriate. Certainly, regular visits to the nurse specialist for support and encouragement, plus access to a telephone helpline, is the least that must be offered. In addition, stressing to patients that what is being experienced is no different from that experienced by most who are afflicted in the same way, often helps patients to see things in a positive light. Otherwise, they imagine themselves to be the only ones to experience depression and/or anxiety because of the illness. It is possible that by arranging a meeting with a fellow patient who has 'weathered the storm' a positive attitude may ensue. The patients' partners and families need to be made aware of the acute depression or anxiety state, so that they too can provide the appropriate support.

(2) Lack of appropriate medical knowledge

Intervention – Description of disease process relevant to the patient: Poor medical knowledge, and the gradual realisation that there is no cure for the illness, affect most people in much the same way. They crave information in a desire to find answers with which to overcome their new-found fears. As the symptoms associated with the illness begin to take their toll, so doubts are casts upon how they will cope

HAD Scale

Name: Date:

Doctors are aware that emotions play an important part in most illnesses. If your doctor knows about these feelings he will be able to help you more.

This questionnaire is designed to help your doctor to know how you feel. Read each item and place a firm tick in the box opposite the reply which comes closest to how you have been feeling in the past week.

Don't take too long over your replies: your immediate reaction to each item will probably be more accurate than a long thought-out response.

Tick only one box in each section

I feel tense or 'wound up':
- Most of the time
- A lot of the time
- Time to time, Occasionally
- Not at all

I still enjoy the things I used to enjoy:
- Definitely as much
- Not quite so much
- Only a little
- Hardly at all

I get a sort of frightened feeling as if something awful is about to happen:
- Very definitely and quite badly
- Yes, but not too badly
- A little, but it doesn't worry me
- Not at all

I can laugh and see the funny side of things:
- As much as I always could
- Not quite so much now
- Definitely not so much now
- Not at all

Worrying thoughts go through my mind:
- A great deal of the time
- A lot of the time
- From time to time but not too often
- Only occasionally

I feel cheerful:
- Not at all
- Not often
- Sometimes
- Most of the time

I can sit at ease and feel relaxed:
- Definitely
- Usually
- Not often
- Not at all

I feel as if I am slowed down:
- Nearly all the time
- Very often
- Sometimes
- Not at all

I get a sort of frightened feeling like 'butterflies' in the stomach:
- Not at all
- Occasionally
- Quite often
- Very often

I have lost interest in my appearance:
- Definitely
- I don't take so much care as I should
- I may not take quite as much care
- I take just as much care as ever

I feel restless as if I have to be on the move:
- Very much indeed
- Quite a lot
- Not very much
- Not at all

I look forward with enjoyment to things:
- As much as ever I did
- Rather less than I used to
- Definitely less than I used to
- Hardly at all

I get sudden feelings of panic:
- Very often indeed
- Quite often
- Not very often
- Not at all

I can enjoy a good book or radio or TV programme:
- Often
- Sometimes
- Not often
- Very seldom

Do not write below this line

Figure 5.1 Hospital Anxiety and Depression Scale (HAD)

both now and in the future. The inevitable questions are: 'How will I manage?'; 'Will I have to stop work?'; plus the all-important question, 'Will I end up in a wheelchair?'. Because of this distressing situation it is essential to provide information as quickly as possible, that is before well-meaning friends and neighbours confuse the patient even further. In addition, the patient will hear of, and read, many articles which will give conflicting advice. It is therefore essential to arrange to spend time with the patients as soon as possible, in order to explain the implications of their particular disease and in a way that is easily understood. Booklets and information sheets can also be provided. The patient should be advised to take the written information home and to share it with the rest of the family. In this way everyone concerned with the patient on a day-to-day basis will understand the condition better, and as a result be more willing to provide the required support. Questions should be answered as they arise, without being too concerned at this juncture as to the amount of information actually being understood or retained, as the nurse will reinforce the relevant information at each session. Many booklets are provided free by the Arthritis and Rheumatism Council and by Arthritis Care. They can be obtained by using the appropriate ordering sheets. The addresses are supplied later in the book.

(3) Drug compliance

Intervention – explain the use of drugs used in rheumatology and supply relevant drug information sheets (DIS): Drug therapy plays a vital role in the treatment of most rheumatic diseases. Therefore, compliance with drug therapy becomes paramount (Fisher, 1992). To aid compliance, drug information sheets (DIS) should be provided. They are of enormous advantage to both the patient and health professionals though in particular to nurses. Almost every rheumatology department now uses them, and if they do not then the nurse specialist can instigate their use. Patients are given the DIS for future reference. With all patients, though particularly with the elderly and confused, the sheets provide information for the relative, neighbour, general practitioner, practice nurse and district nurse to work from. Certainly, if self-medication is contemplated then DIS's are vital for the success of the programme and will greatly enhance patient care and professional knowledge. DIS's should be supplied for every drug used in rheumatology, including all drugs used on the periphery and likely to be dispensed, e.g. anticoagulants, antidepressants, diuretics, etc. In addition to the DIS, dosette boxes can be provided for the elderly and also for the younger patient taking multiple drugs as they help significantly towards compliance. Each DIS should contain the following information:

- name of patient and start date;
- name of drug – both generic and where possible the trade name;
- reason for taking the drug;
- description of drug – this may not always be possible, as there are now different brands of the same drug;
- dosage of drug – including how to take the drug;
- possible side-effects – and instruction on what to do should they occur;
- special instructions – e.g. may change the colour of urine;
- additional information – e.g. on pregnancy;
- instructions with regard to safety and children;
- a telephone helpline number;
- revision date – they must be updated on a regular basis. The responsibility for this could lie with the nurse and/or pharmacy.

When first discussing drug therapy with a patient, put time aside to explain the four different groups of drugs we use in rheumatology, i.e. analgesics, non-steroidal anti-inflammatory drugs (NSAIDs), disease-modifying anti-rheumatic drugs (DMARDs) and steroids (see Chapter 6). This helps clarify why we prescribe the different drugs and what their individual benefits are. It will also give a rational explanation to the patient, as to why so many drugs are being given, and this should aid compliance. This of course will help to empower the patient. It is widely understood that wastage of medication results from misuse on the part of the patient (Haynes, Wang and Gomes, 1987). This can almost always be directly attributed to lack of, or misunderstanding about, 'information'. As a result, overdosing or underdosing occurs. Another danger is that of the patient who has been inadequately informed and stops medication for fear of imagined or actual side-effects. If someone suffers from a chronic illness there is a strong possibility that drug therapy will be necessary for life. Because of this factor, as each drug is introduced its use should be carefully discussed with the patient to enable an informed decision to be made about whether or not to accept the drug concerned. This is particularly important when it is considered that the drugs prescribed are not curative, or life dependent; indeed, the DMARDs, among the most toxic of all the drugs we use, are known only to hold or dampen down the disease.

Liaison with the practice nurse: The actual monitoring of DMARDs is an ongoing problem for most rheumatology departments and also for most GPs. Monitoring of DMARDS can be time consuming and up to a point costly in terms of time involved (see Chapters 4 and 6). Most consultants would prefer GPs, together with their practice nurses (PNs), to monitor their own patients. Unfortunately, many GPs are reluctant to carry out such monitoring, feeling that this responsibility should lie with the consultant. This may be because of the GPs' limited knowledge of such drugs and reasonable fear of side-effects, hence education for all concerned and not only the patient is necessary. GPs also express a reluctance to put yet more responsibility on their PNs. The problem of monitoring, should the GP refuse to do so, can mean a tremendous burden on the nurse specialist in outpatients. She could well find herself monitoring some hundreds of patients, which would be impossible; what is more it is not the nurse's primary role (see Chapter 2). *Monitoring of DMARDS is all about patient safety* and therefore it is not going to go away. Ideally, the NS should liaise with the PN and between them a programme of care can be organised for the individual patient. All PNs seem more than happy to move along this road providing they can secure permission to do so from their GP employer. They too can use the telephone helpline, now provided by most rheumatology departments, should they have any concerns.

(4) Mastering pain control

Intervention – discuss the many and varied forms of controlling pain, plus pain monitoring: Factors which influence pain in rheumatic disease are discussed below:

- As many of the rheumatic diseases are systemic, the disease process is described as *inflammatory*. This results in hot, swollen joints, the consequence of which is pain.
- This inflammation can eventually lead to *destruction of soft and hard tissue*, and deformity may result leading to more pain. Non-inflammatory arthritis can result in bone and cartilage destruction producing deformity, also resulting in pain.
- Such destruction can lead to *bone erosion*, which can produce pressure on nerves, and may add neurological pain.
- At any time there can be *stiffness*, the description of which defies definition; even so, the result is pain.
- Because of joint involvement, *movement aggravates* the condition, and the result is yet more pain.

- The amount of *anxiety and stress* experienced by the patient will influence the degree of pain.
- Our *failure to communicate* is a major source of distress to patients, increasing their pain.
- The presence of pain can *impede communication*, therefore the patient will not seek to reveal their pain and fears to anyone.

Pain, if allowed to, will control the patients, and will dominate their life. The following observation has been attributed to two separate people, McCaffery (1979) and Sternbach (1974). No matter who said it first the message is quite clear: 'pain is whatever the experiencing person says it is, existing whenever he says it does'. In a more superficial vein it has also been said that pain, like love, is a feeling most people understand but have difficulty describing. They are both subjective and unique to each person. Because of this, each individual person has a different pain threshold. The *pain threshold* has been described as the point at which we first notice pain, and *pain tolerance* as the upper limit of endurance. Both of these differ with age, sex, race, religion, cultural upbringing and pain experience. In chronic pain, such as is seen in the patients with whom we deal, complete pain relief cannot be guaranteed. Instead, we aim for temporary or partial relief. Conveying this message to patients is extremely important otherwise their expectations of what we as professionals can achieve on their behalf will be totally unrealistic. By helping the patient towards reasonable pain relief we can hope to avoid anxiety, depression and even anger developing; the latter in particular can have disastrous results for the immediate family (le Gallez, 1993).

Discussing pain control with the patient: Because of pain patients will find it difficult to comply with the treatments suggested; therefore pain control must be a priority. When discussing pain control with patients remember that an element of depression usually accompanies pain. You may already have asked patients to fill in an HAD questionnaire to assess their mood if you were at all suspicious of their mental state. You will therefore take any results you have into account before continuing. Always tell patients the results, as it helps both patients and nurses to be open and frank with each other.

Provide a peaceful and private atmosphere – a room where you will be undisturbed. Listen to the patient; we do not do this often enough and always think we know best. Also, relatives, unintentionally, sometimes talk down to an ill person, thinking it is for the best.

Sleep is essential for its restorative benefits. Often night pain is felt to be the worst kind, so discuss sleeping arrangements. A king-size bed, with two single duvets, is far more suitable than a conventional 4' 6" bed and one double duvet. Also, couples need to sleep together, not split up into separate rooms. Two single beds pushed together may be the solution if space is at a premium (see 'Sexual relationships and arthritis' later in this chapter).

In order to control pain it is essential to break the cycle of tension and depression interlinked with anxiety as quickly as possible. Though various methods of pain control are available, what is suggested here is that once the correct method of taking drugs has been mastered, alternative methods of pain control can be incorporated with each person choosing the method which suits them best.

As a rule when an analgesic is prescribed the patient is told to take the tablets as and when necessary - PRN - rather than on a regular basis. As a result, many people choose not to take the analgesics. They make this decision because they are already taking many drugs, or because they simply dislike taking drugs, or they are afraid of addiction. They seem to feel there is some virtue in suffering pain and, in their words, 'fighting it' rather than 'giving in' and taking something for pain relief. To overcome this reluctance, we must advise the patient of the key factor in controlling pain, that of acting quickly and not waiting until the situation is out of hand. In this way the patient will be in control rather than the pain. Patients should be advised to take their NSAIDs on a regular basis as prescribed, and then back them up with analgesics as and when the pain breaks through. If they remember to step in early when their pain is moving from mild to moderate, rather than waiting until the pain has becomes unbearable and then taking something as they become desperate, they should gain pain relief. If they are experiencing a flare they should continue taking both drugs together until the flare starts to subside. Eventually, as they gain control they can reduce the analgesics. They should do this cautiously and should not be afraid to return to the full dose if the pain level dictates that they should do so. For some people, following these guidelines will not result in the desired effect and pain will continue, in which case a change in analgesic will be required. *Antidepressants* are occasionally prescribed to help break the stress–pain–depression cycle. The drug used is usually dothiepin hydrochloride 25–50 mg nocte. This helps to modulate the pain, and when taken at night can help to induce sleep.

Additional methods of pain control: Any of the following can be used in conjunction with drug therapy, or alone:

- application of heat or cold (see Chapters 2, 7, 8);
- massage: the laying on of hands to heal pain and sickness goes back to biblical times and, indeed, is one of the most potent forms of pain relief. Patients should be advised never to massage without using a medium such as a cosmetic oil, otherwise the skin can easily be damaged. Aromatherapists, of course, use massage as part of their treatment.
- relaxation: when in pain, relaxation is the most difficult state to achieve but it is not impossible. Many tapes are available, though it is worth noting that relaxation is something that needs to be learned; it does not occur automatically as the tape is switched on. Most people find it easier to learn to relax in a group, rather than alone. Many health professionals are now offering this service.
- diversion: this is yet another form of pain control. Advise patients to develop a hobby or to immerse themselves in an established hobby. Many pastimes can be achieved with considerable success, e.g. embroidery, sewing, painting, jigsaws, listening to music or the radio, reading, etc. These pastimes are suitable for both sexes. In addition, maintaining an active social life is a bonus as often agreeable company can very successfully divert thoughts away from pain.
- acupuncture: this has varying degrees of success, though is well worth a try if the patient can afford the cost. Often sustained improvement lapses when treatment is stopped. Some health professionals are now trained and offer this form of treatment.
- reflexology, Shiatsu and hypnotherapy are also available if patients wish to try them.

Assessing/monitoring pain: Pain diaries can be used to monitor pain if it is required to do so. Certainly, if a patient is suffering acute pain post-operatively, a pain diary may be of benefit. However, as we deal with chronic pain, using a diary, unless it is for a research project, may simply over-emphasise the pain to the patient's disadvantage. There is considerable literature on the methods of pain measurement; the following may be of use when deciding on the appropriate tool: Baillie (1993); Bird and Dixon (1987); Buckelew and Parker (1989). A base-line pain score is always a useful measurement to obtain on admission to a ward. However, do wait and allow the patient time to overcome the trauma of travelling to the hospital or an invalid score will be registered. Further scores can be obtained during the stay either daily or at two- or three-day intervals, and these scores will give some indication of the success of treatment or drug therapy.

Never trouble the patient to record assessments of *any kind* unless you intend acting upon the findings.

(5) Coping with everyday tasks both at home and at work

Intervention — planning, pacing and prioritising these tasks, together with an OT referral and assessment: If the patient is exhibiting physical difficulties, however minor, it is at this point that a Health Assessment Questionnaire (HAQ) could be filled in to procure a base-line reading of the patient's physical abilities (Fries et al.,1980) (see Chapter 2). With the results to hand the patient should be referred to the OT as soon as possible (see Chapter 8). Patients who have problem joints require help before deformity has developed. In order to provide this help the patient will be assessed by the OT. The assessment is known as an ADL or 'activities of daily living'. The assessment is carried out in far greater depth than the HAQ and will determine each individual patient's special physical needs and the appropriate aid or adaptation will be recommended and in many cases also provided. If the patient is fairly newly diagnosed it is often very difficult for him or her to accept this form of help. As a result, careful education and counselling on the part of the nurse will be required in order to persuade them to accept the referral as being of benefit to them.

As patients will need help to cope with the day-to-day problems caused by their disease, they should be taught the concept of planning each day ahead, and pacing each activity according to its priority, so helping themselves to derive significant pleasure and satisfaction from life.

In the home, a housewife can plan so that periods of physical activity are followed by periods of rest. Housework should only be continued if the patient feels sufficiently rested. By this method patients will achieve a regular workload with which they can cope, thereby preventing undue physical strain and mental stress developing. Once patients realise it is possible to achieve positive results, i.e. a tidy home and meals cooked, they will also benefit psychologically. With the cooperation of an employer, patients who are at work can learn to plan their workload so that periods of physical activity are followed by periods which are more sedentary. In some instances this can be accomplished with help from the OT and the Disability Training Officer (DTO) who is part of the placing, assessment and counselling team (PACT) (see Chapter 11). The OT and the DTO can visit the place of work and advise accordingly. Also, if the patient is unable to continue to work in the usual environment, either redeployment within the company can be sought, or a reduction in hours or a request for an assessment can be made to the DTO, whose job it is to assess and then recommend retraining for more suitable employment. In these days of increasing public awareness of the problems of the disabled, much can be achieved. Generally it is the nurse's role to reinforce the guidelines associated with joint protection, and check that a referral to the OT has been made.

(6) Maintaining mobility and preventing deformities

Intervention – referral to the physiotherapist for assessment and the development of an individualised exercise programme: Each patient should be referred to the physiotherapist, for an assessment and exercise programme, at the earliest opportunity after diagnosis. The physiotherapist will advise and guide the patient in this very important aspect of treatment. However, it is up to the nurse to reinforce and encourage the patient to continue the daily exercise routine and to reinforce the importance of exercise generally. Patients should be informed of the possible progression of the disease and the need to avoid flexion contractures developing. Most patients find exercise programmes painful, time consuming and boring. The nurse can explain that dedicated athletes spend hours in daily exercise in order to increase muscle tone and to strengthen muscle power to improve their chosen performance. Providing patients continue their daily exercise programme then they too should find a similar improvement in their activities. Certainly a daily exercise programme will help to maintain a normal range of movement within each joint. This in turn will help to sustain a strong supporting muscle and so improve muscle tone (see Chapter 7).

Ideally a booklet should be compiled by the physiotherapy department, which should include the range of exercises patients may need to perform. These exercises should not take too long to perform, otherwise patients will become discouraged and will stop doing them. Each patient's needs will differ and so the advice is not set in stone. It should however contain active, assisted and isometric exercises. Once the patient has made contact with the physiotherapy team an open helpline number should be given to enable immediate contact should a flare in the condition be experienced.

(7) Surviving a flare

Intervention – identify a flare and explain the different forms of treatment: Provide each patient with a booklet which describes a flare and gives an explanation of how to cope should one occur. The aim of the booklet would be to keep the patient and family in control of a difficult situation without having to call out the GP or to seek admission to hospital. The patient would be advised to keep the booklet by the bed as a flare is often apparent first thing in the morning on waking.

The content should cover how to deal with painful, stiff and hot swollen joints as already described under 'pain' and how to take sufficient analgesics and NSAIDs to control pain without endangering life. It should also discuss how to use heat treatment (both dry and moist), cold treatment and rest as restorative therapy. A telephone helpline number should also be provided, for both the patient and the family to use. If a patient lives alone, then coping with a flare becomes more difficult and heavy demands can be made on the nurse specialist in these circumstances. Advising the patient and the family on how to master a flare can prove to be a very cost-effective exercise. Demands on the GP and hospital consultant's time are reduced and inpatient admissions can often be avoided. The nurse specialists, however, may find more demands are made on their time but that is one of the reasons why they are employed in the first place.

(8) Reduced social isolation

Intervention – discuss the past and present social situation and work out a solution, together with the patient and family, where possible: It is well known that patients, in the initial stages of their disease, do not wish to socialise (Bury, 1982) and because of the pain and fatigue they sometimes refuse to go out at all. It is a period of grieving – for the loss of a way of life they once knew. Robinson (Robinson et al., 1972) is quoted as saying 'a person who reacts to a chronic, painful disease with anxiety and depression may not be making desirable adjustments, but it is one which common sense would predict'. The social support which the patient may have access to, at this period, is very important indeed. If the patient is lucky and has family, friends, neighbours and perhaps work colleagues to turn to, then the chances of adapting to the illness and accepting a different lifestyle are good. Without good social support the outlook can be bleak, and adapting to the illness can take much longer. As a result, the first five years can be an exceptionally miserable and difficult period for anyone to experience. It is a state of affairs which most people should have little difficulty empathising with.

When encountering a newly diagnosed patient it is useful to determine, quite soon, exactly what social support is in place. On close questioning you will find most patients, whether male or female, have reduced or will have virtually stopped all previous social activities and even family outings will have been put on hold, though children in the family will still be provided for (le Gallez, 1993) by the well partner or their siblings. Husband and wife may no longer go out together. In addition, owing to the presence of constant nagging pain, coupled with extreme exhaustion, fatigue and uncertainty about the future, patients are often depressed.

By teaching pain control, together with the other components of the education programme, the nurse will be supporting the patient through a very difficult patch and encouraging the patient to see some light at the end of what looks like a very black tunnel. If there is one in the area, a support organisation can play a role here. If not, the nurse can form one herself. Arthritis Care will willingly provide organisational support. Of course, not everyone wants to join a support group, though they may be willing to meet a fellow patient on a one-to-one basis. Simply by joining Arthritis Care the minimum a member will receive will be the quarterly News Bulletin packed with very useful information. Patients should be persuaded, and if necessary bullied, into going out with their spouse, with an explanation as to how important it is to consider their partner's needs in addition to their own.

(9) Sexual adjustments

Intervention − sexual counselling: The very important though sensitive subject of sexual activity can be dealt with successfully by the nurse specialist, though it may be a good idea for the subject not to be broached until a rapport has developed between patient and nurse, and also providing the nurse has sufficient confidence to tackle the subject. If in doubt, do not attempt to tackle this. Instead, refer to a colleague who has the relevant experience or training (Dale, 1996).

With the systemic advancement of rheumatic disease, and possible subsequent development of joint deformity, repercussions on sexuality and sexual activity seem inevitable. The literature suggest sexual problems do exist for people with a mixture of rheumatic diseases (Blake et al., 1987, 1988; Cochrane, 1984; Currey, 1970). All of these studies agree that following the development of the disease a deterioration in sexual function, satisfaction and frequency occurs, when compared with normal controls. As might be expected most difficulties are a result of mechanical or physical problems such as diseased joints resulting in pain, stiffness, fatigue and depression, all aspects of active disease.

Of those problems most likely to occur, and which could prevent the patient or partner from enjoying sex, pain/stiffness is by far the most frequently mentioned. Partners say they are also afraid of inflicting unnecessary pain on the patient if they attempt sex. Tiredness experienced by the patient is also mentioned. Lack of opportunity is said to be a problem for some partners, the waking hours and also some of the night being taken up with medication, dressing, toileting, exercise and generally trying to keep one's head above water! Depression, as already stated, can be experienced by both patients and partners. Peck et al. (1989) found that many RA patients who were depressed were not disabled and many who were disabled were not depressed. This may well apply to early RA when disability is limited and patients are in the throes of a new and chronic illness with which they are still trying to come to terms, and as a result become depressed.

By providing a suitable information booklet aimed at both patient and partners a great deal of embarrassment can be overcome when attempting to deal with this delicate subject (see 'Sexual relationships and arthritis' later in this chapter).

(10) Coping with concomitant illnesses occurring as a result of medication or as a direct result of the principal disease

Intervention – counselling, support, open access via the telephone helpline to the nurse specialist, extra clinic visits, family involvement: Many of the drugs we give to the patient can result in unwanted and permanent damage. The lungs, kidneys, skin and to a lesser extent the liver may be damaged, and the patients have to cope with these additional problems as well as the principal illness. Some of these side-effects may go after a short while, but others will remain, resulting in yet another illness the patient must learn to accept and come to terms with. Many middle-aged or elderly patients may have been taking a moderate dose of corticosteroids for a considerable length of time, or a high dose for a short length of time. As a result, they may develop side-effects to such drugs. The side-effects may be numerous but those most likely to concern us are thinning of the skin and subsequent chronic leg ulcers, together with the more sinister development; osteoporosis. A number of young people with juvenile chronic arthritis will have been given corticosteroids to treat their illness.

Had this not been given to them their life would have been at serious risk. Unfortunately, some of these young people may also go on to develop osteoporosis. Rheumatology patients are more susceptible to other illnesses, in particular the autoimmune diseases such as myxoedema, diabetes mellitus and myasthenia gravis. Certain others will develop Sjögren's syndrome, vasculitis or severe skin conditions.

These patients will require additional support over and above that traditionally meted out. Telephone helplines, open access clinics and smooth emergency admissions will be their lifeline and will help patients and their families to survive.

(11) Eating sensibly so as to maintain a balanced diet

Intervention – discuss alternative diets with the patient, and the effect they have on the disease, and refer to the dietician: As there is no known food or diet which can cause or cure any of the many rheumatic diseases, the task of explaining the implications of diet for the disease should be an easy one. Unfortunately, this is not so. Together with the many alternative therapies which patients can now avail themselves of, diet comes high on the list of priorities. If someone chooses to try a particular diet or alternative therapy it is advisable to give support whether or not your personal inclinations are in sympathy. There is a growing body of patients whose instinct is to avoid drug therapy if at all possible, and they should be permitted to take that decision, without feeling guilty, if that is their wish, though only after they have been made aware of the consequences of delaying conventional treatment. Their unconventional approach is as a result of the scare stories they read in the media with regard to drugs and their side-effects and who can in fact blame them? Most patients, once having tried the alternative methods, be it a diet or some form of therapy, eventually return to clinic ready to try conventional treatment. They go through a process of searching for the elusive 'cure' and having found it has eluded them they are then ready to try the drug treatment we have to offer.

The real challenge for the health professional arises when trying to persuade those patients who are grossly overweight how important it is for them to lose weight, and as quickly as possible, otherwise they will sustain permanent damage to the joints. Weight Watchers or Slimmers World seem to have a good success rate in this direction, providing the patient can be persuaded to join them.

The patient who is systemically ill and or physically incapacitated may also be undernourished or of low body weight, and for a number of reasons. If patients are unwell then they will have a poor appetite, and if they also live alone, and are physically unable to prepare meals, then they will not bother to feed themselves. If they are elderly and incapacitated they will be unable to get out of the house to do any shopping. Many housebound elderly people rarely get out into the fresh air and sunshine and quickly become deficient in vitamin D. Certain social services exist to help the elderly overcome these problems, though it may take an alert nurse or OT to pick up the clues and ensure the necessary services are provided.

In the Asian community many of the female members are restricted to wearing clothing which covers the whole of the body, and in some instances even the face, leaving little or no exposed skin. As a result, they suffer from vitamin D deficiency and osteomalacia. As some of these women are also vegans, poor diet may also be a contributing factor.

Conclusion

The following quotation expresses, in very few words, the philosophy behind patient education. We should always try to keep this message in mind when dealing with patients and their families:

> The chief business of the chronically ill person is not to just stay alive or keep his symptoms under control, but to live as normally as possible despite his symptoms and disease (Strauss, 1975).

Following are two examples of education/information leaflets:

1.   sexual relationships and arthritis
2.   pregnancy and arthritis

The copyright has been waived in regard to these leaflets only, and they may be copied by the reader if they wish. An acknowledgement to the author and publisher is requested.

1. Sexual Relationships and Arthritis

Introduction

Arthritis affects people of *ANY* age, and from *ANY* social or cultural background. This pamphlet therefore is not only for the very young or the sexually liberated, it is for *anyone who has arthritis*. Partners should also be encouraged to read it.

Because osteoarthritis, rheumatoid arthritis and ankylosing spondylitis are among the most common of the arthritic complaints, the likelihood is that you will have one of these conditions or even a combination of two, or, you may have a non-specific arthritic condition, such as low back pain, fibromyalgia or a painful neck or shoulder joint. No matter which condition you are suffering from, each one can have a significant effect on your sex life and, in the more damaging forms of arthritis, can have a lasting effect upon sexuality. The purpose of this pamphlet is to highlight sexual problems which may develop and to discuss a number of solutions to them. These questions and answers are designed to cover a multitude of problems and not all of them will apply to you. It is also important to remember that everyone's sexual needs and attitudes are different and they change with time and experience, regardless of whether arthritis is present or not, and therefore we need to adjust our sexual expectations with advancing years.

How will arthritis affect my sex life?

As someone with arthritis you will be experiencing a variety of problems, among them pain, stiffness, tiredness and perhaps a reduced desire for sex, together with a change in your appearance, described as self-image. This is not to suggest that you are experiencing all of these problems or, indeed, if you are, that you experience them all at the same time or all of the time. Nonetheless, because of these distressing symptoms, arthritis can have a serious effect on your sex life. Still, it is important to realise that having arthritis does not *directly* affect your ability to be aroused sexually, or to be satisfied sexually. Where a caring and loving relationship exists, a rewarding and satisfactory sex life can still be achieved and aimed for. When you are feeling particularly low it is worth remembering that many couples who do not have a painful illness to struggle with can also experience sexual difficulties.

The extent of your illness will determine the effect it has on your sex life. Short, minor bouts or exacerbations involving few joints may have an unfavourable effect on your sexual activity, which may cause a temporary loss of self-esteem, but this will soon be regained. However, prolonged severe flares involving many joints may be more disabling, and may cause someone to feel sexually unattractive and depressed. As a result, sexual activity may well decrease or even stop, which could be harmful to your self-esteem, and this in turn may have a severe impact on your partner's sex life also.

Good communication means talking to each other, sharing your feelings

Establishing good communications with your partner is perhaps the most useful advice to give to anyone who wishes to avoid sexual problems developing. Unless you talk to each other and share with your partner those private thoughts and feelings which relate to your sexual needs, then misunderstandings will very quickly develop and barriers will be erected which may prove very difficult to break down.

Surprisingly, even in our enlightened society, many people find discussing sex an embarrassing experience. This applies to married couples as well as to single people. Also, many health professionals shy away from the subject when it is broached and certainly avoid introducing it even though they may recognise that a sexual problem exists.

Some of the people reading this pamphlet may have been married for many years, and may find it easy talking to their partners, in which case coping with the problems which arthritis may bring will be made easier for them. Sadly, some couples, no matter how many years they have been together, may find communicating with each other difficult.

A loss of self-esteem, and in some cases a loss of self-respect, can quickly occur in someone who is unwell and experiencing a painful illness. As a result, when one member of a partnership develops arthritis a number of important changes have to take place, and these will require a special understanding from the well partner which he or she may not previously have considered. Not only will alternative positions need to be considered, but also alternative ways to have sex. Consequently, a great deal of patience and tolerance will be required of the well partner. Providing a stable relationship exists most couples not only weather the rough times but may indeed find their relationship strengthened in spite of them.

What if my sex life was not all that good before I developed arthritis?

If someone had an unsatisfactory sex life before the arthritis developed, then their sex life may actually deteriorate even further. In this situation, it is never too late to start sharing your concerns and your private feelings with your partner.

Why should having arthritis cause sexual problems to arise?

It takes little imagination to appreciate that sexual problems can arise when painful, stiff, unstable or deformed joints have developed, regardless of whether the person is male or female. The very act of love-making can be extremely physical, and damaged painful joints may not respond as the couple would wish.

Conventionally, sex takes place in the morning and/or the evening. Unfortunately, for someone who has arthritis, the morning or evening can prove to be most unsuitable for sexual activity. Often the ill person is extremely tired, particularly towards the end of the day, and though this can be for a variety of reasons it is generally the result of suffering from chronic pain and experiencing sleepless nights. Stiffness too can be a problem as this can be much worse first thing in the morning.

One significant comment made by partners of people who have arthritis is the sudden lack of special or free time to indulge in sexual activity, and for a variety of reasons. Not only does the ill person now have to cope with the pain and stiffness already mentioned, but time may also need to be set aside during the day for periods of rest as well as for a daily exercise routine. In addition, simple routine tasks like washing and dressing may take much longer and are therefore a further drain on available time. Even taking medication, often three or four times a day, can make inroads into whatever time is left available between caring for the family and maybe going out to work. If we consider these facts it is easy to see why partners may well feel excluded and neglected.

What advice can you give to help overcome some of these problems?

As good sex does not have to be spontaneous, the advice would be as follows.

1. *Take advantage of the time of day or night during which pain is at its lowest level*, and, if at all possible during this special time, leave the 'arthritis' on the other side of the door. You may find this is all you need to do. It is of paramount importance to try and remember always to take into account your well partner's sexual needs, as well as your own. Providing sexual problems are mechanical, that is, due to painful joints and muscles, and not psychosexual in origin, then the following advice may also help. Of course, sex without a partner is also a possibility and more will be said about this later.

2. *Take painkillers* (analgesics) if sex is anticipated. Take prescribed painkillers, for example paracetamol, at least 30 minutes before sex. If there is time, have a warm bath, or shower, together with your partner if you both so wish. The warm water will help to relax painful muscles. Remember, painkillers do not have to be taken with food.

3. *Try relaxation.* Having taken the painkillers, or immediately following the bath, consider resting in the room you intend to use, arranging pillows or cushions to support the more painful joints. Now is the time to relax and listen to your favourite music or a relaxation tape. If you fall asleep, don't worry, you will probably enjoy sex even more having had a short nap beforehand.

4. *Massage.* The laying on of hands to ease pain goes back to biblical times and, indeed, is one of the most potent forms of pain relief. If your partner is willing, allow him or her to GENTLY massage any painful areas using a non-greasy oil. Never try to massage without using some form of oil, otherwise the skin can be stretched and possibly broken. You don't have to massage someone for hours; just a few minutes massage can prove most beneficial and is of course excellent foreplay to sex.

5. *Alternative positions.* If, when having sexual intercourse, you have always used the conventional position of the man on top of the woman, then it is possible you may now have to consider alternative positions, or indeed alternative ways to have sex. Remember to discuss beforehand how you will respond if making love becomes too painful to continue. Once you and your partner are in the 'throes of passion', it could be too late.

6. *Sleeping arrangements.* Occasionally, some people will complain about difficulties with sleeping and this affects their relationship. The ill person, who may often be disturbed because of pain during the night, may be particularly concerned at disrupting the well partner's sleep pattern. What frequently happens is for

the well partner to move into a separate bed which can often be in a spare room. This solution, even if it is suggested by the ill partner, is not to be recommended, even on a temporary basis. Too often the temporary situation becomes a permanent one, to the detriment of the ill partner. It is during the night when pain appears to be at its worst that the reassuring arm of the well partner can provide an invaluable source of comfort. In addition, the closeness of the well partner will help to reinforce the positive feelings the couple have for each other. One solution is to check the size of your bed. If a couple are struggling to share the conventional 4' 6" bed then the purchase of a king-size bed, with two separate mattresses and two single duvets rather than one double, could go a very long way towards relieving the problem. If two single beds are available these can be pushed together, again using two single duvets rather than a double. A single duvet is much lighter, and for someone with painful joints is easier to handle, and will cause far less disruption to the well partner's sleep. Females who are experiencing menopausal symptoms, and in particular night sweats, will greatly benefit from the use of a separate duvet, as indeed will their partners.

What if certain of my joints are so severely damaged that I cannot manage any of the above positions or I simply feel too ill?

There may be times when it becomes impossible to achieve vaginal penetration because of damaged hips or knees or owing to certain back disorders, and yet you will still wish to achieve sexual satisfaction. In these instances *alternative ways* for sexual satisfaction can be explored. If you already have a fairly liberated attitude to sex then the alternative methods about to be discussed will already be well known to you. Mutual or self-masturbation is of course one of these. The drawback to this method arises if the person with the arthritis has swollen and painful hands; these can occur with osteoarthritis, or repetitive strain injuries, as well as with the inflammatory forms of arthritis. If the ill person is a female then the use of a hand-held vibrator is a possibility, held either by the well male partner or the female with the complaint. This method can quickly achieve an orgasm for the female, thereby relieving the hands of too much stress. As these machines can produce a strong vibration, care should be taken when first experimenting with them. One suggestion is that a condom is slipped over the vibrator to buffer the vibrations. Vibrators are available from Anne Summers local agents or Disability

Centres or by mail order. It is also possible that on other occasions the person who is ill may not have the energy to enjoy personal satisfaction but would nonetheless derive great fulfilment from providing pleasure for the partner he or she cares for. The solution is for the well person to self-masturbate, while the ill partner provides a loving embrace and encouragement. Of course there is no reason why this should not work in reverse should a couple feel so inclined.

My joints are so damaged I know I cannot achieve sexual intercourse!

For those people whose disability renders sexual intercourse a physical impossibility, a partnership in which vaginal penetration will not take place can also be satisfying, providing both parties fully understand and accept the situation before a permanent commitment is made. Good communication is essential in this situation, and the affected partner, should only one be disabled, should not take for granted the prospective partner's agreement to the lack of vaginal penetration within the marriage or partnership. A relationship between two people without vaginal/penis involvement can be successful providing both are fully aware of the limitations and the risks. Holding, hugging, touching, caressing, kissing and licking are all actions that can prove to be satisfying between two people who care for each other.

I do not want a sexual relationship; does that make me some kind of freak?

There are of course many couples living absolutely full and contented lives in which neither partner wishes to resume sexual relationships and there is no suggestion here that such people are anything other than perfectly normal, or that they should make an effort to do something they feel is entirely unnecessary for them.

I seem to be on my own these days, what about sex for me?

At certain times in our lives, whether we are disabled or not, there may come a time when we are unable to attain a satisfactory and permanent relationship. If this is the case then a life of celibacy need no longer apply. Engaging in sex with a responsible attitude outside marriage or a partnership is considered to be socially acceptable and though some people may still think that sex on one's own is unacceptable, this need not be so. After all, why should it be that sexual stimulation, and therefore satisfaction, is acceptable only if you are in the company of one other person? Surely everyone is entitled to responsible sexual satisfaction if that is their wish? Self-masturbation, providing the state of the hands allows for this, can therefore prove useful in this situation, or the use of a mechanical vibrator, as previously mentioned, is an alternative.

Because I am young and have a physical disability my family do not accept I also have sexual needs!

Young people who have disabilities may encounter prejudices from their well-meaning relatives when it comes to establishing themselves in a sexual relationship. It is very hard for some parents to let go of their children whether they have disabilities or not. If this applies to you then perhaps showing your parents this pamphlet may help to smooth the path; and of course, joining groups such as Young Arthritis Care will provide opportunities to meet others in a similar situation. While there you can gain from the experiences of other young people. They also produce a booklet called *The Ruff Guide to Sex*. (Young Arthritis Care, Telephone 0171 1916 1500.)

What is sexuality?

Whilst sexuality is difficult to define, it is nonetheless an important part of our personality. It has been described as the energy or life-force which enables us to experience love, affection and friendship. A positive sexuality can provide a feeling of well-being and vitality. If you feel good about your personal self-image then you will respond favourably to others. If you have a poor self-image then you may respond to others in a negative fashion. Of course there are people who, though they do not have a physical problem, are nonetheless very unhappy with their own self-image. These people usually have unrealistic ideas of what is considered to be beautiful or acceptable and, because of this, they may go through life feeling very unhappy with themselves. Perhaps the key lies within us and so, regardless of how we look on the outside, we need to be happy with ourselves on the inside. Therefore, if you like yourself the chances are you will be liked by others, and this will give you confidence in the image you project.

How do I cope with an altered body image?

What sometimes happens when a person develops an arthritic condition is damage to the joints and the surrounding muscles, resulting in an unstable or deformed joint. Sometimes many joints are affected involving the hands, feet and knees in particular. As males and females customarily perform different roles within our society, and in addition society has different expectations of the sexes, the reduction in the use of a particular joint is quite likely to affect people differently depending on whether they are male or female. For example, the loss of physical strength, as a result of damage to a joint, may be more important to a man than it would be to a woman, whereas the unsightly appearance of a joint may be more distressing to the female than the problem of reduced physical strength.

Occasionally, because of these very damaging effects a wheelchair may have to be used. This can have a devastating effect on self-image, and the outcome is often a feeling of low personal self-esteem. In some instances, the individuals concerned becomes angry and then depressed at what is happening to them.

Not surprisingly, many people have great difficulty in coping with physical changes should they occur, because these can further rein-force the poor self-image they may already hold, and further compound their loss of self-esteem. The advice given in such circum-stances comes not from the professionals but from people who have arthritis. They suggest that if you have a poor self-image as a result of the arthritis *you should try to accept your body as it is, with all its limitations, and at the same time acknowledge the possibility of developing a full and useful life*. Yes, your body will have its limitations but, unless you are careful, the limitations you experience may well be governed by your personal attitude to your illness, rather than to the physical restrictions imposed by the arthritis itself.

Will surgery help improve my physical limitations and as a result my sex life?

Surgery of the hip joint can give some people dramatic relief from pain, and at the same time give greater hip movement which means greater freedom during sexual intercourse. If someone is experienc-ing problems during intercourse because of painful hips, he or she should discuss this with a surgeon. Such problems can be considered significant enough reason for deciding to operate. Some people may worry in case they cause damage to the hip following an operation should they have intercourse. Yet their fears are unfounded provid-ing they follow a few simple rules, it is usually possible to resume intercourse within six weeks of the operation. Still, it should be borne in mind that they must avoid bending the hip too far towards the chest, particularly while lying on the back, a movement they may be tempted to use during intercourse. Bending from the hip and also squatting are best avoided for some time. As different surgeons have different polices, guidelines can vary.

Hand surgery may also help improve dexterity, which in turn may enhance your sexual performance. Shoulder, elbow or knee surgery may help to reduce pain and allow for greater movement and enjoyment during sexual activity. Whether or not a surgeon would consider these reason enough to operate needs to be challenged. As joint replacements are now carried out on younger and younger people the suggestion is thought provoking.

In conclusion

Having read this pamphlet, we hope you will have found it of some benefit. However, if you remain unconvinced then the suggestion is that you return to the section on 'communication' and read it through slowly once again. Having done this, approach your partner, and unless you have done so already, persuade him or her to read this pamphlet too.

2. Pregnancy and arthritis

Introduction

The questions and answers which follow have been written for young women who have an arthritic condition, are pregnant, or are thinking of becoming pregnant. They may also prove useful to men who have an inflammatory arthritis, and who, whilst hoping to start a family, are concerned about the drugs they are taking. It is hoped that well partners will also find this pamphlet of interest.

We are thinking of starting a family; do you think this is wise?

Many problems face the young, male or female, when they are considering starting or increasing a family, particularly so when they also have a chronic arthritic condition. Couples question the need to have children at all, and ask should they leave well alone? If they already have children, should they increase the family? Or would it be better to stop at those children they already have? Understandably, they also worry in case the drugs they are taking will damage the baby. In addition, they are concerned in case the disease they have is passed on to the baby. Young women worry in case they cannot cope physically with a new baby, both at the time of the delivery and later when they take their baby home.

The decision to have a baby is usually taken because the mother-to-be is well, and the disease is under control. Consequently, perhaps the most difficult hurdle most couples have to face is knowing that either one or both will have to stop taking their drugs in order to conceive without damaging the baby. This means their condition may well deteriorate, and therefore it is a great sacrifice for them to make.

As drugs are perhaps the most pressing concern, they will be considered first of all.

I know taking drugs can be dangerous if you are pregnant. What should I do?

As a chronic illness requires taking drugs continuously, it is important to think carefully about which drugs to take not only while pregnant but also before becoming pregnant, and again for some time after the pregnancy if breast feeding is intended. Thinking about which drugs to take is equally as important for a man as for a woman, and particularly so if they wish to increase their family, though this only applies to the period *before* they intend starting a baby.

How will my baby be affected by the drugs I take?

Drugs taken during pregnancy are always taken because of the needs of the mother and not because of the needs of the unborn baby. The mother and the unborn baby will respond differently to the drugs taken by the mother and, because of this, the drug may prove to be of benefit and *harmless* to the mother and yet may prove to be *harmful* to the unborn baby. Hence the risks associated with taking drugs have to be considered very seriously. Some people think the placenta (the afterbirth) will stop the drugs passing from the mother to the unborn child but this is not so, with the possible exception of heparin and insulin. These are drugs used in heart disease and diabetes.

What happens if I take drugs and start a baby?

Certain drugs are known to be teratogenic (this is pronounced exactly as it is written). This means they can cause the baby to be born damaged in some way. However, not only drugs are teratogenic. Damage to the unborn baby can be caused by other means which are also teratogenic, for example, alcohol, tobacco or environmental pollutants such as waste products from certain factories.

It is well known that damage to the mother's eggs can occur even *before* the baby is conceived, and again to the unborn baby at *any time* during the pregnancy. Damage can also occur at any time to the sperm from the father, which is why men may have to stop the drugs they are taking *before* they start a baby. Even so, the period during which damage is *most likely* to occur to the unborn baby is during the *first three months of pregnancy*, known medically as the first trimester. As many women do not realise they are pregnant until they reach this stage, it is wise to plan a pregnancy, then certain drugs taken by the mother or the father can be stopped *before* starting the baby. A sensible attitude to contraception, by both the mother and the father, is therefore advisable.

What drugs can I take before and during the pregnancy?

Painkillers: Should you require a painkiller while pregnant then paracetamol is recommended. Certainly, try to avoid aspirin and co-proxamol because they are known to cause side-effects both in the early and late stages of pregnancy, and may also affect the baby after delivery. Many painkillers bought over the counter contain aspirin, so beware!

Non-steroidal anti-inflammatory drugs (NSAIDs): Examples are Brufen, Indocid, Voltarol, Piroxicam, Naprosyn and many others. These are best avoided if at all possible, especially during the early stages of pregnancy, though, if you are pregnant and suffer with ankylosing spondylitis or severe back disorders, painkillers alone may not be sufficient to control the pain. As a result, as the baby grows and puts extra strain on the muscles around the hips and shoulders, severe pain can become a problem. In these circumstances your doctor may prescribe a low-dose NSAID for you, possibly ibuprofen (Brufen). If at all possible NSAIDs should also be avoided towards the end of the pregnancy, and particularly during labour, because of possible complications occurring during the delivery, or to the baby after delivery.

Whilst painkillers and NSAIDs may be required by *anyone* with an arthritic condition, certain drugs – *steroids and disease modifying anti-rheumatic drugs (DMARDS)* – will only be prescribed for those people who have an inflammatory arthritis, for example juvenile chronic arthritis, rheumatoid arthritis, ankylosing spondylitis, scleroderma, psoriatic arthritis or lupus (SLE), all of which are known to affect young men or women in particular.

Steroids: Prednisolone is an example of this group of drugs, and is considered safe if taken in low doses of between 5 and 10 mg daily. High doses are to be avoided. It is important to note that if your doctor stops your steroids within two months of your baby being delivered (for whatever reason) then you will be required to take steroids again as you go into labour in order to help the body cope better with the stress of the delivery.

Disease-modifying anti-rheumatic drugs (DMARDs): These are Myocrisin (gold injections), Auranofin (gold tablets), sulphasalazine, penicillimine, hydroxychloroquine, methotrexate, azathioprine, cyclosporin, cyclophosphamide and Tigason, though Tigason is not strictly a DMARD but is prescribed for people with psoriatic arthritis. DMARDs will almost certainly be prescribed before pregnancy but their use during pregnancy is best avoided if at all possible. This is because some of these drugs will damage the unborn child as already described, whilst for the remainder the effect they may have during pregnancy is still unknown, and therefore the recommendation is that all DMARDs are stopped. Ideally, you will be advised to come off all DMARDs *before* becoming pregnant, and in some instances as early as six months before starting your pregnancy, particularly so with methotrexate, cyclophosphamide and Tigason, as these drugs are known to damage the mother's eggs. On account of this danger, *you must use a contraceptive during this six-month period.* If, however, your arthritis is active, then a DMARD may be continued, though in a very low dose. This is because, in some instances, your life, or that of the baby, could be at risk. The possibility of having to take DMARDs while pregnant applies in particular to young women who are known to have SLE (lupus). (More on lupus later.)

Men with arthritis who take methotrexate, cyclophosphamide or Tigason will also be advised to come off these drugs six months before attempting to start a family, Once again, because of the damage that could occur to the sperm, *contraceptives must be used over this six-month period*. Some doctors are suggesting three months may be long enough to come off the drugs but until an agreement is reached, you will have to be guided by your consultant. Men who are taking sulphasalazine will have a decrease in the number of sperm they produce. Though this will reduce their ability to start a child, the sperm count will return to normal on stopping the sulphasalazine.

What should I do after the baby is born?

The first week after the baby's birth can be a time when the mother is in need of many drugs. The most commonly used drugs, taken by all mothers immediately after their baby is born, are painkillers, sedatives and antibiotics. In addition, women suffering from an arthritic conditions may also need to take a DMARD, NSAID or steroids. Therefore if you intend breast feeding you will need to take care.

What safeguards can I take if breast feeding?

All drugs taken by the mother when feeding her baby, and this includes alcohol, will pass into the breast milk, though in most cases only in small amounts. Even so, if you intend breast feeding it is better to take only those drugs which are essential to maintain your health, and to take only a minimum of alcohol.

There are two important points to remember if you wish to breast feed and you also have to take drugs. The first is the baby's health, and the second is how often you will feed the baby. The healthier the baby is, the greater are the chances that it will cope with any drugs passed on to it in the breast milk. Also, as the baby grows, because it is becoming stronger, it will cope more easily with any drug passed on to it. Finally, as the baby grows older breast milk will be given less frequently or in smaller quantities, so there is less chance of the drugs taken by the mother passing on to the baby.

Are there any special do's and don'ts while breast feeding?

If you must take a drug, take it soon *after* you have breast fed the baby, which will allow plenty of time for the drug to clear from the breast milk before the next feed is due, so reducing the chances of passing the drug on to the baby. If you are in pain, try to remember the following: in most instances though not all, many drugs, and in particular the painkillers and some of the NSAIDs, will be at their highest levels in your blood if taken 30 to 60 minutes *before* breast feeding. In these situations you would be advised to delay taking the drug until after the baby has been fed. If your baby is being fed on demand rather than regular three or four hourly feeds, and you are taking an NSAID, then a slow-release (SR) NSAID may be more suitable for you, and consequently also for your baby.

The following are drugs which may be taken, and some which should be avoided, during breast feeding. They may be taken in order to control pain and the progression of the disease. They should be used with caution and in the lowest dose possible AND ONLY ON THE ADVICE OF YOUR DOCTOR.

- Painkiller paracetamol   AVOID aspirin and coproxamol
- NSAID   ibuprofen   AVOID indomethacin, naproxen and tenoxicam, and possibly certain others
- DMARDs   hydroxychloroquine, AVOID all other DMARDs.
  methotrexate and
  azathioprine, though
  only in the smallest
  possible dose.

I have heard your arthritis gets better when you are pregnant

All women need to take extra care of themselves when pregnant and particularly so if, in addition to their pregnancy, they have one of the arthritic conditions previously mentioned. Though a number of such women will have some remission from the arthritis while pregnant, others may get worse. Most important of all, despite the fact that you have an arthritic condition, and with the exception of lupus, there is no danger to the unborn child.

The following guidelines relate to specific diseases.

Rheumatoid arthritis and juvenile chronic arthritis

In such women as many as 75 per cent will experience a remission which occurs gradually during the first three months of their pregnancy. At first, they may notice a decrease or a complete end to early morning stiffness, followed by a further decrease in joint tenderness and swelling. Eventually, they may begin to carry out certain daily tasks which they have been unable to do for some time. Even so, such young women will need to plan their day carefully exactly as they did before the pregnancy; this makes certain they have adequate periods of rest and exercise. If young children are already members of the family, then finding time to rest obviously becomes more difficult, and more will be said about this later. Sadly, it is a well-known fact that any remission will come to an end after the baby is born, in some instances within a week or two, though for some mothers not for six months or more. The degree to which the activity returns is variable and there is no way of predicting this. Having enjoyed a temporary relief from symptoms, mothers, and indeed their partners, will need to prepare themselves psychologically for the return of the active disease. However, for such women the time when the baby is delivered is usually no different than for anyone else. Only if there are problems with the hips, and/or the neck joint, and this may apply in particular to young women who have juvenile chronic arthritis, will special precautions need to be taken. If there is restricted hip movement, a caesarean section may be performed, and for neck problems a collar should be worn throughout the operation or throughout labour.

Other arthritic conditions including ankylosing spondylitis and chronic back pain

For those women who have an arthritic conditions which does not go into remission, being pregnant may make the condition worse, and a difficult few months can follow. Some mothers may feel a slight improvement early in the pregnancy but for most, as the baby increases in size, the additional weight puts an extra strain on the back and the shoulders which results in an increase of pain. Because of the increased pain many daily tasks become extremely difficult to carry out, and therefore domestic support should be arranged well in advance, either from within the family or through social services.

Because these arthritic conditions will have remained active throughout the pregnancy, such young women may require considerable help and support at the time of the delivery, as giving birth can, for them, be an uncomfortable ordeal, stiffness being a particular problem. Fortunately, the obstetrician will, in all probability, take a special interest in their case and the midwife will be aware of their special needs. Consolation lies in the fact that the problems only last around four or five months, after which, you will have your baby as compensation, and though the arthritis will still remain, you will no longer be pregnant.

Systemic lupus erythematosus (lupus)

Though many women with lupus have successful pregnancies, there is an added risk, though this usually only applies if the disease is active and difficult to control. If the disease is not active and you are feeling well generally, and there is no kidney involvement, then there are usually no difficulties. Pregnancy is normally safe, and without complications, and generally there is no great risk to the infant. There may be a greater risk of a flare-up of the lupus after delivery, in which case the advice already given in this pamphlet should be followed.

Is there any additional help I may need?

Two very important health professionals will need to be involved in your care, the *physiotherapist* and the *occupational therapist*. Make certain that you have contact with a physiotherapist (PT) as soon as possible after becoming pregnant. With luck, you will already be in touch with a physiotherapist through the hospital rheumatologist. If this is the case, advance notice should be given to the PT of the impending birth, so that you can be advised on posture, exercise and rest throughout the pregnancy. Contact should also be made, on your behalf, with the maternity hospital, so that a physiotherapist can be involved in your care as soon as possible after the baby is born. Some mothers require instant support, individual joints having become rather stiff and painful following labour. Women with ankylosing spondylitis are particularly vulnerable and need additional help and understanding at this point. Most midwives are quite happy to hand over certain aspects of care to other experts once the baby has been delivered.

The occupational therapist (OT) should also be contacted at some point during the pregnancy, even though the need for her expertise will not arise until soon *after* the baby is born. Nonetheless, you need to meet the OT well beforehand so that your family situation can be assessed and advice given on all aspects of coping with the new baby. Whilst certain problems will present themselves almost immediately following the birth, by planning ahead well before the baby arrives, together with the OT, they can usually be resolved. The actual mechanics of dealing with the new baby will present the first hurdle. Holding, dressing, washing and feeding the baby may well be more difficult for a mother with an arthritic condition. Hands, elbows, shoulders, neck and back joints are going to give rise to the main problems. By planning and pacing each day exactly as before becoming pregnant, you too will be able to experience the joys of motherhood exactly the same as everyone else.

I am easily tired now. How will I cope once the baby is born?

A good night's sleep is essential to all, and is just as important during pregnancy as it is afterwards. Lack of sleep at any time can lead to irritability and depression, a consequence of which is the inability to cope with our daily lives. Night feeds can present difficulties, mainly because of stiffness. Just trying to pick the baby up, once you have been to sleep for a short while, can present difficulties. But there are ways round the problem and once again the OT will be able to advise. Partners can take over the night feeds, even if you are breast feeding, as the milk can be expressed in advance. If young children are already a part of your family then help caring for these children needs to be considered. As the young mother in question you will require additional support from your partner in every aspect of daily life. Your family and also social services should be called in to help where appropriate. If friends and neighbours are also available to help, then do not hesitate to take advantage of their generosity.

My arthritis developed soon after having my baby

It is possible that some young women reading this pamphlet have been unfortunate enough to develop a form of arthritis immediately following the birth of their babies. The shock of this happening, on what should be a joyous occasion, can prove very difficult to cope with. If this is what has happened to you, request an immediate referral, via your GP, to an occupational therapist, a physiotherapist and the nurse specialist as soon as possible, even if you are still waiting to see a rheumatologist at this point.

Should I be X-rayed during pregnancy?

The short answer is no. Yet, as you have arthritis, your doctor may request an X-ray at any time to check on the progress of the arthritis, or even to diagnose a particular form of arthritis. Therefore, if you are pregnant, or even if you only suspect that you might be pregnant, it is very important that you tell your doctor. You are advised to avoid *ALL* X-rays during the first three months of pregnancy as there may be a risk to the baby.

Can arthritis be passed on?

There may be a slight tendency for some forms of arthritis to appear more common within families, for example rheumatoid arthritis, ankylosing spondylitis and psoriatic arthritis. The medical word used to describe this is 'familial'. This does not mean these conditions are hereditary. Hence, the chance of passing on these diseases to your children is very small indeed.

Is there someone I can turn to for advice if I find I am not coping?

Most hospitals these days, if they have a rheumatologist, will also have a nurse who specialises in rheumatology who is known as the nurse specialist, who will usually run a telephone helpline. Make sure you have the number so that you can call for help and support at such times. Also, the physiotherapist and occupational therapist should give you a telephone number so that you will have open access to them should you require it. Finally, Arthritis Care may well have the number of the Young Arthritis Care contact in your area. Some of the members will have experienced exactly what you are going through and are most willing to offer their support.

By planning your pregnancy carefully you will avoid many problems. If a pregnancy occurs which you did not intend then the information in this pamphlet should go some way towards not only helping you with your problems, but may also help you achieve a joyful and happy pregnancy. (Arthritis Care, tel: 0171 9161500.)

References

Baillie L (1993) A review of pain assessment tools. Nursing Standard 7(23): 25–9.

Bellman L (1994) Principles of educating patients. Surgical Nurse 7(1): 8–10.

Bird HA, Dixon JS (1987) The measurement of pain. Baillière's Clinical Rheumatology 1(1): 71–89.

Blake DJ, Maisiak R, Alarcon GS, Holley L, Brown S (1987) Sexual quality of life of patients with arthritis compared to arthritis free controls. Journal of Rheumatology 14: 570–6.

Blake DJ, Maisiak R, Koplan A, Alarcon GS, Brown S (1988) Sexual dysfunction among patients with arthritis. Clinical Rheumatology 7: 50–60.

Buckelew SP, Parker JC (1989) Coping with arthritic pain: a review of the literature. Arthritis Care and Research 2(4): 136–45.

Bury M (1982) Chronic illness: a biological disruption. Sociological Health and Illness 4: 167–81.

Cohen JL, van Houten Sauter S, De Vellis RF, McVoy De Vellis B (1986) Evaluation of arthritis self-management courses led by laypersons and professionals. Arthritis and Rheumatism 29(3): 388–93.

Close A (1988) Patient education: a literature review. Journal of Advanced Nursing 13: 203–13.

Close A (1992) Strategic planning in patient education. Nursing Standard 6(43): 32–5.

Cochrane M (1984) Sex and disability. Nursing Times 80: 28–34.

Currey HLF (1970) Osteoarthritis of the hip joint and sexual activity. Annals of the Rheumatic Diseases 29: 488–93.

Dale KG (1996) Intimacy and rheumatic disease. Rehabilitation Nursing 21(1): 38–40.

Fisher RC (1992) Patient education and compliance. Patient Education and Counselling 19: 261–71.

Fries JF, Spitz P, Kraines RG, Holman HR (1980) Measurement of patient outcome in arthritis. Arthritis & Rheumatism 23: 137–45.

Hawley DJ, Wolfe F, Cathey MA, Roberts FK (1991) Marital status in R.A. and other rheumatic disorders: a study of 7293 patients. Journal of Rheumatology 18(5): 654–60.

Haynes RB, Wang E, Gomes MD (1987) A critical review of interventions to improve compliance with prescribed medication. Patient Education and Counselling 10: 155–66.

Hilbourne J (1973) On disabling the normal. British Journal of Social Work 2: 494–504.

Hill J, Bird HA, Hopkins R, Lawton C, Wright V (1991) The development of a patient knlowledge questionnaire in RA. British Journal of Rheumatology 30(1): 45–49.

Hilton S (1992) Does patient education work? British Journal of Hospital Medicine 47(6): 438–40.

le Gallez P (1993) Rheumatoid arthritis: effects on the family. Nursing Standard 7(39): 30–4.

Lindroth A, Bauman A, Barnes C, McCredie M, Brooks PM (1989) A controlled evaluation of arthritis education. British Journal of Rheumatology 28: 7–12.

Lorig K, Feigenbaum P, Regan C, Ung E, Chastain RL, Holman HR (1986) A comparison of lay taught and professional taught arthritis self-management courses. Journal of Rheumatology 13(4): 763–67.

Lorig K, Fries JF (1980) The Arthritis Helpbook. Reading, MA, Addison-Wesley (4th edn 1995).

Lorig K, Konkol L, Gonzalez V (1987) Arthritis patient education: a review of the literature. Patient Education and Counselling 10: 207–52.

Lorig K, Lubeck D, Kraines RG, Seleznick M, Holman HR (1985) Outcomes of self-help education for patients with arthritis. Arthritis and Rheumatism 28(6): 680–85.

Lorish CD, Parker J, Brown S (1985) Effective patient education. Arthritis and Rheumatism 28(11): 1289–97.

Manne SL, Zautra AJ (1992) Coping with arthritis: current status and critique. Arthritis and Rheumatism 35(11): 1273–80.

McCaffery M (1979) Nursing Management of the Patient with Pain 2nd edn. Philadelphia: JB Lippincott 10–21.

Meenan R, Yelin EH, Nevitt M, Epstein WV (1981) The impact of chronic disease. Arthritis and Rheumatism 24: 544–9.

Peck JR, Smith TW, Ward JR, Milano R (1989) Disability and depression in RA. Arthritis and Rheumatism 32: 1100–6.

Reisine ST, Grady K (1989) Work disability among women with RA. Arthritis and Rheumatism 32(5): 538–43.

Robinson H, Kirk RF, Frye RL, Robertson JT (1972) The psychological study of patients with RA and other painful diseases. Journal of Psychosomatic Research 16: 53–6.

Scott DL, Symmons DPM, Coulton BL, Popert AJ (1987) The long term outcome of treating rheumatoid arthritis: results after 20 years. Lancet i: 1108–11.

Spector TD (1996) Epidemiology of rheumatic disease. In Snaith ML (Ed), ABC of Rheumatism. London: BMJ 82–5.

Sternbach RA (1974) Pain Patients. Traits and Treatment. New York: Academic Press.

Strauss AL (1975) Chronic Illness and the Quality of Life. London: CV Mosby/Henry Kimpton.

Wiener C (1975) The burden of RA: tolerating the uncertainty. Social Science and Medicine 9: 97–104.

Zigmound AS, Snaith RP (1983) The hospital anxiety scale. Acta Psychiatrica Scandinavica 67: 361–70.

Chapter 6
Drugs in rheumatology

MARGARET SOMERVILLE

Introduction

Rheumatology covers a wide range of rheumatic diseases many of which are characterised by inflammatory changes resulting in damage to the surrounding structures. These conditions appear to be mulifactorial in origin but many have been precipitated by some exogenous challenge which then initiates a pathological process in genetically predisposed subjects. The factors predisposing susceptibility vary according to the disease and the individual. Rheumatology covers such conditions as rheumatoid arthritis, osteoarthritis, spondyloarthropathies, psoriatic arthritis, connective tissue disease, polymyositis, dermatomyositis, systemic lupus erythematosus and infective arthritis.

Specific aetiology and pathogenesis are as yet unknown, but it is thought an agent, or agents, precipitate an immune response which is perpetuated by antigens present in the synovial compartments. There is increasing evidence that 'T' lymphocytes play a pivotal role in the initiation and propagation of such diseases. Autoimmune disease can be either organ-specific or systemic.

The following are examples of non-rheumatological organ-specific autoimmune conditions and will not be discussed further: thyroiditis, Addison's disease, Type 1 diabetes, myasthenia gravis, primary biliary cirrhosis.

Below are examples of systemic, non-organ-specific autoimmune conditions frequently encountered in rheumatology:

(1) rheumatoid arthritis;
(2) dermatomyositis;
(3) systemic lupus erythematosus;
(4) scleroderma.

The spectrum of autoimmune disease is wide and as complicated as is the treatment. Rheumatoid arthritis is the most common of the chronic inflammatory diseases. Primarily involving the synovium, it also has the potential to affect other organs. Data produced by the Norfolk Arthritis Register show an incidence of 36 cases per 100 000 adult women per year and 14 cases per 100 000 adult men per year (Symmons, 1994). Without more specific information concerning the aetiology of these conditions, treatment has to be aimed at (1) symptom relief; and (2) disease modification.

At present there is no cure for most of the rheumatological conditions and it is extremely important that any therapies undertaken are done so in the light of the most up-to-date research available. Objective measures of outcome should be set to enable both physicians and patient decide whether a treatment is successful or otherwise. Any therapy has a cost–benefit ratio which needs to be adequately balanced. The equation should include both the effects of uncontrolled disease progression on the patient and family, as well as the ongoing costs which disability entails, versus the safety and efficacy of specific treatments, including long-term cost implications. Economic resource utilisation and quality of life measures will increasingly be used in assessing diseases' impact and treatment, when determining the distribution of health resources. Evidence-based medicine and nursing practice have never been as important as they are today in the highly politicised arena of the National Health Service.

To enable treatment to occur as early as possible, accurate and early diagnosis, as with all the systemic illnesses, is paramount. Unfortunately, the early symptoms of RA quite often mimic other arthritides and we lack a conclusive biochemical test to enable an accurate and early diagnosis to be made. The American College of Rheumatology (ACR) (Arnett et al., 1988) has therefore devised the following list of criteria which a patient has to fulfil in order to be labelled with the diagnosis of RA. Similar criteria are presently being prepared for other rheumatological conditions.

American Rheumatism Association Criteria for RA:
(1) morning stiffness in or around joints exceeding one hour in duration;

(2) arthritis (pain and swelling) of at least three joint areas;
(3) arthritis of hand joints;
(4) symmetrical arthritis (simultaneous involvement of the same joint areas bilaterally);
(5) rheumatoid nodules;
(6) serum rheumatoid factor positive;
(7) erosive changes.

For a diagnosis of RA to be made, four of the above seven criteria must be fulfilled and have been in existence for a minimum of 6 weeks.

Drugs and Therapeutic Interventions in Rheumatology

Whilst there are 200 different rheumatological conditions, treatment nonetheless is directed to three primary areas.

(1) analgesia;
(2) symptomatic relief of inflammation using NSAIDs;
(3) disease modification in the absence of cure.

The first two are usually undertaken by the GP, the third by the rheumatologist.

Analgesia

Pain management

The one symptom common to all 200 rheumatic diseases is pain. Patients experience varying degrees of pain, depending on their condition, time of day, and some say even the weather. Pain management is therefore of vital importance to the patient's well-being. Uncontrolled pain can set up a vicious circle resulting in reduced physical ability, anxiety and depression. This negative bio-feedback can perpetuate and exacerbate the pain, reinforcing a feeling of lost control. Education regarding the safe, regular use of analgesia in conjunction with an element of self-management will enable the patient to gain control once more. Most people will have experienced pain and will have become accustomed to a quick response from an analgesic such as paracetamol. In conditions such as rheumatoid arthritis the pain is often unremitting and therefore difficult to alleviate, and as such requires a different approach and in some instances stronger medication, which in turn may cause a variety of side-effects further adding to the distress experienced by patients with a chronic condition.

Table 6.1 gives a list of non-opioid analgesics commonly used, aspirin and paracetamol being predominant among them, and which work by blocking the synthesis and secretion of prostaglandins, preventing noiceptor sensitisation.

All of the following analgesics are suitable when used alone and in the early stages of treatment for most of the rheumatological conditions ranging from mild backache to peripheral joint pain. They are also particularly useful in musculoskeletal conditions, for example sports injuries. However, for the pain caused by the more severe systemic conditions, the list of opioid analgesics given in Table 6.2 will be required. These work by fitting into the opioid receptors of the brain and spinal cord, also used by endorphins, the body's own opioids.

Tables 6.1 and 6.2 reflect the variety of analgesics available to treat chronic pain. They are centrally acting analgesics which reduce the perception of pain, but, as seen by the side-effect profile have a variety of secondary and unwanted side-effects. One of the least serious but often most distressing side-effects is that of constipation. This

Table 6.1: Commonly used non-opioid analgesics

Generic preparation	Proprietary name	Side-effect profile
Paracetamol	Panadol	Rare: rashes, blood disorders Following overdose: liver damage
Acetylsalicylic acid	Aspirin	Common: high incidence of GI irritation, bronchospasm, skin reactions in hypersensitive patients
Co-codamol (codeine phosphate 30 mg, paracetamol 500 mg)	Solpadol, Tylex Kapake	Rare: rashes, blood disorders, constipation, nausea, vomiting, drowsiness, respiratory depression Following overdose: liver damage
Co-dydramol (dihydrocodeine tartrate 10 mg, paracetamol 500 mg)		As above
Co-proxamol (dextropropoxyphene hydrochloride 32.5 mg, paracetamol 325 mg)	Distalgesic Fortagesic Lobak	As above
Nefopam hydrochloride	Acupan	Rare: Nausea, nervousness, light-headedness, blurred vision, sweating, tachycardia, headaches, confusion, hallucinations

Table 6.2: Opioid analgesics

Generic preparation	Proprietary names	Dosage	Side-effect profile
Dihydrocodeine tartrate 60 mg or 30 mg 40mg	DHC continuous DF118 Forte	Up to 240 mg daily in three or four divided doses	Nausea, vomiting, constipation, drowsiness. Large doses produce respiratory depression and hypotension, headaches, bradycardia, vertigo, palpitations, etc.
Meptazinol 200 mg	Meptid	200mg every three to six hours	As above
Buprenorphine	Temgesic	200/400 μg 8 hourly	As above
Tramadol	Zydol	50–100 mg 4/6 hourly	As above
Fentanyl patches	Durogesic	50–75 mg changed every 72 hours	As above

is compounded by the inability to exercise regularly as functional ability is often significantly impaired. When considering suitable analgesia, this therefore becomes an important element to consider. Fentanyl patches are particularly useful for vertebral fractures due to osteoporosis, but are discontinued once pain is under control.

The early symptoms of systemic arthritis – hot, swollen, painful joints, early morning stiffness (EMS) and fatigue – can often be alleviated with the use of analgesia. It is preferable to treat chronic pain by taking analgesia on a regular four-hourly basis rather than waiting for the pain either simply to go away, or hoping it will not occur at all. When pain has been persistent and unremitting, as often occurs in a 'flare', regular use of an analgesic should help attain reasonable pain relief. Prescribed analgesia as listed in Tables 6.1 and 6.2, if taken on a regular four-hourly basis, should help maintain pain relief. However, analgesics alone are often insufficient to control the severity of the problem, and the addition of a non-steroidal anti-inflammatory drug (NSAID) is usually given as a supplement.

Non-steroidal anti-inflammatory drugs (NSAIDs)

Action and use of NSAIDs

The inflammation experienced by patients suffering from a systemic illness is often evident in the small peripheral joints of the hands and feet as well as such large joints as the knees, and often at the same time. As everything we do entails the use of these joints, functional ability is reduced significantly, and the need therefore to reduce this inflammation becomes paramount.

Inflammation is characterised by swollen, hot and painful joints, and is one of the main symptoms experienced by patients suffering from many of the rheumatological conditions. NSAIDs are the means by which they obtain relief from these symptoms. NSAIDs are amongst the most frequently prescribed drugs in the world (CSM, update 1986) and their ability to reduce pain, swelling and heat makes them an invaluable therapy in the management of all rheumatological conditions.

They are particularly helpful in controlling the early morning stiffness of rheumatoid arthritis and also the stiffness or gelling described by patients with osteoarthritis and experienced after sitting or resting for a long or short period of time. NSAIDs are often used in conjunction with analgesics to obtain maximum benefit.

Mode of action

Following any form of tissue injury there is a release of prostaglandins, the product of the enzymatic oxidation of arachidonic acid. The release of these hormones appears to cause signs of inflammation such as redness and heat. Drugs have therefore been targeted to cause interference with this inflammatory pathway and to work by inhibiting the synthesis of some of the prostaglandins, in particular the enzyme cyclo-oxygenese, thus inhibiting inflammation. The inflammatory cascade is a complicated one with prostaglandins possessing both pro-inflammatory and anti-inflammatory properties.

The earliest anti-inflammatory was aspirin (salicylic acid). This drug unfortunately has the potential to cause severe gastric irritation and as a result vast amounts of money have been spent by the pharmaceutical companies endeavouring to produce a drug with the established efficacy of aspirin but without the side-effects.

Choosing an NSAID

The results of their endeavours can be seen in Table 6.3. The variety and availability of present-day NSAIDs is now vast and ever increasing. When physicians are choosing an appropriate NSAID they will consider the age of the patient, previous gastrointestinal history, evidence of previous renal impairment and any difficulties in swallowing medications which the patient may have. Many of the preparations are now available on a once per day regimen. Also, many are available as either rectal suppositories, intramuscular injections or in the form of a topical application. Patients like to rub creams and ointments into affected areas but in general it is doubtful whether sufficient absorption occurs to warrant the extra expense for this sort of preparation. Many patients will need to try a variety of NSAIDs before they find one which is suitable. When deciding on a NSAID, doctors will in general use the criterion of efficacy in conjunction with the specific drug's side-effects profile, and weigh these against the cost of the medication. Comparisons of anti-inflammatory activity among the different NSAIDs are in general small, but there is considerable variation in individual patient response.

NSAIDs have both analgesic and anti-inflammatory properties. Most NSAIDs should produce a response within a few days, but if used for their analgesic properties alone, as perhaps for osteoarthritis or soft tissue injury, then they should be changed if no response is obtained within a week. If in addition to their analgesic properties they are also used for their anti-inflammatory component, as in RA, then they should be changed, if no significant response has been achieved, after three weeks.

NSAID side-effects profile

NSAIDs account for 5 per cent of National Health Service prescriptions but also account for 25 per cent of the reports sent in of adverse reactions. Of these adverse reactions to NSAIDs, 75 per cent were experienced by people over the age of 60 (Committee on Safety of Medicines update, 1986).

It is wise, then, to note that although present-day NSAIDs are extremely helpful in the treatment of rheumatic disease, they are not without their side-effect profile. Even the least toxic of them can cause a degree of gastric irritation, causing both nausea and/or gastric reflux. Because of this, some of the current NSAIDs on the market incorporate gastric protection as part of their formulation (see Table 6.3, Napratec). This method of presentation is presently causing some controversy. The debate revolves around whether or

not it should be mandatory to provide prophylactic gastric protection when prescribing NSAIDs. One drawback to this form of
prescribing is that patients are often unhappy about having to take
further medication purely to alleviate the possible side-effects of
exisiting medications. At present most physicians use their discretion
and, in view of the potential damage which NSAIDs can have on the
gastric mucosa, various forms of gastric protection are often
prescribed concomitantly. These include such drugs as cimetidine
(Tagamet), ranitidine (Zantac) and nizatidine (Axid), all H2 receptor
antagonists. They heal gastric and duodenal ulcers by reducing
gastric acid output. Maintenance treatment using half the usual dose
prevents ulcer relapse. Treatment of undiagnosed dyspepsia is sometimes acceptable in younger patients but less desirable in the elderly
where it may mask a diagnosis of gastric cancer. In most rheumatology units, severe dyspepsia usually warrants an endoscopy in order
to confirm the diagnosis of gastric ulceration prior to the commencement of an H2 receptor antagonist. In the main, and in spite of the
controversy, in many units an H2 receptor antagonist is prescribed
prophylactically and concomitantly with NSAID therapy. It should
also be noted that an H2 blockade is not without its own side-effect
profile of which dizziness, fatigue and rash are but a few, but all have
occasionally been reported. As these also occur with the use of
NSAIDs it is preferable to discontinue either the NSAID or the H2
receptor antagonist in order to determine which is the culprit.

Another group of therapies useful in the prevention and treatment of gastric ulceration is the 'proton pump' inhibitors such as
omeprazole (Losec) and lansoprazol (Zoton). Gastric acid is
produced and secreted by parietal cells in the oxyntic glands of the
gastric mucosa. The parietal cells are stimulated to produce acid by
activating receptors. The three most important receptors are activated by histamine, acetylcholine and gastrin. A cascade event
occurs following the activation of receptors which stimulate an
enzyme known as the proton pump to secrete acid. Effective control
is therefore achieved by blocking the hydrogen–potassium adenosine
triphosphatase enzyme system (the proton pump) of the gastric parietal cells, and stopping acid production. H2 receptor antagonists, by
contrast, inhibit acid secretion by selectively blocking the histamine
receptors only and are unable to control acid secretion by other
routes. Misoprostol (Cytotec), a synthetic prostaglandin analogue,
has both anti-secretory and protective properties which promote
gastric and duodenal ulcer healing.

Gastric reflux is quite a common problem with patients who require

NSAID treatment. It responds well to Gaviscon 10-20 ml given prn after meals and at bedtime. Cisapride 10 mg 3–4 times daily with a maintenance dose of 20 mg nocte is helpful in improving impaired gastric motility which is often secondary to conditions such as systemic sclerosis. Domperidone (Motilium)10-20 mg every 4–8 hours is useful in treating functional dyspepsia, nausea and vomiting and particularly helpful when patients become nauseated after receiving cytotoxic drugs which are commonly used in the treatment of rheumatoid arthritis and other arthritides.

Many patients are found to have *helicobacter pylori* on gastroscopy examination. Duodenal ulcers are known to have a strong association with infection from *helicobacter pylori* and this usually responds to a two-week course of amoxycillin and metronidazole given concurrently with ranitidine or alternatively giving amoxycillin concomitantly with omeprazole.

Elderly, frail patients are at particular risk as their diet is often inadequate and irregular, which allows for potential problems to arise when taking NSAIDs on an empty stomach. Most nurses will be aware of the numbers of admissions to Care of the Elderly Units of patients suffering from severe anaemia, or worse gastric haemorrhage, following repeated ingestion of medications similar in nature to aspirin.

Whilst the greatest potential hazard with an NSAID is its effect on the gastric mucosa, NSAIDs may also affect renal function and hepatic function. In addition, particular caution is required with patients who have a known history of hypersensitivity to aspirin or other NSAIDs, as bronchospasm or angio-oedema may be precipitated. Furthermore, all drugs have the potential to interact with one another and it is therefore important for the side-effects profile of any drug which the patient is receiving to be reviewed and potential interactions noted. This does not preclude the use of such medication, but obviously careful monitoring will be required.

Early morning stiffness (EMS) is also a major component of RA. Fortunately, NSAIDs are helpful in alleviating this symptom too. Often, EMS can last between 4 and 12 hours per day, and its persistence can be both disabling and extremely depressing. With EMS in mind, it is preferable to take the NSAIDs late at night, in order to achieve maximum benefit early in the morning.

More recently there has been research into the effects of NSAIDs on the development of infertility, an area which will need significant long-term research (Akil, Amos and Steward, 1996). Careful and repeated education of patients on the safe taking of all medications, let alone NSAIDs, is imperative and something in which all staff can play a part.

Table 6.3: Some of the most common NSAIDs in use

Generic name	Trade name	Dosage	Side-effect profile
Diclofenac	Voltarol	75–150 mg daily in divided doses	GI disturbances, nausea, diarrhoea, bronchospasm, rashes, headaches
Ibuprofen	Brufen	1.2–2.4 g daily in divided doses	As above. Contra-indicated in patients with a history of hypersensitivity to aspirin
Ibuprofen	Brufen Retard	1.6 g nocte SR (preferably given in the early evening)	As above
Naproxen	Naprosyn	0.5–1 g daily in two divided doses	As above
Naproxen plus Misoprostol (NSAID + gastric protection)	Napratec	Naproxen 500 mg tablet + 200 µg Misoprostol given bd	As above. Side-effect profile of misoprostol includes diarrhoea, abdominal pain Intramenstrual bleeding and postmenopausal bleeding
Indomethacin	Indocid, Flexin	75–200 mg daily in divided doses given bd. May be given rectally as suppositories at 100 mg bd	Equal in action or possibly superior to Naproxen but with a higher incidence of side-effects including headaches, dizziness and GI disturbances
Ketoprofen	Oruvail, Orudis	100–200 mg once daily. May be given orally, rectally or by IM injection	As above. With the addition of pain at the injection site; suppositories may cause rectal irritation
Nabumetone	Relifex	1 g nocte in severe conditions and 0.5 to 1 g in the morning	As above
Piroxicam	Feldene	10–30 mg daily, either in single or divided doses. Also available as Feldene Melt, a sublingual version	As above
Sulindac	Clinoril	200 mg bd	As above
Tenoxicam	Mobiflex	20 mg daily	As above
Azapropazone	Rheumox	1.2 g daily in two or four divided doses, or given 300 mg bd in the elderly to avoid severe renal impairment	As above and particular caution with the elderly or those with evidence of renal impairment

Alternatives to the Bio-medical Model

There is a vast array of information available to patients about both complementary medicines and alternative therapies. Magazines and newspapers contain advertisements for miracle treatments which are often extremely costly and available by post from specialist pharmacists only. There may well be a place for some of these preparations, but patients should be encouraged to discuss their use and nurses should be available to counter the extreme claims of efficacy of such preparations with scientific evidence. It is entirely reasonable for patients to seek alternative therapies in view of the extensive side-effect profile already discussed. However, their choice should be based on scientific proof rather than advertising hype. There are some preparations which can be of use if taken in sufficient quantities. Fish oils have been promoted as a cure of arthritis for numerous years. They do not effect a cure, but if used in sufficient quantities do have anti-inflammatory properties (Geusens et al., 1994). It may be suggested to patients that they can either take their fish oils as a capsule or by simply having a regular intake of any oily fish. There are a number of preparations which contain oil of evening primrose which have similar benefits (Geusens et al., 1994). If the patient has been experiencing significant problems with indigestion connected with NSAIDs then this may, in the future, be a possible way to help alleviate their symptoms. Further research is needed. In general if patients are keen to try an alternative therapy or a new diet which they believe might be beneficial, it is helpful if they try it rigidly for at least a month to try to establish whether any benefits are felt. There is no evidence-based research to suggest that any diet can alleviate symptoms, but simply telling patients is often less effective than allowing them to experience something for themselves.

Alternatives to bio-medicine in relief of pain

There are some simple techniques that individuals can utilise to alleviate symptoms of pain if used in conjunction with analgesics. The use of heat and cold is particularly helpful. The use of warm-water soaks to specific areas of the body, such as the hands or feet, may be sufficient to ease those aching peripheral joints. We are all aware of the comfort of luxuriating in a hot bath, and the addition of aromatic bath oils is found useful by some people. Hydrotherapy and wax baths are often initiated by the physiotherapists in a hospital setting. Wax baths can also be utilised at home providing the correct equipment is available, otherwise they are too dangerous to contemplate. The use of covered hot-water bottles or the newer gel packs which can be heated and then applied to specific areas of the body such as the neck are also known to be helpful. Gel packs can be used either hot or cold. The application of cold compresses can be as beneficial as that of heat. The gel pack applied cold can quickly take on the shape of the particular joint which is hot, inflamed and painful, and its application can be extremely soothing (see Chapter 7).

The use of a TENS machine (transcutaneous electrical nerve stimulation) can be particularly helpful and although often initiated by the physiotherapists, patients can borrow them from the depart-ment or buy them for approximately £40.00. The machines emit an electrical stimulation which is often helpful in reducing pain, enabling the individuals to have control over their pain management (see Chapter 7).

Alternatives to conventional therapy

As we have seen there are a variety of therapies other than those which adhere strictly to bio-medicine. These include the use of heat and cold as well as nerve stimulation through a TENS machine. The anti-inflammatory properties of fish oils and oil of evening primrose have been shown to be effective as long as taken in large quantities (Geusens et al., 1994). Psychosocial elements of establishing self-management models can be extremely helpful in breaking the vicious pain circle that sometimes ensues with a chronic condition. Self-management groups and self-support groups are both being run within rheumatology units throughout the country.

As with all medications there is a cost–benefit ratio and most patients could not function at all without the use of NSAIDs. Even so, we must always remember that all of these medical conditions produce side-effects solely as a result of having the illness, and not exclusively as a result of the medications used to alleviate them.

Corticosteroids

Corticosteroids, or steroids as they are more commonly known, have a part to play in the treatment of inflammatory arthritides. They are the most powerful of all the anti-inflammatory agents and, like the NSAIDs and analgesics, purely treat the symptoms rather than the cause of the underlying pathological process. However, they also suppress the picture of inflammation by reducing the heat, swelling and pain present in inflamed tissues. Corticosteroids can be given in a variety of ways including orally, by intra-articular injections or intra-muscular injections and also by intravenous infusion. The dose which is used is totally dependent upon the patient's condition, the severity of the symptoms, and the requirement for local or systemic effect. Patients generally respond quite dramatically to steroid therapy with a rapid reduction in inflammation. This improvement often poses potential problems in that this miraculous response increases the demands of the patient for continuous steroid treatment. It is therefore imperative that the potential long-term side-effects of such therapies are discussed prior to treatment.

The side-effect profile has been well documented over the years, with most patients being aware that steroids may, in the short term, induce diabetes, hypertension, skin and subcutaneous tissue atrophy as well as purpura. There are also significant long-term effects of high-dose steroids on bones, including the development of osteoporosis and aseptic necrosis. Steroids may also precipitate hypertension owing to their ability to increase fluid retention.

In the past, because of known long-term side-effects, steroids have been used quite late in conditions such as rheumatoid arthritis. They are the drug of choice in such diseases as polymyalgia rheumatica (PMR) and giant-cell arteritis. PMR occurs in the older age-group, median age 65, and responds dramatically to between 15 and 20 mg of steroids daily, reducing the dose as the ESR gradually decreases until eventually over approximately two years the patient is weaned off completely. Giant-cell arteritis is a form of vasculitis which may occur alongside PMR and is a medical emergency as it can precipitate blindness if not treated quickly. The drug of choice is again prednisolone with doses of between 50 and 70 mg per day given if there are any indications of ocular involvement. Once control is achieved a gradual reduction of steroids of 2.5–5 mg daily is undertaken until 20 mg daily is reached. Each centre will have its own specific regime for the tailing off of steroids from that point onwards.

Intra-muscular corticosteroids

Patients who have rheumatoid arthritis or other systemic illnesses will often experience a flare in their symptoms. This flare consists of inflammation and pain in numerous peripheral and large joints in the body. This may well respond quite dramatically to a one-off intra-muscular (IM) injection of Depo-Medrone 40–120 mg, or Kenalog 40-100 mg. The decision to give IM steroids is usually made either prior to the initiation of disease-modifying agents, or at a time when these agents are no longer working, and an alternative second-line agent is being considered. Most of the second-line agents take between 10 and 12 weeks to become established and the intra-muscular injection will give cover during this period of time. It is important to give the injection with a one-and-half inch needle deep into the muscle, otherwise muscular atrophy may occur.

Intra-articular injections of corticosteroids

Patients suffering from a variety of inflammatory arthropathies may also require intra-articular injections when they are experiencing an acute inflammatory episode. The decision for an intra-articular injection will depend upon the severity of the symptoms, the location of the inflammatory process and the numbers of joints involved. Quite often the majority of joints may be under control but the patient may have specific problems with only one or two joints, which are better treated with a localised injection rather than an intra-muscular or oral preparation which would have a systemic effect. Large joints such as the knee, which may have significant effusions, are usually aspirated prior to an intra-articular injection with a steroid preparation. The dose used is dependent upon the site and mostly a local anaesthetic of lignocaine is given either concomitantly or around the joint margin prior to administration of the steroid. The drugs used tend to be one of the following: hydrocortisone, triamcinolone or methylprednisolone. Some centres still use IV pulse steroids though they are less favoured now because the effect, though excellent, is extremely short term.

Mode of action

The effect of corticosteroids on the inflammatory process is complicated but it is believed that they inhibit the release of arachidonic acid from phospholipids and therefore decrease the formation of prostaglandins. They can also exert a suppressive effect on the adrenocortical function which may inhibit a response to stresses of all kinds. They are, however, extremely useful if used in the right dose for the right condition at the right time.

Side-effect profile

(1) Steroids have an effect on the endocrine system and may precipitate the development of diabetes if used in large quantities. Patients may develop symptoms of Cushing's syndrome with the characteristic moon face, obesity and an increase of fine body hair (hirsutism).

(2) They may suppress growth in children and cause amenorrhoea. They are known to cause skin and subcutaneous tissue atrophy as well as purpura and acne.

(3) They have the potential to mask the symptoms of gastrointestinal

disturbances whilst at the same time an exacerbation of peptic ulceration continues.

(4) In muscles, they may cause a myopathy.
(5) In the eyes, glaucoma and subcapsular cataract as well as papilloedema may occur.
(6) In the central nervous system, intra-cranial hypertension, depression and mood swing may become apparent.
(7) In bone, osteoporosis is a common consequence of long-term steroid use. Aseptic necrosis is a possibility.
(8) Electrolyte disturbances may occur resulting in fluid and sodium retention, hypertension and hypokalaemia.
(9) They reduce resistance to infection.

Summary of corticosteroid therapy

Despite the long list of potential side-effects which have a high incidence of occurring with high-dose oral steroids, these drugs still have a significant role to play in a variety of rheumatological conditions. If used sensibly at the lowest possible dose to induce reduction in the inflammatory process together with careful monitoring, they can be extremely beneficial in reducing pain. **All patients on long-term steroid treatment should carry a STEROID CARD.** The Bristol Group in their study (Kirwan, 1995) suggest that early in the disease and over a short term, i.e. over two years, low-dose steroids of 7.5 mg daily were relatively safe, as they were when used in combination with second-line agents, and may actually have a disease-modifying effect by reducing the erosive changes so characteristic of rheumatoid arthritis. Research into the long-term effects, however, has yet to be carried out. The alternative anti-inflammatory agents to corticosteroid therapy are the non-steroidal anti-inflammatories already discussed.

Pregnancy: If the patient's condition warrants this drug then 10 mg daily is considered a safe dose. It is also considered safe during lactation though long-term effects on the baby are uncertain.

Disease modification

Drugs to modify the disease

The first two sections have covered symptomatic relief, which has a major part to play in the management of all 200 rheumatological conditions. The following and final section covers only those drugs used in the treatment of the inflammatory arthritides and autoimmune conditions and not the degenerative arthropathies. At present there is no known cure for any of the conditions mentioned and, in the absence of a cure, disease modification has become the cornerstone of treatment.

Past and present terminology

(1) Second-line agents.
(2) DMARDs: disease-modifying anti-rheumatic drugs.
(3) SAARDs: slow-acting anti-rheumatic drugs.

DMARDs and SAARDs = second-line agents.

All three of these terms are used throughout the world in rheumatology. The term second-line agent was used for a number of years as in general the 'first-line agents' were the analgesics and NSAIDs. First-line agents were often initiated at the first visit to the GP's surgery and continued for many years until the patient developed signs of erosive changes, when it was then considered appropriate to prescribe potentially therapeutic but toxic medications. These treatments were called second-line agents. More recently, as prescribing has changed significantly, or rather the timing of the prescribing of these agents has changed, so has the terminology, and 'disease-modifying' or DMARD is now more commonly used. SAARD is a term that has also evolved in recent years as the majority of these agents are slow acting as opposed to the immediate response that has been seen with steroids. SAARDs may be used in the place of DMARDs but for clarity in this book DMARD will be used from now on.

Criteria for initiating a DMARD

Prior to commencing any sort of disease modification it is important to consider the following:

(1) Timing: when should DMARDs be initiated?
(2) Choice of DMARD: i.e. which disease-modifying agent should be used and at what stage in the disease.
(3) Combination therapy: not simply combining analgesia, NSAIDs and DMARDs, but considering combining two DMARDs as well.
(4) Duration of therapy: how long should a therapy be tried, and at what dose before we are able to indicate success or failure?

Timing

Until relatively recently, if a patient presented to a GP with painful and swollen joints consistent with an inflammatory process, the GP would normally initiate treatment with a simple analgesic and NSAID. If the symptoms were not controlled with these medications, a GP would at that time refer the patient to a consultant rheumatologist. The delay in seeing a rheumatologist could be anything from a few months to a few years. In many cases, by the time the patient saw a rheumatologist there were already significant signs of erosive changes in a large number of the joints. When the disease was shown to be of a progressive nature, then and only then would second-line therapies, DMARDS, be initiated. The medications were considered to be so potentially toxic that many doctors had considerable anxieties about prescribing them to patients who it was felt may or may not have developed prolonged problems. At that time there were no clear prognostic indicators to enable doctors to evaluate the possible outcome of these conditions. However, we now have a much clearer picture of those patients who will develop severe disease and of those who may have either intermittent or mild disease that is relatively easily managed on analgesia and/or NSAIDs alone. There have been a variety of research projects into early arthritis and the Norfolk Arthritis Register in particular has not only given us a clearer idea of the incidence and prevalence of such things as rheumatoid arthritis, but has also given us some prognostic indicators to highlight those patients who are likely to develop the more severe arthropathies (Brennan, 1996). The following is a list of potentially useful prognostic indicators:

(1) high Health Assessment Questionnaire (HAQ) score at presentation;
(2) positive rheumatoid factor;
(3) knee involvement within the first year (Barrett; 1993);
(4) HLA D24 tissue type – marker of severity;
(5) nodules developing early in the disease.

The appearance of any one of these indicators alone is insufficient to predict outcome, but the more these signs and symptoms are seen together at an early stage in the disease progression, the more likelihood there is of the patient developing more severe disease. This sort of information is particularly useful when deciding which patients to target for early intervention therapy. The rationale for such timing corresponds with the views found in oncology. It would be considered quite inappropriate to wait until the patient has developed metastases before initiating cytotoxic therapies. Equally, it is being considered that we should no longer wait until erosive changes have developed before starting potentially more therapeutic drugs even though they might be considered to be potentially more toxic. In the early stages of any rheumatic condition patients are basically healthy and symptoms are often localised to the skeletal system. They are therefore, at this stage, in the best physical condition to cope with a variety of medications which might be considered toxic. Whereas when they are more debilitated, having endured their condition over a number of years, other systems, i.e. kidneys, lungs, skin, etc., may also have become involved. It is this philosophy which has initiated consideration of the reversal of the 'therapeutic pyramid' (Wilske, 1993). This model introduced NSAIDs and analgesics as the base of the pyramid and continued to introduce only the least toxic disease-modifying agents as the disease progressed. Those drugs which were considered to be potentially more therapeutic but also more toxic were given very much as a last resort. Steroids at that time were at the top of the pyramid. The reversal, thus, would consider giving the most toxic, but equally potentially therapeutic medication first, i.e. methotrexate or cyclosporin, if the patient presented with a combination of the predictors of severe outcome.

Choice of DMARD

There are a considerable variety of disease-modifying agents available. Many of them have been available for between 20 and 50 years, and have often been used for conditions other than inflammatory joint problems. The choice today is based on disease duration, severity of disease and prognostic indicators.

(a) *Mild systemic disease:* Mild disease is characterised by a display of a small number of inflamed joints which do not respond to a simple analgesic or NSAID, and have developed along a mildly unremitting course. Such patients are invariably prescribed either hydroxychloroquine, sulphasalazine, penicillamine or gold.

(b) *Moderate systemic disease:* This is characterised by unremitting polyarthritis with moderate functional impairment. Sulphasalazine seems to be the drug of choice in most centres.

(c) *Severe systemic disease:* This is characterised by unremitting polyarthritis with the addition of severe functional disability and the exhibition of many of the prognostic indicators of severe disease as listed above. Methotrexate has become increasingly the drug of choice, followed by azathioprine and cyclosporin in some centres.

(d) *Very severe systemic disease:* This involves other organs or systems of the body including such conditions as vasculitis, pericarditis and secondary respiratory problems. Systemic disease of this severity would warrant the initiation of such drugs as cyclosphosphamide, often given as pulse therapy initially in combination with high-dose steroids.

Combination therapy

Increasingly, disease-modifying agents are used not only concomitantly with NSAIDs and analgesia, but also in combination with each other. There are a variety of regimes used in these combinations. Some centres will commence therapy with one DMARD, then when the standard dose has failed to precipitate a response after a specified length of time, usually three to six months, the second DMARD is introduced, and increased until its standard dose is achieved and hopefully efficacy established. Failure to achieve efficacy at this stage in some centres prompts the initiation of a third DMARD. It is not uncommon now to find the use of two DMARDs, plus NSAIDs, plus analgesics.

Duration of therapy

Most DMARDs require a treatment period of a minimum of three months prior to efficacy being established. Once the patient is established on a satisfactory regime, treatment can be continued indefinitely as long as a response continues. However, often after a period of time, efficacy is either lost or the onset of side-effects precipitates either a dose reduction, temporary stopping of treatment, or therapy cessation due to unacceptable side-effects. A clear response to treatment is not a reason for stopping a drug. In some cases, once the therapy has been stopped, it becomes increasingly difficult to achieve efficacy when restarted. Flares in symptoms often occur within a two- to four-week time-scale following cessation of treatment. The majority of patients remain on a specific DMARD for a minimum of a year with others able to tolerate individual DMARDs for five years plus. It is very much idiosyncratic, and as yet impossible to predict, those patients who will respond and continue to respond over any particular length of time. In view of this relatively short duration of treatment with an individual DMARD, it does not take much time to run out of all the available options. This has provided the impetus to discover new therapies and just as importantly to reassess available therapies by using them differently or more appropriately. It had been hoped that with the introduction of a DMARD, patients would gain control and treatment would be stopped. A small number of patients do go into remission with or without treatment. Most others achieve a considerable degree of control over their illness. This consists of periods of control followed by periods called flares during which the disease becomes active again. Others have such severe unremitting disease that no matter what treatments they have, the outcome remains unaltered and severe destruction of joints continues.

Specific disease-modifying anti-rheumatic drugs (DMARDS)

It is important to state that all doctors have their own dose range and drug-monitoring regimen. However, where possible those shown here follow the guidelines recommended by the British Society for Rheumatology.

It is important that all patients on disease-modifying therapy should have blood results and urinalysis recorded in a monitoring booklet. Serial data recorded in such a way are more helpful in detecting decreasing or increasing trends in blood results, as well as alerting the monitor to any nephrotoxicity detected through a regular urinalysis.

DMARDS in regular use:

- hydroxychloroquine (Plaquenil) HCQ;
- penicillamine (Distamine) DPA;
- IM gold (Myocrisin) and oral gold (auranofin);
- sulphasalazine (Salazopyrin) SASP;
- methotrexate (Matrex) MTX;
- azathioprine (Imuran) AZP;
- cyclosporin (Neoral) CyA.

DMARDs for mild disease

Patients presenting with mild symptoms, but which are persistent, are often prescribed one of the following: hydroxychloroquine (Plaquenil), penicillamine (Distamine), auranofin (Ridaura).

Hydroxychloroquine (Plaquenil) HCQ

HCQ has some disease-modifying properties which can induce control in mild rheumatoid arthritis. It is a drug which is rarely used these days as other DMARDs are considered to be more efficacious. It is used for the treatment of systemic lupus erythematosus (SLE) and discoid lupus, in which it is considered the drug of choice. It is also used in the treatment and chemo-prophylaxis of malaria.

Though beneficial in treating mild rheumatoid arthritis, it has the very rare potential to cause hepatic and renal impairment, though more frequently gastrointestinal problems may occur. It is known to exacerbate the skin condition in psoriasis. However, the main concern with its long-term use is the effect on the eyes. Prior to commencing treatment it is therefore important to establish any evidence of pre-existing retinal disease. Ocular toxicity is usually dependent on the dose and the length of time someone has been on the drug; the longer the time and the higher the dose the more likely ocular problems are to occur.

Dosage: not exceeding 6.5 mg per kg per day, or 200/400 mg daily is considered safe.

Side-effects and what to do

Minor side effects:

- **gastrointestinal disturbances:** take tablets last thing at night;
- **headaches:** try taking tablets last thing at night;
- **skin reactions:** may exacerbate psoriasis.

Major side-effects (these rarely occur):

- **hair loss:** very rare though serious, particularly for females;
- **visual disturbances:** corneal opacities, potentially irreversible retinal damage. Should they occur HCQ must be STOPPED.

Monitoring: In view of the potential eye toxicity pre-existing retinal disease should be excluded. The eyes must be tested *before* starting the drug and six-monthly thereafter while on the drug. The eye test can be carried out by certain high street opticians, though a charge will be made. Amsler testing (see Figure 6.1) should be performed in order to detect pre-macularopathy (visual disturbance in absence of ophthalmoscopically visible macular changes. Changes detected by Amsler are frequently reversible.) Despite the potential ocular retinopathy, toxicity is quite rare, and in general hydroxychloroquine is well tolerated and effective in mild disease. Bloods are usually tested at clinic visits only.

Pregnancy: HCQ should be avoided in pregnancy as there are known teratogenic problems in the first trimester. It may be possible to take chloroquine during lactation as this has not been detected in measurable amounts in breast milk.

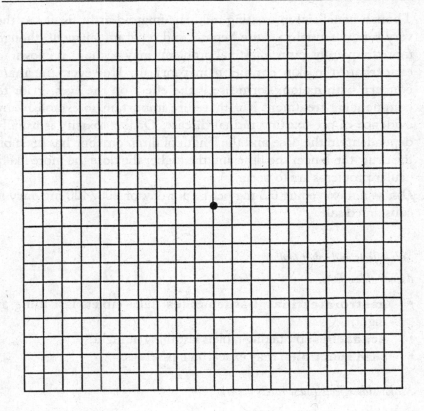

Figure 6.1. Amsler recording chart. A replica of chart No. 1, printed in black and white for convenience of recording. Reproduced by kind permission of Keeler Ltd of Windsor.

Penicillamine (Distamine) DPA

Effective in the treatment of mild to moderate rheumatoid arthritis, penicillamine has disease-modifying properties which have the potential to induce and maintain control in rheumatoid arthritis. It is one of the few drugs which should be taken on an empty stomach, at least one and a half hours before or after food. It does interact with iron and antacids and these should therefore be taken with meals or at different times of the day. It has the advantage of being taken just once a day.

Dosage: Start with 125 mg per day, increasing by 125 mg daily for four weeks to 500 mg per day. If no response after 24 weeks increase by 125 mg every 4 weeks to 750 mg per day. If no response by 36 weeks increase by 125 mg every four weeks to 1 g per day. If no response at 48 weeks stop treatment. Maximum recommended dose is 1 g daily. Efficacy normally is established within 10 to 12 weeks.

Side-effects and what to do

Minor side-effects:

- **loss of taste:** patients should be warned that a loss of taste may occur early in treatment, but usually returns after about six weeks irrespective of whether or not treatment is discontinued;
- **nausea:** may occur but is usually not a problem if the penicillamine is taken just before going to bed. If preferred it can be taken during the day; mid-morning is most suitable.

Major side-effects:

- **bone marrow suppression causing thrombocytopenia and neutropenia:** this is a potentially serious problem and patients should be warned to tell the doctor or nurse immediately if they develop sore throats, mouth ulcers, bruising, fever or rashes; WBC $<3.0 \times 10^9/l$, caution. Repeat in one week. $< 2.0 \times 10^9/l$, STOP treatment;
  Platelets $<150 \times 10^9/l$, caution. Repeat in one week. $<120 \times 10^9/l$, STOP treatment.

- **renal toxicity:** indicated by a proteinuria or haematuria on urinalysis. Trace of protein, ignore. 1+ on two occasions, wait one week then recheck. If still present, STOP, check MSU and 24-hour urinary protein. If in excess of 2 g protein, treatment should be stopped. Proteinuria associated with immune complex nephritis occurs in up to 30 per cent of patients but may also resolve despite continuation of treatment. Treatment may therefore be continued as long as renal function tests remain normal, and there is no evidence of oedema. Haematuria is less likely to occur. If 1+ request MSU and wait one week then recheck. If WBC or RBC present on microscopy, STOP drug;
- **rashes:** may occur in the first few months of treatment, usually disappear when the drug is stopped and treatment may then be reintroduced at a lower dose later on. Rashes which occur later on in treatment are more resistant and often necessitate discontinuation of treatment. Check for other causes, if these are in the clear; try reducing dose. If severe, STOP medication.

Very rarely febrile reactions or **drug-induced lupus** may occur.

Monitoring:

(1) FBC with differentials fortnightly for the first eight weeks and thereafter monthly. Abnormal trends in any direction of any value should prompt caution and vigilance.
(2) Urinalysis weekly for around first three months then monthly as bloods move to monthly. Carried out by the patient using dipsticks.
(3) Monitoring booklet should be provided.

Look for a fall in WBC, neutrophils and platelets. Protein and blood in urine.

Pregnancy: Because of the known side-effects which may occur to the mother DPA is not recommended. Difficult to assay therefore avoid during lactation.

Auranofin (Ridaura) oral gold

Has not been found to be as efficacious as Myocrisin and is therefore reserved for mild RA only. Auranofin is obviously easier for patients to take as it does not require repeated visits to the surgery for injections. It does, however, require the same degree of monitoring as Myocrisin because of the potential for bone marrow suppression. Patients should therefore be warned to report if they develop an infection, mouth ulcers, bruising or fever, all of which might indicate bone marrow suppression. The most common side-effect though is diarrhoea, with or without nausea, together with abdominal discomfort. These side-effects may respond to bulking agents such as bran or a temporary reduction in dosage.

Dosage typical regimen: 3 mg bd increasing to 3 mg tds after four to six months if no improvement. Discontinue treatment around six months if no response.

Monitoring: Monthly FBC and urinalysis. Otherwise the same as IM Myocrisin.

Pregnancy: Not recommended though according to the manufacturer's data 13 healthy babies have been born to mothers taking this drug. Avoid during lactation.

DMARDs for moderately severe disease

Sodium aurothiomalate (Myocrisin IM gold)

Gold therapy has been used for 40 or more years and is particularly useful in the treatment of rheumatoid arthritis, juvenile chronic arthritis (Still's disease) and palindromic rheumatoid arthritis. Gold may be given either intramuscularly (IM) as Myocrisin or orally as auranofin (see above).

Administration and dosage: Myocrisin should be given by deep intramuscular injection into the buttocks or deltoid muscle following a test dose of 10 mg. Thereafter increase to 50 mg weekly until up to a maximum dose of 1 g. If no response has occurred at this point STOP treatment. Benefit is not anticipated until between 500 mg and 1 g have been given. In patients who do respond, the interval between injections can be gradually increased to monthly 50 mg injections. Myocrisin which has darkened in colour must be discarded. Once efficacy has been reached treatment should be continued. People may stay on the drug for as long it appears to be helping them.

IMPORTANT: Guidelines from the manufacturers are insisting on a 30-minute surveillance of all patients following ALL IM Myocrisin injections because of possible anaphylactoid effects. This will cause problems for many nurses, particularly district nurses. Patients who have to work will also find it an encumbrance.

Side-effects and what to do

Major side-effects:

- **rashes with pruritis or mouth ulcers:** these can occur at anytime during treatment, and may require dose reduction or discontinuation. Rashes are important and must be taken seriously;
- **bone marrow suppression** causing thrombocytopenia and neutropenia; these are potentially serious side-effects;
  WBC <3.0 × 10⁹/l, caution. Repeat in one week. <2.0 × 10⁹/l, STOP treatment;
  platelets <150 × 10⁹/l, caution. Repeat in one week. <120 × 10⁹/l, STOP treatment;
- **eosinophilia:** this may precede skin rash. Reduce Myocrisin dose or frequency and monitor more frequently.
- **renal toxicity:** indicated by a proteinuria or haematuria on urinalysis. Trace of protein ignore. 1+ if found on two or more occasions, wait one week then recheck. If still present, STOP, check MSU and 24-hour urinary protein. If in excess of 2 g protein, treatment should be stopped but may also resolve despite continuation of treatment. Treatment may therefore be continued as long as renal function tests are normal, and there is

no evidence of oedema. If haematuria more than 1+ check MSU and test again one week later. Depending on results may have to stop Myocrisin.

Monitoring:

(1) A full blood count (FBC) with differentials is required before each weekly injection, and the week *before monthly* injections. Abnormal trends in any direction of any value should prompt caution and vigilance.
(2) Urinalysis weekly for around first three months then monthly before each injection. Carried out by the patient using dipsticks. Nurse to check for blood.
(3) Pre-treatment chest X-ray followed by a yearly chest X-ray.
(4) Monitoring booklet should be provided.

Look for a fall in WBC, neutrophils and platelets and a rise in eosinophils. Protein and blood in urine.

Pregnancy: As with DPA, because of the known side-effects which could occur to the mother, gold is not recommended. Not recommended during lactation.

EC sulphasalazine (Salazopyrin) SASP

Sulphasalazine was used many years ago in the treatment of rheumatoid arthritis, but lost favour when it appeared to fail to achieve the remission which had been intended. It has been reintroduced over the last 10 years and re-evaluated. It is now fully established in the treatment of rheumatoid arthritis and in some centres also for ankylosing spondylitis which exhibits peripheral joint involvement. It is also used in the treatment of Crohn's disease and ulcerative colitis. It is given orally as an enteric-coated (EC) tablet. At present this is the only form of SASP with a product licence for use in RA. The majority of patients respond extremely well without experiencing any major side-effects. It is helpful to inform patients that their urine may take on an orange colour following treatment with sulphasalazine, and soft contact lenses may also become discoloured.

Dosage: Typical regimen may be 500 mg per day increasing by 500 mg weekly to 2.0 g daily. Maximum of 3 g daily. Efficacy is normally established between 8 and 12 weeks.

Side-effects and what to do

Minor side-effects:

- **nausea, abdominal discomfort, headaches, dizziness:** these often respond to a reduced dose, later increased without side-effects.

Major side-effects (less common):

- **rash:** sometimes very severe, STOP drug. If mild may persevere;
- **bone marrow suppression:** thrombocytopenia, leucopenia, neutropenia;
  WBC $<3.0 \times 10^9/l$, caution. Repeat in one week. $<2.0 \times 10^9/l$, STOP treatment;
  platelets $<150 \times 10^9/l$, caution. Repeat in one week. $<120 \times 10^9/l$, STOP treatment;
- **hepato-toxicity:** elevation of liver enzymes ALT, ALK PHOS, AST to twice the upper limit of normal warrants stopping therapy;
- **macrocytosis:** Check B12 and folate levels and initiate treatment with folic acid. SASP quite often precipitates a folate deficiency.

Monitoring:

(1) FBC and differentials two-weekly and LFTs four-weekly for the first 12 weeks and subsequently repeated on a three-monthly basis. Although these are the guidelines from the BSR most centres check FBC, differentials and LFTs four-weekly for 12 weeks then as above. Abnormal trends in any direction of any value should prompt caution and vigilance.

(2) Patients should be asked to report to a doctor immediately if they develop a persistent sore throat, fever, malaise or non-specific illness.

Look for a fall in WBC, neutrophils and platelets; a rise in AST, ALT and alkaline phosphatase.

Pregnancy: Thought to be safe during pregnancy as there is no evidence of teratogenesis, even so rarely used. Could be useful as a substitute for Methotrexate during six months prior to conception, then discontinued as soon as first pregnancy test is obtained. Should be avoided near to term because of risk of jaundice in the neonate (le Gallez, 1988). Could be safe during lactation.

All the previous disease-modifying agents are slow-acting and beneficial in mild to moderate disease. In general they are well tolerated, and less potentially toxic than the following drugs, but equally they are not found to be particularly beneficial in the more severe and unremitting type of disease.

DMARDs for severe disease

In the more recent past the following drugs were used only as a last resort, for example when patients had failed to respond to those drugs thought to be less toxic, as listed above. However, in the last two or three years the general consensus of opinion has been that potentially effective treatment should not be withheld until, as in the case of rheumatoid arthritis, joint erosions have become so severe that further treatment may prove to be unsuccessful. Damaged joints will not repair, therefore replacement becomes the only option. Although the following drugs are by implication more toxic, it is now felt that the 'side-effects of the disease' are potentially more devastating than the drugs themselves even when carefully monitored. The rationale behind such thinking coincides with that of the oncologists. They do not wait until metastases have occurred before considering treating with potentially life-saving cytotoxic drugs despite the known toxicity. Once erosive changes have occurred in a patient with rheumatoid arthritis and the joint becomes destabilised, the only effective treatment becomes arthroplasty. The solution therefore is to find a deterrent to prevent the erosive changes occurring in the first place. The major difficulty is in deciding when to commence treatment, which drugs to use, and on which patient to initiate treatment. This decision depends on our present knowledge of prognostic indicators. Research such as that undertaken by the Norfolk Arthritis Register is increasingly able to help in such decision making. It could be argued that there is no comparison between treating a condition which has a high mortality rate as in malignancies and in treating the various rheumatological conditions. However, the mortality rate of patients suffering from rheumatoid arthritis can be equated with non-Hodgkin's lymphoma (Symmons, 1991) and the morbidity rate is substantial. The prospect of enduring a condition which so debilitates an individual, causing severe pain, disability and loss of self-esteem, warrants careful consideration before therapeutic decisions are made. Therapy which has the potential to stop this disease progression is therefore being considered much earlier. However, all of the drugs under discussion here have the potential to be extremely dangerous unless properly monitored. Even so, the following drugs are therefore being used much earlier in the disease and often within the first few months of diagnosis if the patient's condition warrants it.

Methotrexate

Methotrexate is a cytotoxic agent used for many years in the treatment of malignant disease. It is found to have major disease-modifying properties, not only reducing the signs and symptoms of inflammatory joint disease, but also reducing any extra-articular manifestations including vasculitis. It is thought that it slows down or prevents erosive damage from occurring in the joints and is used extensively in North America and increasingly in this country for patients with severe rheumatoid arthritis. It is potentially hepatotoxic, nephrotoxic and in rare cases can cause pneumonitis.

Dosage: Typical regimen may be to start with 2.5 mg to 7.5 mg orally once per week increasing by increments of 2.5 mg weekly until a maximum of either 10, 15 or 20 mg weekly is reached, depending on clinical response. Maximum dose 25 mg weekly. Clinical response is usually established within four to six weeks. Lower doses should be used in the frail elderly or if there is significant renal impairment. Folic acid 5 mg given three days after each dose may reduce the incidence of side-effects. Some centres give 2.5 mg to 5.0 mg of folic acid daily. Others suggest not taking the folic acid on the day of the MTX dose. There is a great deal of discrepancy surrounding the recommended dose of folic acid, though not its use.

IM Methotrexate is given in doses between 5 mg and 25 mg weekly. All the necessary precautions when handling cytotoxic drugs should be taken.

Side-effects and what to do

Mild side-effects:

- **nausea, abdominal discomfort and diarrhoea:** often prevented by adding folic acid 5 mg daily or alternatively on the day before, the day of and day after taking the weekly dose of methotrexate. If this fails, then splitting the dose and missing out one day some times works, i.e. 5 mg Monday, miss Tuesday, 5 mg Wednesday;

- **mouth ulceration:** unless very mild, STOP the drug;
- **headaches:** unless mild, STOP the drug.

Serious though less common side-effects:

- **bone marrow suppression:** precipitating thrombocytopenia or neutropenia.

  WBC $<3.0 \times 10^9/l$, caution. Repeat in one week. $<2.0 \times 10^9/l$, STOP treatment.

  platelets $<150 \times 10^9/l$, caution. Repeat in one week. $<120 \times 10^9/l$, STOP treatment.
- **hair thinning:** will depend on the patient's response whether or not treatment is stopped.

Rare but potentially serious side-effects:

- **hepatotoxicity causing fibrosis or cirrhosis:** elevation in liver enzymes to twice the upper limit of normal, STOP treatment. In North America patients are told categorically that they should not drink any alcohol whilst on methotrexate as this is known to increase the risk of hepatotoxicity. In the UK patients are advised not to drink or to drink in moderation only. Where alcohol has been avoided, evidence of fibrosis or cirrhosis has been rare. Equally it is important to exclude pre-existing liver disease prior to initiating treatment with methotrexate;
- **pulmonary conditions:** with the development of acute pneumonitis or pulmonary fibrosis. In view of the potential serious consequences of toxicity occurring, once on methotrexate therapy, it is important to establish a pre-treatment chest X-ray to note any existing problems as pulmonary fibrosis may occur for other reasons. If patients develop any symptoms of chest involvement including dry cough, dyspnoea or fever, a chest X-ray should be requested and treatment stopped;
- **hair loss:** this will depend on the patient and his or her response to the drug. If there is a good response, the patient may choose to wear a wig. Hair will grow once again if drug is stopped for any reason.

Drug interactions

Trimethoprim or co-trimoxazole (Septrin) may interact with methotrexate, and therefore should be avoided; deaths have been recorded on Septrin. There should also be caution with the use of anti-convulsants, and live vaccines should not be given. Although the concomitant use of NSAIDs and aspirin is advised with caution, it is suggested that because the dose of MTX used in rheumatoid disease is so small the risk is subsequently reduced.

Monitoring:
(1) FBC with differentials every one to two weeks for the first four to eight weeks and thereafter monthly. LFTs, ALT, bilirubin and alkaline phosphatase and creatinine every alternate test. Abnormal trends in any direction of any value should prompt caution and vigilance.
(2) Monitoring booklet should be provided.

Look for a fall in WBC, neutrophils and platelets and a rise in AST, ALT, alkaline phosphatase and creatinine.

Patients should be counselled with extreme care prior to commencing methotrexate therapy, and the necessity to give this medication only once per week cannot be over-emphasised. As with all second-line agents a monitoring programme should be established as soon as the patient commences therapy and patients should always bring the shared-care monitoring booklet with them to clinic and to the GP's surgery to ensure that blood results are updated and trends which can indicate toxicity are carefully noted and acted upon.

Pregnancy: Methotrexate is teratogenic to ova and sperm and therefore patients of either sex should be counselled about appropriate contraception during treatment. There is conflicting advice as to the length of time females and males need to be off the drug. It is recommended for females to stop from two to six months before attempting to conceive and males should be off for three to six months before attempting to impregnate their partners. In low dose may be safe in lactation; more work needs to be carried out.

Azathioprine (Imuran) (AZP)

Azathioprine (Imuran) is an immunosuppressant used extensively in the field of transplant surgery. The rationale behind its use in rheumatology is based on the knowledge that these conditions are auto-immune in nature. In rheumatoid disease much lower doses are used than in transplant surgery, averaging approximately 2.5 mg per kg per day. Azathioprine has disease-modifying properties sufficient to induce and maintain control in patients who have such conditions as rheumatoid arthritis or dertmatomyositis. The drug is metabolised to mercaptopurine and the dose should thus be reduced when concurrent therapy with allopurinol is prescribed.

Dosage: Start with 50 mg daily for the first week. Increase to 2.5 mg per kg per day if tolerated with an average dose of between 100 mg and 150 mg per day. Clinical response established at between 8 and 12 weeks.

Side-effects and what to do:

Minor side-effects:

- **nausea, abdominal discomfort or headaches:** these usually respond to either treatment with an anti-emetic or dose reduction.

Less common side-effects:

- **bone marrow suppression:** precipitating thrombocytopenia and leucopenia;
  WBC $<3.0 \times 10^9/l$, caution. Repeat in one week. $<2.0 \times 10^9/l$, STOP treatment;
  platelets $<150 \times 10^9/l$, caution. Repeat in one week. $<120 \times 10^9/l$, STOP treatment;
- **hepatotoxicity:** elevation of liver enzymes, ALT, alkaline phosphatase, AST to twice the upper limit of normal, STOP treatment.

Risk of atypical infection including herpes zoster, if large doses are required.

Drug interaction

Allopurinol potentiates the effect of azathioprine and therefore increases its risk of toxicity. The dose of azathioprine should therefore be reduced. The use of live vaccines should be avoided.

Monitoring:

(1) FBC and LFTs should be checked two-weekly for the first four weeks and thereafter monthly.

Look for a fall in WBC and platelets with a rise in AST, ALT and alkaline phosphatase.

Pregnancy: There is no evidence that azathioprine is teratogenic if used appropriately as evidenced by its use in the transplant world. However, most patients contemplating pregnancy would be advised to stop therapy. Nonetheless, it is used during pregnancy in rheumatic disease if the patient's condition warrants the use of such medication. It is felt the benefits outweigh the risks, especially for the mother.

Cyclosporin (Neoral)

Cyclosporin is an immunosuppressant. It acts upon the 'T' lymphocytes known to play a part in the pathogenesis of rheumatoid arthritis. It was first used in the transplant world, but in much larger doses. In the rheumatic diseases only 2.5 mg–4.0 mg per kg per day are used when treating auto-immune diseases such as rheumatoid arthritis. It has been used since the start of the 1990s in rheumatology units. It is effective in a variety of conditions aimed at inducing and maintaining control and is presently licensed to be used for the treatment of psoriasis as well as severe rheumatoid arthritis when conventional therapy is considered to be either inappropriate or ineffective. It has been used experimentally in this country to treat a wide variety of auto-immune conditions including uveitis, scleroderma, Behcet's, enteropathic arthropathy and psoriatic arthropathy.

Dosage: Start with a dose of 2.5 mg per kg per day. Increase by 25 mg at four-weekly intervals after six weeks' treatment to a maximum of 4 mg per kg per day. Clinical response normally established between 8 and 12 weeks. There is a dose sensitivity at between 3 mg and 3.5 mg per kg per day, when efficacy is normally established without evidence of toxicity. Slow, low increases are preferable in order to establish efficacy without precipitating toxicity.

Side-effects and what to do

Minor side-effects:

- **nausea, abdominal discomfort, hand tremor, paraesthesiae or headaches and gum hyperplasia** are sometimes experienced in the first few weeks of treatment. These usually subside as the patient becomes established on the treatment.

Major side-effects:

- **hypertension, nephrotoxicity.**

Rare side-effects but particularly important to female patients:

- **hirsutism.**

Side-effects and what to do

(1) If the serum creatinine exceeds 30 per cent of pre-treatment baseline on more than two consecutive occasions, the dose should be reduced by 25 mg.

(2) If serum creatinine exceeds 50 per cent of baseline on two consecutive occasions, dose should be reduced by 50 per cent.

(3) If serum creatinine fails to return to acceptable levels following dose reduction, discontinuation of treatment should be considered. A sliding scale ruler is available from the manufacturers to aid safe monitoring of this drug.

(4) Hypertension should be treated with anti-hypertensive therapy such as nifedipine and cyclosporin should be stopped only if the hypertension remains uncontrolled. Nausea is normally mild and transient, but if it persists domperidone is useful.

(5) Hirsutism or gum hyperplasia are rare and if efficacy has been established it is often better to discuss either the use of facial depilatories in the case of hirsutism or improvement in oral hygiene in gum hyperplasia.

Monitoring:
Cyclosporin is potentially nephrotoxic though it is used at at least three to four times this level in renal transplants. Problems experienced with treating patients who have a rheumatological condition occur because of a variety of factors which may be unconnected with the drug therapy. These include age of patient, duration of disease and effect of previous therapies, including NSAIDs, on renal function.

Pre-treatment: Initial baseline renal function should be established prior to initiating treatment.

(1) Creatinine clearance to establish normal renal function.

(2) An average of three recent serum creatinine levels prior to treatment. The average must be within the normal range.

(3) Establish pre-treatment blood pressure level and treat any hypertension prior to commencing cyclosporin.

Ongoing monitoring:

(1) FBC, differentials, urea and electrolytes, blood pressure, urinalysis, every two weeks for the first three months then monthly thereafter; LFTs rarely elevated but should be included in the monthly monitoring.

Look for raised serum creatinine, raised blood pressure.

Drug interactions

There should be particular caution when using concomitant NSAIDs as some may potentiate the potential toxicity of cyclosporin. Combination with compounds known to be nephrotoxic including aminoglycosides, amphotericin B, ciprofloxacin, melphalan or trimethoprim should be avoided.

Pregnancy: As with azathioprine not thought to affect fertility and may be considered safe in pregnancy. Avoid during lactation.

For severe systemic disease

Cyclophosphamide

There is now considerable evidence to suggest that cyclophosphamide, which is a cytotoxic drug which interferes with cell replication, is helpful in the treatment of severe systemic disease associated with such conditions as rheumatoid arthritis, systemic vasculitis and other connective tissue diseases. Every rheumatology unit will have its own regime for the administration of this drug, and often doses are initiated at a fortnightly then monthly intervals according to clinical response and haematological monitoring. Cyclosphosphamide is widely used in the treatment of chronic lymphocytic leukaemia, lymphomas and tumours. It is inactive until metabolised by the liver and there is a danger that the urine-metabolised effects of cyclophosphamide may cause haemorrhagic cystitis. In view of this risk patients are encouraged to increase their fluid intake for at least 24 to 48 hours following intravenous injection to help avoid the complication. Cyclophosphamide is a cytotoxic agent which has disease-modifying properties. It acts by damaging the DNA, thus interfering with cell replication. It has the ability to achieve control in such conditions as sytemic vasculitis. In line with all other cytotoxic drugs it has the ability to cause major side-effects.

Dosage in the treatment of systemic vasculitis:

(1) Intravenous cyclophosphamide 10–15 mg per kg plus methylprednisolone 1 g which is given first. Both drugs are to be given slowly over a period of 30–60 minutes each.

(2) Oral cyclophosphamide 5 mg per kg per day is given for three further days in addition to prednisolone 100 mg daily for three days.

Patients who are systemically ill with active inflammatory lesions such as scleritis, pleurisy, pericarditis, etc., often require 20 mg of oral prednisolone which should be gradually reduced and stopped after the first 3 months. Not all patients require oral prednisolone at this time.

Pulse therapy of cyclophosphamide should be given every two weeks on six separate occasions. Between the first and second pulsed therapy, the white cell count should be measured at 7, 10 and 14 days.

Precautions:

(1) if low WBC <3.0 (polymorphs <2.5), reduce dose for the next pulse and repeat white cell count at 7, 10 and 14 days;
(2) if white count at 14 days is lower than 10-day value, delay treatment for up to a week;
(3) if white cell count is acceptable, look for lymphopenia to indicate some immuno-suppression. For future pulses measure WBC on day of treatment only.

Extra precautions

Cyclophosphamide should be reduced if there is evidence of renal impairment. H2 antagonists such as ranitidine 150 mg bd should be given throughout treatment. Patients should be encouraged to drink at least three litres per 24 hours during treatment and for 24 hours afterwards.

Six pulses of cyclophosphamide are normally given IV and then therapy is transferred to oral treatment. In milder cases oral treatment may be initiated much earlier. Some patients tolerate IV treatment better than oral, particularly if severe nausea occurs, in which case IV can be given throughout.

A minimum of six pulses of therapy at two-weekly intervals is the standard maintenance therapy initiated, if response is good.

Maintenance therapy

The interval between cyclophosphamide pulse therapy is gradually decreased and often monthly pulses are sufficient for one year. If remission has occurred after a year, most patients may be converted to azathioprine or methotrexate.

Conditions treated

- Wegener's granulomatosis;
- Churg-Strauss syndrome;
- systemic sclerosis;
- systemic vasculitis.

Pregnancy: Known teratogen, therefore recommend avoidance before and during pregnancy. Also avoid during lactation. Can cause permanent sterility: counselling and possible sperm storage should be considered.

Conclusions

At the present time there appears to be no cure for most of the rheumatological conditions. In the absence of a cure, disease modification with the use of DMARDs is extremely helpful in reducing the speed at which joints may be eroded in conditions such as rheumatoid arthritis.

Experimental therapies

Presently a variety of new preparations are being developed which may be of use in treating auto-immune diseases such as rheumatoid arthritis. Synovial cultures obtained from patients who have active rheumatoid arthritis, exhibit high levels of cytokines including interleukin-1, interleukin-6, Tumour necrosis factor (TNFα), and interleukin-8, monoclonal antibodies and interleukin receptor antagonists as well as anti-TNFα antibodies are presently undergoing clinical trials to evaluate their effect. Biological agents aimed at interfering with the complicated immune response are being investigated by a number of centres throughout the world. Rheumatology has never been as exciting as it is at the present time, with novel agents being developed as well as new combinations of existing therapies. At the same time research into the pathogenesis and aetiology of these diseases is constantly under review.

Disease-specific treatments

Arthritis

Osteoarthritis: Osteoarthritis is characterised by a progressive destruction of articular cartilage. At present management of the condition is aimed at relief of pain.

Drug management: Analgesia such as paracetamol and NSAIDs are useful in controlling symptoms. Occasionally intra-articular steroid injections are helpful in reducing inflammatory exacerbations of the condition. In major disease, with severe joint destruction; joint replacement maybe indicated.

Rheumatoid arthritis: Rheumatoid arthritis is a chronic inflammatory disease primarily involving the synovium, but often associated with systemic and extra-articular involvement including rheumatoid nodules, vasculitis or such conditions as Sjogren's syndrome.

Drug management: Effective management of this condition depends upon the severity of the disease and will include analgesia, NSAIDs and DMARDs. All three may be necessary to alleviate pain and symptoms of inflammation including stiffness, and to enable control of the disease progression. Steroids are often used as an adjunct to therapy in situations where there is a major flare, and the efficacy of DMARDs has not had sufficient time to become established. In early RA the addition of low-dose steroids may be effective in reducing the incidence of erosive changes if combined with a DMARD (Kirwan, 1995). Intra-articular injections of steroids are useful, particularly if only one joint is causing specific problems such as a knee effusion. Long-term therapy requires a multidisciplinary approach comprising a variety of therapeutic interventions, not all of which are part of the biomedical norm, for example acupuncture.

Ankylosing spondylosis: Characterised by a loss of lumbar lordosis and increased kyphosis, management is heavily reliant upon physiotherapy and exercise regimes.

Drug management: NSAIDs, particularly of the slow-release variety, are often effective in relieving pain at night and early morning stiffness. Sulphasalazine is also useful to gain long-term control of the disease where peripheral joint involvement is seen.

Reiter's syndrome: A condition in which a reactive arthritis occurs in conjunction with a non-specific urethritis and conjunctivitis. Infection with shigella, salmonella or chlamydia have all been implicated in this reactive arthritis.

Drug management: NSAIDs are usually effective but in chronic cases sulphasalazine or azathioprine are sometimes useful. The arthropathy usually responds within a few months, but some patients continue to have recurrent arthritis.

Psoriatic arthritis: This is a sero-negative arthropathy which may occur in conjunction with psoriasis.

Drug management: Analgesia and NSAIDs are helpful, but if the arthropathy is uncontrolled, DMARDs are useful. Cyclosporin and methotrexate are particularly helpful and reduce the signs and symptoms of psoriasis faster than reducing the polyarthritis associated with it.

Septic arthritis: This occurs as a result of a joint infection with a pyogenic organism, often staphylococcus aureus. This is a medical emergency which requires treatment with antibiotics often given parenterally initially.

Connective tissue disease: This term covers (1) systemic lupus erythematosis (SLE); (2) Polymyositis and dermatomyositis; (3) systemic sclerosis.

Systemic lupus erythematosus: Characteristics of this condition include asymmetrical arthralgia and non-specific features of fever, malaise and depression. A facial rash following a butterfly distribution is often exacerbated by contact with sunlight.

Drug management: Dependent upon severity of symptoms but will include NSAIDs and the use of DMARDs if symptoms are uncontrolled. Corticosteroids are often required in moderate to severe disease and immunosuppressants such as azathioprine or cyclophosphamide may be necessary if there is any renal involvement. The drug of choice in mild SLE is hydroxychloroquine.

Polymyositis and dermatomyositis: This is a muscle disorder of unknown aetiology which is characterised by myalgia, muscle wasting and photosensitivity as well as a purple periorbital skin rash. Other features may include dysphagia and Raynaud's phenomenon.

Drug management: As there is a wide variety of symptoms, management is aimed at symptomatic relief. In active disease a dose of very high steroids, i.e. 60 mg daily is used, in conjunction with immunosuppressant therapy such as azathioprine or methotrexate.

Gout: There is an abnormality of the metabolism of uric acid which results in the deposition of sodium urate crystals in joints and soft tissues, often causing tophi and tenosynovitis. Acute attacks of gout are extremely painful and are characterised by swelling, most frequently in the metatarsal phalangeal joints of the large toe, but can present in any of the peripheral joints. Attacks may be precipitated by dietary or alcoholic influences as well as use of certain diuretics.

Drug management: Acute attacks often resolve with NSAIDs, with indomethacin being particularly useful. Oral colchicine may be useful if NSAIDs are contra-indicated. Allopurinol inhibits xanthine oxidase, which is an enzyme in the purine breakdown pathway and is particularly helpful in the long-term treatment of gout. Once initiated, allopurinol should be given indefinitely.

Systemic sclerosis: This may be a multi-system disease affecting both skin and internal organs. Cutaneous manifestations are characterised by thickened, tight skin affecting a variety of areas around the body. Common areas include the face, characterised by a fixed expression as the skin tightens around the facial structures. Often fingers taper and the skin around the wrists tightens to form restrictive bands. This is a complicated disease which may have systemic involvement. Therapeutic management is therefore aimed initially at symptom relief and immunosuppressant treatments in specialist centres when evidence of severe systemic involvement occurs.

Drug treatment: This includes such drugs as cyclophosphamide or cyclosporin.

Outcome measures – response to therapy

Therapeutic intervention should always be accompanied by baseline information concerning the disease activity and criteria set for achievement of therapeutic response. In rheumatoid arthritis the following are useful criteria to judge response.

(1) early morning stiffness (EMS): this should reduce significantly if treatment is effective;
(2) articular indices: the number of joints which are swollen and painful should reduce;
(3) health assessment questionnaire (HAQ): functional ability should improve;
(4) pain level: visual analogue scale (VAS). The score on a VAS should reduce;
(5) C-reactive protein (CRP) and erythrocyte sedimentation rate (ESR): either one or both of these are usually elevated in active disease, therefore should reduce;
(6) haemoglobin is often reduced in active rheumatoid arthritis and often returns to normal when disease activity is under control;
(7) platelets elevated in active disease; usually return to normal level.

Serial data are important when assessing biochemical and haematological results as the trend is more indicative of response rather than actual levels.

Case history

Rheumatoid arthritis

A 48-year-old lady presented to her GP in April 1995 with sudden onset polyarthritis involving MCPs (metacarpophalangeal joints), elbows, shoulders, knees and feet. She was already experiencing severe stiffness in all joints; this was present on waking and lasting in excess of three hours. She felt as if she had flu, but as the symptoms had not subsided after a two-week period, she contacted her GP. He arranged routine blood tests including an FBC, ESR, CRP and rheumatoid factor. The results were as follows: Hb 11.5 g/dl; ESR 90 mm/1h; CRP 228 mg/100ml; normal urea and electrolytes; normal LFTs. She was rheumatoid positive with an RF titre of 1280 (range 0–40).

The GP prescribed co-proxamol two qds and piroxicam 10 mg–20 mg daily to alleviate the pain and help reduce the early morning stiffness. The patient improved moderately over a period of two weeks, but an urgent referral to a consultant rheumatologist was made. Her symptoms were exceptionally severe and he felt that second-line therapies might be appropriate. On admission to hospital, she was still experiencing three–four hours of EMS and on examination she had active synovitis of both shoulders, both elbows, all MCPs and the right wrist. Her hips were normal but there was a large effusion of her right knee. Her right ankle was warm and she had significant pain and swelling of several MTP joints.

Medical history
Nothing of significance.

Social history
Mother has osteoarthritis. Smoker until three months ago. Enjoys the occasional alcoholic drink. Lives with her husband in a second-floor flat, and at present unable to climb the stairs without enormous difficulty.

Arrangements were made for an intra-articular injection of her right knee, and for her to be assessed by the physiotherapists and occupational therapists to learn about exercise and joint protection. General education about her disease and treatment came from the nurse practitioner.

Her condition demonstrated several of the prognostic indicators suggesting severe disease (see page 159). Early treatment with methotrexate was suggested. Plans were made for her to commence oral methotrexate 2.5 mg weekly later that week increasing to 7.5 mg weekly over three weeks. Prior to commencing therapy she would have an opportunity to discuss her treatment with the nurse practitioner and arrangements would be made for a chest X-ray to exclude pre-existing respiratory problems. By the end of the first week the patient was feeling significantly better following a period of general rest and aspiration and intra-articular injection of her right knee. The occupational therapist made her a resting splint for the right wrist, and gave her general information about joint protection. The physiotherapist gave her a full assessment and went through a range of appropriate exercises with her. By the end of the first week she was able to exercise easily in the hydrotherapy pool with assistance from the physiotherapist and as a result was beginning to feel much better. Baseline bloods, in particular LFTs, were recorded in her shared-care monitoring booklet and arrangements made for her to be followed up in the GP monitoring clinic on a monthly basis once she was discharged home. An appointment would be made for her to return to the rheumatology outpatient clinic in three months' time.

Methotrexate was gradually increased to 15 mg weekly in increments of 2.5 mg weekly after six months as she was still experiencing significant problems and it was felt appropriate to introduce low-dose steroids at this time. Prednisolone 7.5 mg daily was therefore prescribed. She was experiencing some nausea the day after taking the methotrexate, and folic acid 5 mg daily was subsequently prescribed.

In December 1995 she was seen in the outpatient clinic, early morning stiffness was reduced to 30 minutes and joint activity was also significantly reduced. CRP was now 30 and ESR 50. Functional ability as assessed on the HAQ had improved, although she was still finding difficulty in gripping and opening certain objects. Serial data unfortunately indicated an upward trend in her liver function tests to double their pre-treatment level, and methotrexate was therefore reduced to 12.5 mg weekly. Bloods would be repeated on a monthly basis and as long as liver function tests stabilised she would remain on the 12.5 mg of methotrexate, and the prednisolone 7.5 mg was to be continued.

In April 1996 she was again seen in the outpatient clinic. Early morning stiffness had increased to one hour and she had active synovitis of MCPs and PIPs of both hands. X-rays of hands and feet were repeated and compared with those taken when first diagnosed. There were early erosive changes of two MCPs of the right hand, but otherwise nothing abnormal detected. She no longer required co-proxamol, although continued to take piroxicam without any evidence of indigestion. At that time it was agreed to commence cyclosporin (Neoral) at 2.5 mg per kg per day in addition to the methotrexate, because of the erosive changes, suggesting that the methotrexate was not entirely controlling the disease progression. Nodules remained on the elbows and the ESR was 50. She was given both written and verbal information about cyclosporin, and monitoring protocols were sent to her GP as she would require blood checks to be repeated two-weekly for the first three months, while waiting for an efficacious level of the cyclosporin to be established. This normally occurs at approximately 3.5 mg per kg, although it is individual to each patient. Pre-treatment creatinine clearance was arranged in order to establish her normal renal function.

In July 1996 she returned to the clinic. Joints were now quiescent with a reduction also in ESR from 50 to 12 and CRP from 30 to 20 mg per hour. She was not experiencing any new problems and her renal and hepatic functions remained within normal parameters. She will continue to be followed in clinic on a 3–6 monthly basis and will require blood checks monthly at her surgery.

References

Akil M, Amos RS, Steward P (1996) Infertility may sometimes be associated with NSAID consumption. British Journal of Rheumatology 35(1): 76–8.

Arnett FC, Edworthy SM, Block DA McShane DJ, Fries JF, Cooper SN, Healey LA, Kaplan SR, Liang MH, Luthra HS, Medsger TA Jr., Mitchell OM, Neustadt DH, Pinals RS, Schallar JG, Sharp JT, Wilder RL, Hunder GG. (1988) The American Rheumatism Association 1987: Revised criteria for the classification of RA. Arthritis and Rheumatism 31(3): 315–24.

Barret EM, Bankhead CR, Bunn D, Galpin L, Langrish-Smith A, Isvins, Somerville M, van Poortvliet P, Scott DGI, Silman A, Symmons DPM (1993) Knee involvement in early rheumatoid arthritis. British Journal of Rheumatology 32.

Brennan P, Harrison B, Barrett E, Chakravarty K, Scott DGI, Silman A, Symmons D (1996) A simple alogorithm to predict the development of radiological erosions in patients with early RA: prospective cohort study. British Medical Journal 313: 4716.

Committee on Safety of Medicines Update (1986) NSAID side effect profile. British Medical Journal.

Fries JF, Spitz P, Kraines RG, Holman HR (1980) Measurement of patient outcome in arthritis. Arthritis and Rheumatism. 23: 137–45.

Geusens P, Wouters C, Nijs J, Jiang Y, Dequeker J (1994) Long-term effect of omega 3 fatty acid supplementation in active RA. Arthritis and Rheumatism 37(6): 824–9.

Kirwan J (1995) The effect of glucocorticoids on joint destruction in RA. New England Journal of Medicine (July).

le Gallez P (1988) Teratogenesis and drugs for rheumatic disease. Nursing Times 84(27). 41–4.

Symmons DP (1991) Review of UK data on the rheumatic diseases. British Journal of Rheumatology 30 (4): 288–90.

Symmons DP (1994) Incidence of RA in UK. Results from NOAR. British Journal of Rheumatology 33(8): 735–9.

Wilske KR (1993) Approaches to the management of RA, rationale for early combination therapy. British Journal of Rheumatology 32(Suppl 1): 24–7.

Chapter 7
Role of physiotherapy in rheumatology

HEATHER SMRUTI RILEY

Introduction

Rheumatic disease is the greatest single cause of disability in the UK today. Primary preventive measures are limited, as research into the aetiology and pathogenesis of many arthritic conditions is still inconclusive (Shipley and Newman, 1994). Thus, the management of most rheumatic diseases is largely reliant on conservative measures based on a multidisciplinary team approach. Most aspects of patient care involve medicine, surgery, educational strategies, therapy, psychology, sociology and significant other. This holistic approach has the potential to reduce disability and restore the patient to a functional lifestyle. Physiotherapy has long been thought to play an important role in the management of the various rheumatic conditions and recent evidence supports this, especially in certain common conditions such as rheumatoid arthritis (RA), ankylosing spondylitis (AS), osteoarthritis (OA) and soft tissue rheumatism, etc. (Robinson, Haldeman and Imrie,1980; Rosen, 1994; Viitanen and Suni, 1995).

The management of rheumatic diseases poses a major challenge, as not only do rheumatic conditions differ in their clinical presentation for each patient, but many conditions can overlap simultaneously, and often follow an unpredictable course. Therefore, to provide patients with good quality care, an in-depth knowledge of the pathophysiology of the various rheumatic diseases and their natural progression, plus a good knowledge of the principles of management, is vital (Hyde, 1980).

The primary role of the physiotherapist is to assess the impact of rheumatic disease on the neuro-musculoskeletal system and its ability to function. Based on assessment, the goal of physiotherapy treatment is to minimise the symptoms associated with inflammation such as pain, stiffness, muscle weakness and loss of function. The overall treatment strategy aims to give the patient an optimal level of functional capacity, despite impairment and disability.

This chapter provides an overview of physiotherapy assessment, and of the therapeutic management, in the common, inflammatory rheumatic diseases. It focuses on describing the rationale of those physiotherapy interventions which are the most relevant to rheumatic diseases. However, the role of physiotherapy described here should be seen as a part of an integrated multidisciplinary approach to the management of patients with arthritis.

Assessment

An appropriate and accurate assessment is essential in designing effective treatment strategies. Selection of the appropriate treatment and adapting it to each aetiology in the various phases of the inflammatory process, i.e. acute, sub-acute and chronic, is important if interventions are to succeed. There are many comprehensive methods of assessing the impact of inflammatory disease on the musculoskeletal system, and many assessments are standardised. A detailed description of the assessment of specific arthritic diseases is cited in other texts (Hyde, 1980; Gerber and Hicks, 1988).

In general, the basic purpose of physiotherapy assessment is:

* to establish a diagnosis, i.e. source of pain and dysfunction, based on examination findings. These findings are important, as they indicate the appropriate therapeutic management;
* to provide the physiotherapist with baseline data which can be monitored continuously in order to assess the improvement or deterioration of function. This enables the therapist to decide when to continue, modify or discontinue the treatment;
* to enable the therapist to communicate to other team members the relevance of the clinical findings. This encourages an integrated approach in setting individual and realistic treatment goals.

Most therapists use a basic framework of assessment that is adapted to assess a specific arthritic condition. The essential components of assessment consist of a careful and accurate subjective assessment and objective assessment (Figure 7.1). The clinical relevance of the most common features of subjective and objective assessment is described below.

Subjective assessment

The purpose of subjective assessment is to determine the patient's perception of factors influencing symptoms or causing disabilities. It also involves assessing the relevant information on past and present medical history and drug history which includes drug efficacy. The psychological and/or socioenvironmental circumstances that may have a direct influence on present problems or on physiotherapy intervention are also included.

Pain

Pain is the most important symptom in rheumatic disease and is used as a prime diagnostic indicator of disease activity (Kazis, Meenan and Anderson, 1983). Its assessment is therefore vital. Whilst acknowledging that rheumatic pain is complex in nature with many dimensions to it, identifying the possible source of pain is essential in order to evaluate the need for physiotherapy intervention, e.g. pain due to ligamentous inflammation can be effectively managed with physiotherapy, whereas affective pain may require a cognitive-behavioural approach.

Identifying and clarifying the nature of pain, its site, distribution and severity are important in establishing a clinical diagnosis, and

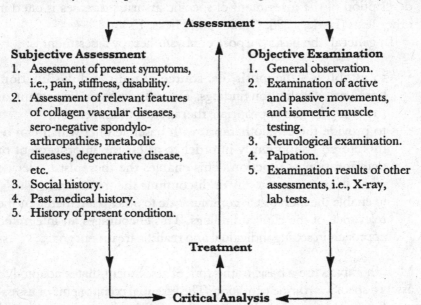

Assessment

Subjective Assessment
1. Assessment of present symptoms, i.e., pain, stiffness, disability.
2. Assessment of relevant features of collagen vascular diseases, sero-negative spondylo-arthropathies, metabolic diseases, degenerative disease, etc.
3. Social history.
4. Past medical history.
5. History of present condition.

Objective Examination
1. General observation.
2. Examination of active and passive movements, and isometric muscle testing.
3. Neurological examination.
4. Palpation.
5. Examination results of other assessments, i.e., X-ray, lab tests.

Treatment

Critical Analysis

Figure 7.1. Assessment

influences the selection of treatment strategies. For example, joint degeneration pain, as in OA, may be deep, boring and diffuse, whereas a superficial precise pain could indicate a soft tissue lesion. Patients with polymyalgia rheumatica (PMR) may complain of pain and tenderness in the proximal muscles rather than the joints.

Exploring factors which exacerbate or ease pain helps to identify various stages of the inflammatory phases (Table 7.1). In the active stage of disease the pain is unremitting, often disturbing sleep, emphasising the value of rest and the importance of pain relief. During the chronic phase of inflammation, pain may be intermittent and mild, indicating a more vigorous intervention to increase tissue length and strength. In certain conditions there may be a typical pain pattern, for example pain in RA and AS is worse in the mornings, whereas in OA the pain usually worsens as the day progresses – it is worse with activity and eased by rest. In patients with fibromyalgia syndrome (FMS), pain is usually described as 'all day', and is typically accompanied by fatigue and muscle tenderness. Each requires a different type of intervention.

Table 7.1. Phases of inflammation and therapeutic management

Phases of inflammation	Acute inflammation	Sub-acute inflammation	Chronic inflammation
Pain	Constant pain, diffuse distribution pain increases active or passive movements, difficult to ease.	Intermittent pain. Pain during movement and/or at the end of range. Increasing with repeated movement.	Pain on forceful repeated movement.
Movements	Severe restriction in both active and passive movements with swelling/pain/ spasm.	Both active and passive limitation of range of movement with pain and tissue tightness.	Active and passive restriction with tissue tightness, weakness and deformity.
Modalities	Ice, TENS, splints.	Ice/heat, TENS, IFT, hydrotherapy.	Ice, heat, TENS, IFT, ultra-sound, pulsed short wave diathermy
Exercises	Rest and passive range of movement exercises, (least gravitational stress).	Balance of rest/ exercises, stretching exercises, isometric/ isotonic exercises as tolerated.	Stretching, strengthening exercises, aerobic conditioning exercises and recreational activities.

Clinical data suggest that the patient's current pain status is a good predictor of subsequent pain and disability status (Kazis et al., 1983). Measurement of pain intensity by various methods, e.g. visual analogue scales (VAS), pain rating scales, or pain description on body charts, etc., establishes a quantitative baseline from which the outcome of treatment can be assessed (Skevington, 1993). The level of pain severity and irritability guides the therapist in advocating the appropriate balance of rest and activity and in prioritising treatment.

Stiffness

Stiffness is a common feature of inflammatory arthritis, and is also used as a significant diagnostic indicator. A long period of stiffness is common in severe, active inflammatory diseases, particularly in RA or AS, and is described as early morning stiffness (EMS). EMS can last three to four hours, or in some severe cases even longer, whereas the stiffness with OA or tendinitis may last only a few minutes, and may worsen again with inactivity. Stiffness affects the quality of movement, thus activities of daily living (ADL) are slow and deliberate. Treatment strategies are modified depending on its severity, e.g. advising the use of hot showers or stretching exercises before starting the day's work. Also, advice can be given on pacing daily activities with periods of rest.

Other relevant features

The diagnosis of a specific rheumatic disease by a combination of biochemical, radiographic or other technical procedures is necessary to eliminate other confounding conditions. However, these findings are often insufficient or inconclusive. For example, the mere presence of rheumatoid factor does not justify a diagnosis of rheumatoid arthritis, whereas the presence of rheumatoid nodules, vasculitic lesions or Raynaud's phenomenon may help to validate a clinical diagnosis of RA. Similarly, in patients with the psoriatic lesions in the presence of ulcerative colitis, iritis or sacroiliitis, such symptoms may indicate seronegative spondyloarthropathies. Physiotherapists need to be vigilant in observing these features, as treatment may need to be modified, e.g. if Raynaud's symptoms are present then ice therapy is contra-indicated. Aortic valve insufficiency in AS may contra-indicate certain types of exercise. General malaise, myalgia, weight loss and joint pains may herald systemic inflammatory disease requiring urgent medical management or a painful gouty joint may benefit from drug therapy rather than physiotherapy.

Disability

Despite the fact that patients may look healthy, the impact of arthritis often affects their daily lives. Symptoms of arthritis, i.e. pain, weakness or stiffness, may require the patient to change his or her daily routine, and the patient may be unable to accomplish certain tasks or only perform them with great difficulty. Often the systemic features such as fatigue, feeling unwell or EMS may further compromise the patient's ability to carry out ADL. The ADL assessment evaluates the patient's potential ability, and encourages the therapist to set realistic treatment goals.

The relationship between the underlying disease and the level of functional impairment can be assessed by various standardised health assessment questionnaires. The most frequently used disability measures for arthritis are the Health Assessment Questionnaire (HAQ; see Figure 7.2) (Fries, Spitz and Kraines, 1980) and the Arthritis Impact Measurement Scale (AIMS) (Meenan, Gertman and Mason, 1980). Disability is graded according to the patient's perceived ability, physical difficulties and the need to use assistive devices or personal assistance in carrying out activities. The final scores of these assessments are a good indicator of appropriate and individualised assistance that may be needed by the patient.

Monitoring the disability measurement score over a period of time is a useful tool in measuring overall function, disease activity and the outcomes of intervention. However, the disability measurement tool should be applicable and sensitive to the patient's needs and be relevant to the particular disease being evaluated (Fitzpatrick and Badley, 1996), for example, use of adapted HAQ for assessment of patients with AS.

Social history

Assessing the effect of arthritis on the patient's lifestyle, occupation and personal and social relationships is vital. Some patients may lack the core support of the family or be under pressure to return to a work situation which is clearly unsuitable for his or her condition. The attitude and support of 'significant others' is vital if the patient is to be encouraged to adhere to the treatment plan (Wallston, 1993). In circumstances where the patient is involved in the care of a dependent disabled spouse, joint protection advice is unlikely to be followed. Often a major hindrance in returning to a functional lifestyle is the socioenvironmental factor whereby the patient may have difficulty in accessing transport, place of work or recreational centre, thereby hampering a return to work or recreational activities.

HEALTH ASSESSMENT QUESTIONNAIRE

Name .... Date ....

We are interested in learning how your illness affects your ability to function in
daily life. Please feel free to add any comments at the end of this form.

**PLEASE TICK ONE RESPONSE WHICH BEST DESCRIBES YOUR
USUAL ABILITIES OVER THE PAST WEEK:**

	Without ANY difficulty	With some difficulty	With much difficulty	Unable to do
1. DRESSING AND GROOMING Are you able to:				
– Dress yourself, including tying your shoelaces and doing buttons?	☐	☐	☐	☐
– Shampoo your hair?	☐	☐	☐	☐
2. RISING Are you able to:				
– Stand up from an armless chair?	☐	☐	☐	☐
– Get in and out of bed?	☐	☐	☐	☐
3. EATING Are you able to:				
– Cut your meat?	☐	☐	☐	☐
– Lift a full cup or glass to your mouth?	☐	☐	☐	☐
– Open a new carton of milk (or soap powder)?	☐	☐	☐	☐
4. WALKING Are you able to:				
– Walk outdoors on flat ground?	☐	☐	☐	☐
– Climb up five steps?	☐	☐	☐	☐

Figure 7.2. Health Assessment Questionnaire

PLEASE TICK ANY AIDS OR DEVICES THAT YOU USUALLY USE FOR ANY OF THESE ACTIVITIES:

☐	Cane	☐	Devices used for dressing (button hook, zipper pull, long handled shoe horn, etc.)
☐	Walking frame	☐	Built-up or special utensils
☐	Crutches	☐	Special or built-up chair
☐	Wheelchair	☐	Other (specify) ....

PLEASE TICK ANY CATEGORIES FOR WHICH YOU USUALLY NEED HELP FROM ANOTHER PERSON:

☐	Dressing and grooming	☐	Eating
☐	Rising	☐	Walking

PLEASE TICK THE ONE RESPONSE WHICH BEST DESCRIBES YOUR USUAL ABILITIES OVER THE PAST WEEK:

	Without ANY difficulty	With some difficulty	With much difficulty	Unable to do
5. HYGIENE Are you able to:				
– Wash and dry your entire body?	☐	☐	☐	☐
– Take a bath?	☐	☐	☐	☐
– Get on and off the toilet?	☐	☐	☐	☐
6. REACH Are you able to:				
– Reach and get down a 5 lb object (e.g. a bag of potatoes) from just above your head?	☐	☐	☐	☐
– Bend down and pick up clothing from the floor	☐	☐	☐	☐
7. GRIP Are you able to:				
– Open car doors?	☐	☐	☐	☐
– Open jars which have been previously opened?	☐	☐	☐	☐
– Turn taps on and off?	☐	☐	☐	☐

Figure 7.2. (Contd.)

8. ACTIVITIES
    Are you able to:

–   Run errands to the shops?   □   □   □   □

–   Get in and out of a car?   □   □   □   □

–   Do chores such as vacuuming,
    housework or light gardening?   □   □   □   □

PLEASE TICK ANY AIDS OR DEVICES THAT YOU USUALLY USE FOR ANY OF THESE ACTIVITIES:

□   Raised toilet seat   □   Bath rail
□   Bath seat   □   Long handled appliances for reach
□   Jar opener (for jars that have   Other (specify) ....
    previously been opened)

PLEASE TICK ANY CATEGORIES FOR WHICH YOU USUALLY NEED HELP FROM ANOTHER PERSON:

□   Hygiene   □   Gripping and opening things
□   Reach   □   Errands and housework

Figure 7.2. (Contd.)

Thus, in encompassing the psychosocial and environmental factors, the treatment approach is holistic, and appropriate help can be sought from within the rehabilitation team (Shipley and Newman, 1994).

Past medical history

A brief but precise assessment of past medical history or any surgical interventions and efficacy of various interventions is relevant. Physiotherapists need to be aware of any illness or treatment that may complicate or affect physiotherapy treatment, e.g. patients who have been on steroids for a long period may need careful mobilisation.

History of present condition

The history of the onset of present symptoms, their variability and severity needs to be established in order to gain an accurate profile of the patient's present condition. A global assessment of all systems – musculoskeletal, respiratory and cardiopulmonary – that may be affected by the disease indicates the level of severity of the disease and the efficacy of present medical management. The goal of the physiotherapy intervention will depend on the present state of the disease and its resultant disability. Uncontrollable active RA may indicate poor outcome with therapeutic intervention, as the treatment in such cases is mainly symptomatic. The history of some clinical signs and symptoms may cast doubt or alert the therapist to refer the patient to a specialist for further investigation, e.g. unremitting nocturnal pain may indicate active inflammation but it can also indicate serious pathology.

Objective assessment

The purpose of the objective assessment is to confirm and to measure quantitatively the severity and extent of a patient's specific disability. A detailed evaluation is vital in identifying a likely source of symptoms, or structures, contributing to the disability, and also helps to shape an appropriate treatment strategy. The basic objective assessments consists of:

- general observation;
- examination of movements;
- neurological examination;
- palpation.

General observation

Observation is a simple, quick way of documenting the patient's deformities, postures, gait patterns and functional difficulties in daily activities which can be specifically examined during assessment. For example, observation of typical swan-neck deformities of hands in RA patients may be apparent whilst observing the patient attempting to undress; valgus deformity of the knees may suggest ligament and articular damage; patients with PMR may exhibit great difficulty in rising from a chair.

Examination of movements

Inflammation of joints, both axial and peripheral, of muscles, tendons, ligaments and bursae, is a common manifestation in a number of rheumatic diseases and as a result functional movements are affected. By testing movements it is possible to determine whether they are normal or abnormal, thus establishing whether there is a link between the patient's symptoms and movements (Corrigan and Maitland, 1988). During the examination of movements, tension is applied in a systematic manner to the joint and its related structures, by active movements, passive movements and isometric muscle contraction.

The ability to perform active movements demonstrates that both the contractile structures (muscles, tendons) and non-contractile

structures (joint surface, capsule) are intact. The various manifestations of rheumatic disease, i.e. acute tendinitis, myositis, joint effusion, capsule contracture or bony ankylosis, may restrict active
movements or precipitate the patient's symptoms. The range within
which these symptoms occur and the type of symptoms produced
are recorded. Observation of the rhythm and quality of movement is
also made. Objective findings are compared with the patient's
subjective history. An analysis of findings may indicate a specific
stage of inflammation (Table 7.1), or reveal typical tissue involvement or a pattern of joint involvement found in specific arthritic
conditions. For example, in acute stages of RA, pain, stiffness and
reduced range of movements in all directions are present, caused by
synovitis, or effusion and reflex pain inhibition. Bursitis often affects
the rhythm of certain movements. A complete loss of active movement may indicate a ruptured tendon, for example extensor tendon
rupture in RA wrist, or indicate neurological involvement. When the
active range is pain-free, it is essential to apply passive over-pressure
to determine an accurate integrity of the structure examined.

Passive movements are performed by the therapist whilst the
patient is relaxed; in this instance there should be no muscle activity.
They primarily determine the integrity of inert structures of the joint
though stress on contractile structures cannot be avoided. Assessment of both the physiological movement and accessory movements
of the joint is made, as limitation in the movement can restrict active
movement of the joint.

The early onset of pain during passive physiological movement,
especially limiting movement in all directions, may signify acute joint
inflammation or severe pathology, whilst pain reproduced at the end
of a range of certain movements may be caused by stretching of
contracted connective or neural tissue or may even be caused by
derangement of joint surfaces. Accessory passive movements, i.e.
'Maitland techniques', reveal the condition of the joint surface and
capsule, and stability of the ligaments (Corrigan and Maitland,
1988). By passively gliding and sliding or compressing the joint
surfaces in different directions, it is possible to determine whether
the movement is normal, excessive or restricted and whether it
contributes to a patient's symptoms (Magee, 1992). In RA, capsule
distension may cause capsulo-ligamentous instability, resulting in an
excessive range, or movements which may be associated with pain
and spasm; in an anklylosed joint there may be no joint movement,
whereas in FMS excessive range of motion may be found due to
hypermobility of tissues. There is a distinct feel at the 'end of range'

movement, described as an 'end feel', which gives valuable information (Cyriax, 1982). A springy type of end feel may indicate a tight ligament or capsule adhesion; there may be an abnormal hard bony end feel signifying reduced space within the joint (OA) or joint subluxation deformity (RA).

Recording the range of movement within which the symptoms occur is described in terms of degrees of flexion, extension, adduction, abduction, rotation, pronation, supination, etc. Peripheral joints are usually measured by a goniometer. The range of the distal joint is often measured by a malleable lead wire. Use of inclinometer or ordinary tape measure is a reliable and validated means of measuring spinal mobility, e.g. Schober's test for lumbosacral flexion or Smythe's test for general spinal mobility in AS. A detailed description of methods of measurement is described in other texts.

Measurement of movement establishes a baseline from which the disease outcome and efficacy of treatment can be monitored. This is especially relevant in rheumatic conditions as many have recurrent fluctuating episodes of exacerbation and remission. Periodic review of movement is a useful indicator of progress or regression of the disease and function (Table 7.2). Deterioration in range and function alerts the therapist to intensify specific therapeutic input, or it could be a useful indicator for surgical intervention.

During isometric muscle testing, the muscle contracts strongly without any movement being produced in the joint. Testing is done in a neutral or resting position of the joint, so that there is minimal stress on the joint surfaces. If the disease involves contractile structures this test may reproduce the patient's symptoms. During the testing, observation is made as to whether the contraction is weak or strong and whether it elicits any pain. Painful weak contraction may implicate a severe lesion in muscle or tendon; a weak painless contraction may

Table 7.2. Baseline measurements of ankylosing spondylitis

Date	9.8.94	24.8.95	23.8.95	14.8.96
Height	173.5 cms	173 cms	174.5 cms	174.5 cms
Chest expansion	4 cms	3 cms	5 cms	5.5 cms
Occiput-to wall distance (Posture)	18 cms	18.9 cms	17 cms	16.1 cms
Finger-tip to floor (General flexibility)	3.5 cms	3 cms	4.5 cms	5 cms
Hip extension	0°	−5°	+5°	8°
Intermalleolar straddle	86 cms	80 cms	110 cms	120 cms

indicate chronic disuse or neurological lesion. Isometric testing also helps in clinical diagnosis, e.g. pain and weakness in proximal muscles is common in polymyalgia rheumatica, whereas medication such as steroids may cause generalised muscle weakness. However, other differential tests are essential to conclude these examination findings, as pain reproduced by this manoeuvre may indicate active joint inflammation or fracture. Also, in the presence of disproportionate pain, a psychogenic factor needs to be ruled out.

Neurological examination

Neurological involvement in rheumatic disease is either due to vasculitis of the nervous system or can be the result of synovitis. In RA, synovitis and tendinitis often cause entrapment neuropathy, i.e. carpal tunnel syndrome. In some inflammatory connective tissue diseases, for example polyarteritis nodosa or mononeuritis multiplexes, polyneuritis may be present. Peripheral neuropathy caused by vasculitis, or cervical myelopathies may be present, caused by atlanto-axial subluxation or vertebral subluxation, as in RA, and needs a careful assessment for the appropriate intervention to be carried out. In patients with systemic lupus erythematosus (SLE) cerebral vasculitis may lead to hemiplegia or epileptic seizures, or neuropsychosis may become a prominent feature, requiring a neurological therapeutic input. Thus, a neurological examination is an essential component of the assessment.

Palpation

Palpation of the joints and surrounding tissues is important in confirming earlier observed abnormality and to ensure joint normality. Palpation helps to localise and to differentiate the exact structure or site of a lesion. The presence of warmth and tenderness at the site of a lesion is common in active pathology. Tenderness on palpation of trigger points is common in FMS. In the presence of joint swelling it is essential to differentiate the type of swelling found. Joint swelling due to synovial hypertrophy has a 'boggy' feel to it, whereas joint effusion is mobile and soft to palpate. A persistent perfuse effusion or synovitis may need aspiration/injection or surgical intervention prior to physiotherapy intervention. A hard bony swelling may signify the presence of osteophytes or joint subluxation which may require a different treatment strategy. There may be localised extra-articular features such as nodules, calcified deposits, tendinitis or bursitis with equal potential to contribute to the symptoms present.

A critical analysis of the subjective assessment and objective examination forms the basis to develop treatment strategies. It is an ongoing process that underpins the therapeutic management of rheumatic conditions (Figure 7.1).

Therapeutic Management

The complexity of the many rheumatic diseases and the varied array of symptoms and dysfunctions requires a broad spectrum of management strategies. A basic concept of management strategy is to provide patients with structured multidisciplinary care. This is achieved by designing short- and long-term treatment strategies (Table 7.3). The short-term strategies are aimed to ease symptoms such as pain, stiffness, muscle weakness, functional disability, etc. These strategies include patient education, stretching and strengthening exercises and mobilising techniques together with judicious use of various physical agents such as ice, ultrasound, transcutaneous nerve stimulator (TENS), etc. Long-term treatment strategies are focused on reviewing disease activity and the functional status of the patient, establishing a safe progressive rehabilitation programme, and above all focusing on those strategies that involve the patient in the active management of his or her own condition.

Table 7.3. Physiotherapy treatment strategies for rheumatological conditions

Short-term goal
Aim
  To alleviate symptoms of inflammation

Strategy
• Accurate assessment of patient's dysfunction
• Patient education and joint protection training
• Judicious use of modalities to alleviate symptoms of inflammation, i.e. use of ice, heat, TENS, IFT, ultrasound, etc.
• Prescription of therapeutic exercises
• Dissemination of assessment to other team members

Long-term goal
Aim
  To restore optimal functioning lifestyles
Strategy
• Periodic review of muscle strength and capsulo-ligamentous stability and modification of appropriate exercises
• Initiate aerobic conditioning and recommendation of recreational activities
• Patient education and prophylactic measures

It is beyond the scope of this chapter to describe the therapeutic management of all rheumatic diseases but this information can be found in other texts (Hyde, 1980; Gerber and Hicks, 1988). The rationale of common interventions used in the management of rheumatic diseases is described here.

Patient Education

Helping patients to cope with their disease by providing information is essential. Increased understanding of the dynamics of the disease, its prognosis and current management reduces anxiety, helplessness and unjustified fears regarding the outcome (Lorig, Konkolk and Gonzalez, 1987). Research supports concepts of information-sharing strategies and suggests doing so encourages positive health behaviour, helping to achieve a greater level of patient satisfaction (Daltory and Liang, 1991; Rosen, 1994; Barlow and Barefoot, 1996).

The aim of the education programme is to encourage the patient to adopt self-management strategies such as effective use of pain-relieving modalities and appropriate safe exercises, the application of relaxation and stress management techniques, effective drug management, use of joint protection and energy conservation methods, etc. Such strategies focus attention away from the patient being the victim of symptoms and enhance independent self-management responsibility.

Explanations regarding the nature of rheumatic pain, which is often benign, the effect of medication and the benefits of exercises or use of assistive devices fosters realistic expectations of the treatment. Improved understanding of disease pathology may enable patients to appreciate the difference between pain symptoms following overuse or abuse of joints, and pain as part of the active disease. Education helps the patient to achieve a balance between activity and rest, and encouraging the adaptation of a lifestyle that does not perpetuate disability.

Many arthritis organisations provide the patient with leaflets and video cassettes containing useful information, essentially aiming to educate the patient about the nature of the disease and its impact. However, the individual patient or a group of newly diagnosed patients with a similar condition may benefit from a structured educational programme. With the mutual support of the group and the multidisciplinary team, patients are less isolated in their suffering and can seek appropriate help. Patients' coping patterns are considered to be significant in determining the outcome of arthritic disease. These are often influenced by the support of 'significant others' and their participation in educational sessions is vital. It not only gives the patient moral support, but also enhances appropriate core support and encouragement. Thus, patient education programmes are paramount in achieving optimal treatment compliance (Wallston,1993). More about patient education may be found in Chapter 5.

Exercise therapy and rest therapy

The role of exercise and rest in the treatment of arthritis is controversial. However, a recent review of the literature suggests that therapeutic exercises are safe and beneficial in restoring muscle strength, joint range and aerobic capacity in patients with arthritis, without exacerbating joint symptoms (Elliott et al., 1990; Ytterberg, Mahowald and Kurg, 1994; Stenström, 1994). These reviews conclude that in the short term at least, appropriately designed exercises improve pain and fatigue symptoms, increase muscle endurance and aerobic capacity and result in improved functional capacity.

However, clinical data also emphasise caution in recommending exercises for rheumatological conditions. This rationale is based on evidence that passive movements and isometric exercises of acutely inflamed joints is shown to cause a rise in the intra-articular pressure, precipitating potentially harmful biochemical changes in the joints (Blake et al., 1989). Some studies indicate that rest and immobilisation can effectively reduce inflammation temporarily (Partridge and Duthie, 1963). Others also advise caution (Jayson, Dixon and Yoeman, 1972) and suggest that, in the presence of marked disruption of joint surfaces or in the presence of osteoporotic bone in RA, attempts to gain movement can result in further pain and disability. Whilst acknowledging the importance of the role of rest as therapy, especially in the acute stages of a disease, the substantial research highlighting the detrimental effects of immobilisation on cartilage, muscle, ligaments and soft tissues cannot be disregarded (Minor et al., 1988; Ekdahl and Borman, 1992). A classical example is the disastrous effect of immobilisation on the posture of AS patients.

Hence, in prescribing exercises or recommending rest therapy, the physiotherapist aims to have a good balance between rest and exercise in an attempt to control inflammation and yet preserve cartilage and muscle strength. The nature of inflammatory disease and its fluctuating symptoms highlights the importance of the role of the physiotherapist in continual assessment of the joint status, in order to recommend appropriate rest and/or exercise.

The rationale for prescribing rest in the active stage of the disease process is to minimise the systemic impact of the disease and to reduce active joint inflammation. Evidence from the literature (Elliott, 1990; Ytterberg et al., 1994) suggest that some patients who are in active flare-up of their disease benefit from judicious rest. However, there is a paucity of controlled trials to validate such statements. Alexander, Hortas and Bacon (1983) observed that patients with less active disease improved with activity whilst those with active disease benefited from rest. Arguably, enforced periods of rest may also provide the patient with an opportunity to benefit from a much needed respite and joint protection, to help reduce fatigue and psychological stress.

In acute systemic disease, when specific periods of rest therapy are prescribed, the physiotherapist instructs the patient to adopt the correct rest posture. This encourages maintenance of a good functional alignment of the joints and surrounding structures. Physiotherapy treatment is aimed at pain relief and the maintenance of range of movement (ROM) to prevent deformities developing. Depending on the individual physician's preference and severity of systemic involvement, the ambulatory and weight-bearing activities of the patient may also be limited. In cases where a prescription for bed rest is not essential, e.g. isolated wrist flare-up, temporary joint rest can be achieved by the use of resting splints. The patient is instructed to observe joint protection techniques and use pain-relieving devices. The aim is to control inflammation and minimise deformity. Most rheumatologists advocate minimal bed rest for inpatients. Complete bed rest is used only where septic arthritis is suspected.

Exercise therapy

Many forms of inflammatory disease are associated with diminished muscle strength, muscle atrophy, decreased joint flexibility and reduced aerobic capacity (Hopkins et al., 1983; Minor et al., 1988; Ekdhal and Borman, 1992). Poor posture, disuse, reflex pain inhibition, medications, myositis, systemic disease, fatigue etc. contribute to the overall deterioration in function (Elliot et al., 1990) The data available suggest that exercise is the vital key to achieving optimal functional capacity. Carefully prescribed exercises such as stretching, strengthening and aerobic exercises are safe for arthritic patients and have therapeutic benefit (Nordemar, Edstrom and Ekblom, 1976a, Berg and Ekblom, 1976b; Lyngberg et al., 1988; Rosen, 1994; Stenström, 1994; Viitanen and Suni, 1995).

However, there is no pre-set form of exercise therapy for patients with arthritis. The prescription for exercise is based on the type of disease pathology and the degree of active inflammation. When devising exercise programmes for various arthritic conditions, physiotherapists utilise different combinations of stretching exercises, strengthening exercises and aerobic exercises for each patient. Each type of exercise has an important role to play in maintaining and improving the overall strength and flexibility of the affected tissue.

Stretching exercises or range of motion exercises

Range of movement (ROM) exercises, such as finger curling and stretching, keep the joints mobile. Movement of joint surfaces which occurs during joint movement spreads the synovial fluid aiding lubrication of the joints (Simon and Blotman, 1981), which is essential to nourish the cartilage. Therapeutic stretches are performed as a slow smooth stretch held for 5–10 seconds at the end of the available range. Initially, during acute stages of inflammation, the repetition and frequency are kept to a minimum and then gradually increased depending on pain tolerance (Gerber and Hicks, 1988). The ROM exercises are either passive, active assisted or active.

Passive ROM exercises are performed by therapists when patients are unable to move the joints themselves due to pain or weakness, e.g. reflex pain inhibition in acute synovitis or during the immediate post-surgery phase. Passive ROM exercises maintain awareness of movement and flexibility of tissues, and relieve symptoms of pain and stiffness, especially when used in conjunction with pain relief modalities such as ice, heat or transcutaneous nerve stimulator (TENS). Use of an inflatable pressure garment such as Flotron or a continuous passive movement machine is another way of applying rhythmic passive movement to gain an early improved range. Serial splinting for example is useful in stretching contractures passively.

During active assisted ROM exercises the patient will move the joint and the therapist will assist with the terminal stretches. These are useful when an acute stage has resolved or during post-operative mobilisation. In scleroderma, gentle active stretching exercises ease tightening of the skin and subcutaneous tissue. Active assistance in mobilisation of the joint reduces the load on the joints thus minimising stress on vulnerable tissues. Hydrotherapy is a good example of active assisted exercise where the buoyancy of the water supports the limb while the therapist assists with the movement of the limb.

During active ROM exercises the patient will move the joint through the full range available to him or her, with or without resistance. A prolonged stretch increases the extensibility of tissue and thus maintains and improves flexibility of the joint, tendons and soft tissues. When heat is used as an adjunct to these exercises optimal tissue extensibility can occur resulting in increased range (Gibson,

1984; Lentall et al., 1992). Often in patients with inflammatory disease, pain can lead to abnormal postural loading, increasing muscle tension, joint stiffness and pain. Stretching exercises can improve posture and ease other symptoms. In a randomised controlled study of AS patients, a daily routine of hip-stretching exercises showed an improvement in the range of movement, in comparison with those who did not exercise (Bulstrode et al., 1987).

During non-acute phases of inflammation these exercises are a major component of warm-up exercises, prior to dry-land strengthening exercises or aerobic exercises. However, caution is indicated when there is reduced joint space as in OA, joint instability as in RA or hypermobility as may be found in FMS, as repeated forceful exercises can induce exercise-related exacerbation of the joint and soft tissue problems (Merritt and Hunder, 1983).

Strengthening exercises

Whilst the aim of stretching exercises is important in maintaining range and flexibility, strengthening weak muscles prevents muscle atrophy and gives the joints the best possible protection by increasing muscle control. Muscles can be stimulated to increase their strength and endurance by therapeutic exercises (Ekblom et al., 1975; Nordemar et al. 1976a, 1976b; Chamberlain, Care and Hairfield, 1982). These include isometric exercises, isotonic exercises and aerobic exercises.

During isometric exercises the muscles contract without moving the joint. Isometric contraction can promote muscle recovery by recruiting progressively larger numbers of motor units. Emphasis is placed on the weakest group of muscles. The practical value of these exercises is in strengthening deconditioned postural muscle. As there is no joint displacement, there is reduced repeated joint irritation and thus these exercises are beneficial during active stages of inflammation or for patients awaiting joint replacement. The patient is instructed to hold for 5–10 seconds, and then relax various groups of muscles at various joint angles throughout the pain-free range (Gerber and Hicks, 1988). Repetition is dependent on the joint status and the aim of exercises, i.e. in the acute stages few repetitions for a shorter duration of contractions is advocated whereas, if the aim is to improve range and strength, frequent longer 'holds' at various angles of the joint are desirable. During the early phases of rehabilitation of rheumatic disease or post-surgical rehabilitation, the use of elastic bands of progressive resistance (1–6 lb) are beneficial in progressing the intensity of isometric exercises. These bands are tied in a loop to a chair or door and the patient is instructed to hold and relax various muscle groups (Figure 7.3).

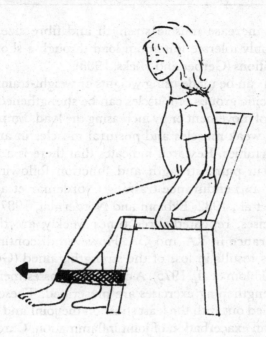

Figure 7.3. Isometric exercises with elastic bands

Proprioceptive neuromuscular facilitation techniques (PNF) are also adapted to the patient's need for progressive rehabilitation (Simon and Blotman, 1981). Techniques such as rhythmic stabilisation, a simultaneous contraction of agonist against the antagonist muscles around the joint, increase joint stability by improving muscular control. Hold-and-relax techniques enhance tissue extensibility by inducing muscle relaxation and thus improve the range. These exercises are incorporated into dry-land exercises for AS patients and for other rheumatic conditions. The use of bio-feedback machines facilitates the efficacy of these exercises. Self-stretching programmes, yoga and relaxation techniques complement these exercises.

Isotonic exercises and isokinetic exercises

Isotonic exercise involves movement of the joint with or without resistance, e.g. lifting weights (closed kinetic chain) or unloaded movement (open chain). Isokinetic exercises require the joint to move at a predetermined speed. These exercises cause the muscle to lengthen and shorten. When the acute stage of inflammation has abated and providing the joint surface is in a condition to accept shear forces, i.e. pain-free active movement, resisted exercises can be prescribed to increase muscle strength and fibre size. Initially, patients may only tolerate minimum load through a short arc and with few repetitions (Gerber and Hicks, 1988).

Progression can be made using weights or weight-training equipment, and specific groups of muscles can be strengthened either by varying speed of movement or by increasing the load. Emphasis is on strengthening weak muscles and postural muscles in an effort to minimise deformities. Research indicates that there is a significant improvement in pain, strength and function following muscle strengthening and endurance training (Nordemar et al., 1976b; Chamberlain et al., 1982; Ekblom and Nordermar, 1987). Regular isotonic exercises, repeated three times weekly, are thought to improve endurance in RA and OA. However, discontinuation of these exercises results in loss of the strength gained (Gerber and Hicks, 1988; Ekblom et al., 1975). A careful joint assessment is essential before strengthening exercises are prescribed. These exercises should be carried out with the least stress on the joint and discontinued if there is an exacerbation of joint inflammation. Careful supervision is necessary as undue pain or fatigue could occur. Forceful repeated movement may cause a further rise in intra-articular pressure and precipitate joint damage (Jayson et al., 1972).

Prescription of any form of exercise is dependent on the patient's particular arthritic condition, level of inflammation, joint status and pain tolerance. For example, the type of exercises for AS patients and RA patients may vary. In AS and related spondyloarthropathies the emphasis is on stretching spinal ligaments, thus flexibility and stretching exercises for the whole spine are of great importance. Stretching exercises are incorporated into the ADL, e.g. pectoral stretches and pelvic tilting exercises. Strengthening exercises specially for the spinal extensors are also emphasised as pain and stiffness can lead to muscle weakness (Viitanen and Suni, 1995). The use of the hydrotherapy pool and a gymnastic ball are invaluable in gaining both general spinal flexibility and strength (Figure 7.4). In RA the capsulo-ligamentous stability is compromised by synovitis and effusion and thus during an active phase judicious use of rest, isometric exercises and passive ROM exercises are imperative. A careful joint assessment before starting strengthening exercises is essential. Exercises should be carried out with the least stress on the joint and discontinued if there is an exacerbation of joint inflammation. In order to improve compliance with exercise regimes, written instruction must be provided. Patients are taught to self-evaluate their joint status and modify their exercises accordingly throughout their rehabilitation programme. Disease activity often varies in patients with inflammatory arthritis and thus a periodic revision of exercises is essential (Lyngberg et al., 1988).

Hydrotherapy

Hydrotherapy is an integral part of the treatment in the management of rheumatic disease (Danneskiold-Samsoe et al., 1987; Minor et al., 1989). It offers varied therapeutic benefits. The raised maintained temperature, 35–36°C, has an analgesic effect. It also reduces stiffness and induces muscle relaxation, thus it can help to increase movements. In painful joint lesions, such as seen in acute RA, AS or OA, the buoyancy of water can help to reduce the joint load and decrease the need for limb support. It encourages the patients to exercise freely. Hydrodynamics can also offer resistance to movement in a practical and safe way. Depending on the level of immersion, the speed of movement, or the use of technical aids, e.g. floats and fins, strengthening exercises can be incorporated into the exercise programmes. Aqua-aerobic exercises are thought to be valuable conditioning exercises (Minor et al., 1989).

Initially the exercises are adapted to the patient's specific needs with regard to his or her pain threshold and level of fatigue. As inflammation recedes, mobility exercises are replaced by strengthening exercises. Techniques such as Bad Ragaz (Figure 7.5) are frequently used by the therapist (Hyde, 1980). The patient is supported by floats and then moves the limbs in a functional pattern from a fixed point, this being the therapist. Research indicates that in RA and OA patients conditioning exercises that include hydrotherapy can improve muscle

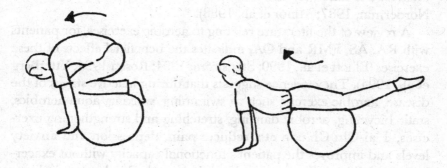

Figure 7.4. Gymnastic ball exercises for ankylosing sponoylitis patients

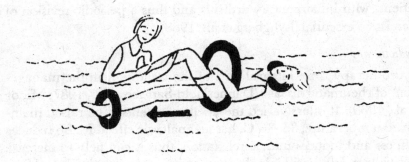

Figure 7.5. Hydrotherapy – Bad Ragaz techniques

strength, aerobic capacity and functional independence without harmful effects on the joints (Danneskiold-Samsoe et al., 1987).

Helliwell, Abbott and Chamberlain (1996), in their randomised control study of AS patients, showed a statistically significant short-term improvement in their cervical range with hydrotherapy when compared with a dry-land exercise regime, thus substantiating the similar findings of other controlled studies (O'Driscoll, Jayson and Badley, 1978). However, careful selection of patients for hydrotherapy is essential. Skin lesions such as psoriasis need not be a contraindication for hydrotherapy, but patients should be screened for contraindications such as unstable cardiac conditions, severe respiratory conditions, open wounds or agoraphobia, etc.

Aerobic exercises

The aerobic capacity of patients with rheumatic diseases is often reduced. Pain, stiffness, muscle weakness and loss of range of motion often lead to inactivity and reduced functional capacity (Ekblom and Nordermar, 1987; Minor et al., 1988).

A review of the literature relating to aerobic exercises, for patients with RA, AS, FMR and OA, indicates the beneficial effects of these exercises (Elliott et al., 1990; Stenström, 1994; Rosen 1994; Ytterberg et al., 1994). The evidence suggests that during inactive stages of the disease, aerobic exercise such as swimming, walking, aqua-aerobics, static bicycling, aerobic dancing, stretching and strengthening exercises, T'ai-Chi Ch'uan etc. reduces pain, depression and anxiety levels and improves the patient's functional capacity without exacerbating the joint inflammation. In patients with OA the data indicate that aerobic exercise improves the endurance for physical activities and thus encourages independent living (Minor et al., 1989).

All aerobic exercises usually have a warm-up phase which takes each joint through a full stretch. However, caution is indicated in stretching unstable joints. A warm-up phase is followed by the aerobic exercises which include exercises aimed to work against a workload that increases the heart rate to 70 per cent of the maximum resting heart rate. Smooth coordinated movements as opposed to jerky movements are vital for joint protection. All aerobic exercises should end with a cool-down phase with relaxation exercises. Programme intensity and duration should be graduated over the weeks and should be reviewed regularly.

The role of the physiotherapist is in devising a safe and specific aerobic exercise programme. The patient's age, sex, habitual physical activity, musculoskeletal status, response to exercise tolerance test, current medication, etc. need to be taken into consideration. For example, a patient with aortic insufficiency or any cardiac involvement should be cleared by the rheumatologist before embarking on an exercise programme. High-impact aerobic activity should be avoided in RA patients with lower limb involvement. Some patients may require adaptive footwear, or splints to protect repetitive loading. A periodic review of all programmes is essential (Lyngberg et al., 1988). Exercise programmes that are adaptable, and enjoyable for the patient, will enhance compliance.

Recreational exercises

Once the flexibility, strengthening and conditioning exercises have been established, a programme of recreational exercises such as weekly swimming, cycling, golf, aerobic dancing, walking and aqua-aerobics, etc. are beneficial to patients with arthritic conditions (Elliot et al., 1990). These activities not only preserve joint range and muscle strength but are also reported to have a beneficial effect on the patient's mood and their self-esteem which decreases social isolation (Nordemar, 1981; Rosen, 1994).

A controlled study on a long-term follow-up of RA patients, not in an active phase of their disease, participating in a variety of recreational activities showed reduced joint symptoms, less need of medication, improved functional capacity and a reduced absence from work compared with those patients who did not exercise (Nordemar, 1981). However, Elliot et al. (1990) recommended caution in the presence of any ligamentous instability or meniscus involvement as in OA, and suggested weight-bearing activities may need to be avoided. Similarly, AS patients can be encouraged to participate in sport that encourages extension and trunk rotation, e.g. volleyball, basketball, swimming (use of snorkels during aquatic sport). However, high-impact or contact sport needs to be discouraged when there is severe ankylosis of the spine (Viitanen and Suni, 1995). Whilst there is a scarcity of controlled study data to substantiate the benefits of recreational activities in rheumatic diseases, careful selection of the type of sport could be pursued.

Superficial Heat and Cold Therapy

The most common therapy used in the treatment of rheumatic disease is that of heat and cold. The aim is to minimise associated symptoms of inflammation such as pain, stiffness, swelling and muscle spasm. Whilst the effect of these modalities on the disease itself is doubtful, the substantial therapeutic benefit is well documented (Lehmann, 1990). There are many different methods used by the therapist to apply superficial heat and ice and the description of its application can be found in other texts (Foster and Palastanga, 1985). The rationale behind the application of heat and cold therapy is discussed in the following section.

Cold therapy

The major physiological benefit of cold therapy is related to the reduction in local metabolic activity, slowing down of nerve conduction velocity and a reduction in the muscle spindle activity. Experimental studies suggest that surface cooling can reduce nerve conduction velocity, especially that of a large diameter, and thus effectively block pain impulses at the spinal cord level altering the perception of pain (Low and Reed, 1990). Ice is also thought to reduce the muscle spindle activity via the anterior horn cells in the spinal cord (Lehmann, 1990). By the application of ice both pain and muscle spasm can be reduced, thus breaking the vicious pain–spasm–pain circle, so restoring normal patterns of movement. As surface cooling also reduces local metabolic activity, ice is useful in reducing post-operative swelling and easing pain. The common methods of cold therapy are cold immersion, the application of crushed ice wrapped in a damp towel, a bag of frozen peas, or gel packs available commercially. However, caution is indicated with the use of cold therapy, especially in inflammatory diseases. In patients with deficient circulation or sensation, e.g. Raynaud's phenomenon, its use is contra-indicated. Above all, it is important to appreciate that pain is a normal protective response; analgesic effects may potentially make the joints more vulnerable to joint stress.

Heat therapy

The major therapeutic benefit to the application of superficial heating is the analgesic effect produced by hyperaemia in the tissues treated. Heat alters neural transmission which in turn elevates pain thresholds and reduces muscle spindle activity (Lehmann, 1990). Hyperaemia is also thought to increase the connective tissue extensibility in muscles and periarticular structures (Lentall et al., 1992). The use of moist heat packs when used as an adjunct to stretching exercises is found to increase range and reduce stiffness (Gibson, 1984). Other methods of applying superficial heat include use of an infra-red lamp, contrast baths, hot showers, heated pool, wax baths, etc. The results of a randomised control trial indicated that the use of wax and exercises in the treatment of RA hands produced a statistically significant improvement in articular index score, range of movement and timed tasks when compared with the application of ultrasound or faradic stimulation with exercises (Hawkes et al., 1986). A further randomised trial also indicated a positive short-term reduction in pain, stiffness and function with the use of wax and exercise when compared with the use of exercise or wax alone (Dellhag, Wollersjo and Bjelle, 1992). However, caution is indicated when superficial heat is applied during active phases of inflammation. Experimental evidence suggests that during active stages of inflammation the hyperaemia associated with heat application can be detrimental (Harris, 1993). Care is also needed in patients with vasculitic skin lesions or skin ulceration, or deficient sensation.

The rationale for the specific use of heat or cold in arthritis is debatable; both heat and cold produce physiological effects which will ease pain and spasm, and increase tissue extensibility. However, clinical studies investigating the effectiveness of heat versus cold on pain and stiffness in arthritis are inconsistent. Patient preferences are also found to be conflicting (Gibson, 1986). Williams, Harvey and Tannenbaum (1986) compared the effects of heat versus cold in RA and concluded that ice was effective in reducing pain, though heat produced a greater increase in movement. Patients, however, preferred heat treatment!

Thus, in the absence of any clear well-defined research on specific use of heat and cold, patient preference is of paramount importance. Some patients may not be able to tolerate ice and prefer heat applications, whilst others may find ice will reduce symptoms of both pain and stiffness. However, clinical experience suggests that heat is effective in the chronic stages of arthritis and can ease pain and also reduce stiffness, whereas ice therapy is beneficial in reducing pain, muscle spasm and swelling during acute stages of inflammation or post-operatively. Whilst the effects of these methods are mostly short term, and they are ineffective in influencing the disease process, they are, nevertheless, both useful adjuncts to exercise or mobilisation techniques (Lentall et al., 1992; Minor and Stanford, 1993).

Electrotherapy and other physical interventions

Electric modalities, such as ultrasound, short-wave diathermy and pulsed short-wave diathermy, TENS, interferential therapy, etc. are frequently used by physiotherapists in the treatment of inflammatory conditions. The analgesic effect and the increased tissue extensibility are both of value therapeutically (Lehmann,1990; Low and Reed, 1990). Once the acute stage of inflammation has abated, deep heat is used as an adjunct to exercise therapy.

Ultrasound

The use of ultrasound is widespread, especially in treating localised inflammatory lesions such as capsulitis, bursitis, tendinitis, enthesis (inflammation of ligaments and tendon insertions), trigger points (in myofascial pain), etc. The selective, deep penetration of sound waves can produce a concentrated heating effect in the deep structures affected by the disease process. As the mechanical sound energy is absorbed by the tissue, they oscillate and cause a rise in tissue temperature. The main therapeutic benefit is the analgesic effect of heat on local tissues. Clinical studies indicate that, following the application of ultrasound, the nerve conduction velocity of large afferent nerve fibres increases with the rise in temperature (Karmer, 1984). This in turn has an inhibitory effect on pain stimuli at the spinal cord level (Wall, 1989). Hyperaemia associated with the application of ultrasound is also thought to increase the extensibility of the connective tissues by enhancing the collagen fibre separation (Lentall et al., 1992).

Whilst ultrasound has no effect on the disease process itself (Goddard et al., 1983), a vigorous rise in tissue temperature in the acute stage of inflammation can be detrimental (Harris, 1993). However, application of ultrasound, in non-acute stages of inflammation, is a useful adjunct to passive therapeutic stretching exercise in improving range (Hayes, 1992). By pulsating the ultrasound beams, the thermal effect can be minimised and the micro-massage effect created by the oscillation of the tissues can give the newly forming collagen a stimulus to align appropriately.

Short-wave diathermy

Short-wave diathermy provides a deep form of heat which is produced by high-frequency alternating current. The heat is produced by the vibration of tissue fluids created by an alternating electromagnetic field. A desired selective heating effect on both the deep and superficial tissues can be obtained by its appropriate application (Foster and Palastanga, 1985). The therapeutic benefits are mainly due to hyperaemia. It is a useful tool once the acute stage of inflammation has abated. The sedative effect associated with hyperaemia can be used effectively in treating osteoarthritic hip, inflamed bursae or deep ligaments (Lehmann, 1990).

The major limiting factor of its use is in the danger of thermal burns and it is also contraindicated in patients with metal implants. However, with the use of pulsed short-wave diathermy (PSWD) there is no danger of thermal injury. By adjusting the pulse length and frequency of current, the non-thermal effect can be used effectively. In a recent double-blind study the application of PSWD has been shown to relieve the pain of OA (Trock et al., 1993). PSWD is a tool of choice when deep heat is indicated, as it can be used safely in patients with artificial joints. However, there are insufficient controlled studies to indicate the efficacy of its use in inflammatory rheumatological conditions.

Transcutaneous electrical nerve stimulator (TENS)

TENS is an electric treatment tool used effectively to modify pain perception, especially in patients with acute and chronic rheumatic conditions. Modulation of pain perception is said to occur by stimulation of the large myelinated nerve fibres which in turn inhibit pain impulses along the small non-myelinated fibres (Low and Read, 1990). Animal studies suggest a possible anti-inflammatory effect of TENS in acute arthritis of peripheral nerve joints when compared with the effect on untreated joints (Levy et al., 1987). Kumar and Redford (1982) have proposed that TENS increases the level of endorphins by stimulating the sympathetic nervous system and brain-stem nuclei and thus modulates pain and inflammation. Several studies indicate that TENS is an effective tool in the treatment of active RA and OA joints. The main benefits are pain relief and improvement in function (Kumar and Redford, 1982; Nienhuis and Hoekstra, 1984; Minor and Stanford, 1993; Aubin and Marks, 1995). The use of TENS in post-operative management such as total knee replacement (TKR) has been shown to improve function, reduce the need for analgesics and reduce the stay in hospital (Harvie, 1979). The application of a TENS machine is simple, and most patients are able to use it safely. Electrodes are placed so as to form a bridge over the painful area or are placed over the peripheral nerve enervating the affected tissue. By adjusting the frequency, intensity and pulse duration, a desired effect can be achieved. Low frequency is thought to give pain relief for a longer duration, whilst high frequency is effective in giving swifter pain relief. The duration of its application can vary as pain relief is often cumulative. Complications are few but an allergic reaction to electrode gel or skin irritation due to adhesive taping requires discontinuation of its application.

Interferential therapy

Interferential therapy (IF) is another form of electrotherapy commonly used in physiotherapy departments as an adjunct to ultrasound and exercise therapy. Interaction of two medium-current frequencies produces a low-frequency current effect in the tissues treated (Foster and Palastanga, 1985). Depending on the range of frequencies and intensity used, it stimulates the tissues in a rhythmic fashion resulting in varying therapeutic benefit i.e., pain relief and muscle contraction. The technique and effects of applying the interferential therapy are described in Low and Reed (1990).

Laser therapy

The use of low-powered laser in the treatment of rheumatological conditions has been reported to ease pain, enhance tissue healing and improve function (Kitchen and Partridge, 1991). However, its efficacy in reducing pain and modulating disease activity has not been clearly established as reviews of the literature show inconsistent findings (Gam, Thorsen and Lonnberg, 1993; Beckerman et al., 1992).

Topical applications

The topical application of anti-inflammatory or neuromodulatory agents is sometimes advocated for rheumatological conditions. The main therapeutic benefit is pain relief. Recent evidence shows promising results. Following a double-blind randomised controlled trial, Deal et al. (1991) concluded that the use of capsaicin cream significantly improved pain in OA and RA. However, the introduction of medication by iontophoresis (use of direct current) or by phonophoresis (use of ultrasound) does not appear to have any superior benefits over topical application (Minor and Stanford, 1993).

Surgical Intervention

When conservative measures are unable to control pain due to arthritis or to restore an acceptable level of function, then surgical interventions are indicated (see Chapter 10).

A detailed rehabilitation programme following specific surgical intervention is described in other physiotherapy texts, and only a brief overview of the role of physiotherapy in surgical management of arthritis is considered in this chapter.

Initially, the role of the physiotherapist, as with all team members, is in patient education. Patient education fosters realistic expectations regarding the outcome of surgery. The final outcome of surgery depends not only on integrated team efforts, but also on the patient's motivation and commitment towards rehabilitation.

Many arthritic conditions have multi-joint pathology and multi-system involvement, and thus require a careful assessment of symptoms by all the team members. It helps to set priorities regarding surgical intervention and to encourage realistic goal setting. Pre-operative assessment of the muscle strength, ROM function, is imperative as it affects the final outcome of surgery. For example, the success of a total knee replacement will depend on the stability and functional status of the hip, foot and ankle joints. In circumstances where both knees are affected, an assessment helps to decide which joint is to be operated on first. Carefully planned and staged surgery reduces the chances of stress on other unstable structures. Hence, lower limb joint replacement would be considered before upper limb joint replacement in order to avoid deleterious effect on the replaced joints of upper limbs should they be replaced first. Immediate post-operative physiotherapy is concerned with chest care and initiating bed exercises. In patients with multiple joint pathology such as rheumatoid arthritis, mobilisation of other joints is essential whilst the patient is on bed rest. Post-operative rehabilitation programmes depend on specific surgical procedures, but the time-frame within which this is initiated often depends on the individual surgeon's views.

The aim of physiotherapy is to ease post-operative symptoms of pain, swelling and stiffness which can be dealt with effectively using ice, elevation and gentle exercises. If pain is limiting active movement, the patient can be advised to use a TENS machine. Following joint replacement, the use of PSWD can be used as a general aid to healing, and in easing post-operative swelling and pain. The onset and intensity of rehabilitation depend on the type of surgical intervention and the individual surgeon's preference. For example, passive mobilisation of the replaced joint begins almost immediately after surgery, whereas the repair of a ruptured tendon may require a longer period of immobilisation. Depending on the patient's response to surgery he or she will be advised regarding the use of modalities and the appropriate balance of rest and exercise.

Provided the patient is adequately screened for any contra-indication, hydrotherapy can be useful for encouraging early, active movements. The heat and buoyancy of water can support the operated limb as the therapist encourages movement. In some cases, e.g. knee replacement or hand reconstruction surgery, the physiotherapist encourages early movement by the use of a continuous passive motion (CPM) machine. Instructing and advising the patient on the use of splints, and modifying them according to the individual's needs, are also integral to the role of the physiotherapist. For example, the tension in the dynamic splints used following small-joint replacement surgery needs to be adjusted daily.

Depending on the stability of the tissue which has been operated on, the type of surgery, the healing time scale and the general abilities of the patient, the rehabilitation programme will progress from passive exercises to active assisted exercises. Later on, strengthening exercises are added to the exercise regime by using elasticised bands, weights and pulleys. Facilitatory techniques such as PNF are common methods used by physiotherapists to improve strength and flexibility.

During the post-operative ambulatory stages, physiotherapists advise the patient in the appropriate use of walking aids, for example use of sticks, crutches or frames. Initially, the patient may need supervision by physiotherapists or nursing staff until safe to ambulate independently. Before discharge the patient's ability to use stairs safely is also supervised by the therapists.

A follow-up appointment to monitor satisfactory progress may be required. In certain operations or in the case of post-operative complications, a supervised progressive exercise programme is necessary. A periodic review of exercises is recommended as patients often show continued improvement between six months and up to a year following surgery. The therapist needs to monitor progress and modify the patient's exercises over several weeks until normal functional use is achieved.

Summary

Physiotherapists are valuable members of the rheumatology team. Their contribution lies in an accurate examination of the neuro-musculosekeletal structures, so as to detect and gauge the patient's dysfunction. The conventional short-term strategy is focused on the treatment of tissues affected by the disease process, in an attempt to ease the symptoms of inflammation and to maintain tissue integrity.

Physiotherapists have a wide array of mobilisation skills and physical modalities to help ease disease symptoms. Due to the chronic nature of many inflammatory diseases, the treatment plan includes a long-term strategy to rehabilitate the deconditioned tissues that are primarily and secondarily affected by the disease process. Physiotherapists are in a strategic position to provide patients with education in self-management of their condition and like other members of the team encourage patients to become active participants in their own care and rehabilitation. The ultimate goal of physiotherapy intervention is to return the patients to a functioning lifestyle.

Despite intervention, many rheumatic diseases follow an unpredictable course and have an equally unpredictable outcome. The psychosocial dimension of chronic rheumatological conditions cannot be underestimated and an awareness of these issues is vital if interventions are to succeed. These problems highlight the importance of a holistic and multidisciplinary perspective on treatment (Rosen, 1994: Shipley and Newman, 1994). A person-focused paradigm of management, as opposed to a traditional disease-focused paradigm of management, enables patients to achieve a functioning lifestyle despite their disease (Frankel, 1994).

Research into arthritis, spearheaded by sophisticated bio-technology, is continuously adding new knowledge and challenges to our present-day clinical perspectives on rheumatic disease and its management. Interpretation and clinical application of such evidence-based treatment is important in justifying intervention and in maximising positive outcomes. Such practices are essential and reflect a good quality of care for patients with rheumatic disease.

Case Study

Mr R, a 25-year-old male, was referred for physiotherapy following a diagnosis of ankylosing spondylitis. His main symptoms were pain and stiffness in the lower lumbar spine and left hip joint. Both were aggravated by inactivity and were eased by hot baths and walking exercises. He complained of extreme tiredness and regular sleep disturbance with early morning pain. The present subjective signs and symptoms were consistent with an inflammatory condition. History of onset of symptoms following an attack of gastroenteritis earlier that year, a previous episode of back pain and family history of ulcerative colitis indicated a spondyloarthropathy. Medical investigations supported this clinical diagnosis. Clinical investigations were as follows: X-ray of the sacroiliac joint was normal, the ESR was slightly raised and the HLA B27 antigen test was positive. He had a history of episodes of back pain since the age of 19 but had not responded to conventional physiotherapy treatment and was also intolerant of non-steroidal anti-inflammatory drugs.

The relevant objective measurements (Table 7.2) highlighted significant reduction in lumbosacral flexion and lateral trunk flexion, occiput-to-wall distance emphasised a stooped posture, and the left hip extension was considerably less than the right hip extension.

The aim of treatment was patient education and the initiation of a safe exercise programme. The patient was invited to join a patient education group. He found the education sessions of tremendous benefit both in raising his morale and helping him to gain confidence via the self-help programmes. Physiotherapy was aimed at easing his symptoms of pain and stiffness and improving his restricted movements. The physiotherapy programme consisted of weekly hydrotherapy, and dry-land gentle active assisted stretching exercises for hip and lumbar spine. Other joints were also exercised. To facilitate movement in the hips, moist-heat packs were used as an adjunct to stretching exercises. As his pain and stiffness eased, progressive strengthening and stretching exercises were included, i.e. the use of floats in the pool, the use of a gymnastic ball, elastic bands and the use of weights, all on dry land. Following improvement in his baseline measurements, he was discharged, and was advised to continue a daily stretching postural exercise programme, and encouraged to participate once a week in some form of cardiovascular conditioning exercises. He was also given the opportunity to join the hydrotherapy sessions organised by the local self-help group.

His yearly review showed there was a general deterioration in his spinal movements, hip joints and posture. He had stopped attending the hydrotherapy sessions with the self-help group due to a change in his working hours, and was also less vigilant regarding his home exercise programme. Symptoms of pain and stiffness had recurred. He was advised to participate in a six-week outpatient AS class to include hydrotherapy, dry-land stretching aerobics and strengthening exercises. At the end of the six weeks his baseline measurement showed some improvement and he was discharged with instructions for a regular home exercise programme. A yearly review since then has shown no further deterioration of his serial measurements. The patient is now a regular user of his local gym and pool, and has resumed active sport.

References

Alexander GJM, Hortas C, Bacon PA (1983) Bedrest activity and inflammation of rheumatoid arthritis. British Journal of Rheumatology 22: 134–40.

Aubin M, Marks R (1995) The efficacy of short-term treatment with transcutaneuos electrical nerve stimulation for osteoarthritis knee pain. Physiotherapy 81(11): 669–75.

Barlow JH, Barefoot J (1996) Group education for people with arthritis. Patient Education and Counselling 27: 257–67.

Beckerman H, De Bie RA, Bouter LM, DeCuyper HJ, Oostendrop RA (1992).The efficacy of laser therapy for musculoskeletal and skin disorders: a criteria based meta-analysis of randomised clinical trials. Physical Therapy 72(7): 483–91.

Blake DR, Merry P, Unsworth J, Kidd BL, Outhwaite JM, Ballard R, Morris CJ, Gray L, Lunec L. (1989) Hypoxic-reperfusion injury in inflamed human joint. Lancet i: 289–93.

Bulstrode S, Barefoot J, Harrison R, Clarke A (1987) The role of passive stretching in treatment of ankylosing spondylitis. British Journal of Rheumatology 26(1): 40–2.

Chamberlain MA, Care G, Hairfield B (1982) Physiotherapy in osteoarthritis of the knee: a controlled trial of hospital versus home exercises. International Rehabilitation Medicine 4: 101–6.

Corrigan B, Maitland GD (1988) Practical Orthopaedic Medicine. London: Butterworths.

Cyriax J (1982) Textbook of Orthopaedic Medicine Vol 1, 8th edn. London: Balliere Tindall.

Daltory LM, Liang MH. (1991) Advances in patient education rheumatic diseases Annals of the Rheumatic Diseases 50: 415–17.

Danneskiold-Samsoe B, Lynberg K, Risum T, Telling M (1987) The effect of water exercise therapy given to patients with rheumatoid arthritis. Scandinavian Journal of Rheumatology 19(1): 31–5.

Deal CL, Schnitzer TJ, Lipstien EL Seibold JR, Stevens RM, Levey MD, Albert D, Reynold F. (1991) Treatment of arthritis with topical capsaicin: a double blind trial. Clinical Therapy 13: 383–95.

Dellhag B, Wollersjo I, Bjelle A (1992) Effect of active hand exercises and wax bath treatment in rheumatoid arthritis patients. Arthritis Care Research 5: 87–92.

Edmonds J, Hughes G (1985) Lecture Notes on Rheumatology. Oxford: Blackwell Scientific.

Ekblom B, Nordermar R (1987) Rheumatoid arthritis. In Skinner JS (Ed), Exercise Testing and Exercise Prescription for Special Cases. Philadelphia: Lea & Febiger 101–14.

Ekblom B, Lövgren O, Alderin M, Fridström H, Satterström G. (1975) Effect of short term physical training on patients with rheumatoid arthritis. A six month follow up study. Scandavian Journal of Rheumatology 4: 87–91.

Ekdahl C, Borman G (1992) Muscle strength, endurance, and aerobic capacity in rheumatoid arthritis: a comparative study with healthy subjects. Annals of the Rheumatic Diseases 51: 35–40.

Elliott L, Semble RF, Loser, Wise M (1990) Therapeutic exercises for rheumatoid arthritis and osteoarthritis. Seminars in Arthritis and Rheumatism 20(1): 32–40.

Fitzpatrick F, Badley EM (1996) An overview of disability. British Journal of Rheumatology 35: 184–7.

Foster A, Palastanga N (1985) Clayton's Electrotherapy. Theory and Practice. Oxford: Blackwell Scientific.

Frankel RM (1994) The secret of good patient care. Hospital Physician 30(5): 45–9.

Fries JF, Spitz PW, Kraines RG (1980). Measurement of patient outcomes in arthritis. Arthritis and Rheumatism 23: 137–45.

Gam AN, Thorsen H, Lonnberg F (1993). The effect of low-level laser therapy on musculo-skeletal pain: a meta-analysis. Pain 52: 63–6.

Gerber LH, Hicks JE, (1988) Syllabus update for joint and connective tissue diseases. In Swezey RL (Ed), Handbook of Rehabilitative Rheumatology, American Rheumatism Association. Scientific basis for use of exercises for rheumatoid diseases. In-course supplement, Vol 1. Atlanta, GA: American Rheumatism Association.

Gibson KR (1984) Effect of manual traction on elbow flexion contractures in RA. Abstract. Physical Therapy 64: 749.

Gibson KR (1986) Rheumatoid arthritis of the shoulder. Physical Therapy 66 (12): 1920–9.

Goddard DH, Revell PA, Cason J, Gallagher S, Currey HL (1983) Ultrasound has no anti-inflammatory effect. Annals of the Rheumatic Diseases 42: 582–4.

Harris ED Jr (1993) Treatment of rheumatoid arthritis. In Kelly WN, Harris ED Jr, Ruddy S, Sledge OB (Eds), Textbook of Rheumatology 4th edn. Philadelphia PA: Saunders.

Harvie KW (1979). A major advance in the control of post-operative knee pain. Orthopaedics 2: 129.

Hawkes J, Care G, Dixon S, Bird HA, Wright V (1986) A comparison of three different physiotherapy treatments for rheumatoid arthritis hands. Physiotherapy Practice 2(4): 155–61.

Hayes KW (1992) The use of ultrasound to decrease pain and improve mobility. Critical Reviews in Physical and Rehabilitation Medicine 3: 271–87.

Helliwell PS, Abbott CA, Chamberlain MA (1996) A randomised trial of three different physiotherapy regimes in ankylosing spondylitis. Physiotherapy 82(2): 85–90.

Hopkins G, McDougall J, Mills K, Insenberg D, Ebringer A (1983) Muscle changes in ankylosing spondylitis. British Journal of Rhematology 22(3): 151–7.

Hyde S (1980) Physiotherapy in Rheumatology. London: Blackwell Scientific.

Jayson MIV, Dixon AS, Yoeman P (1972) Unusual geodes (bone cysts) in rheumatoid arthritis. Annals of the Rheumatic Diseases 31: 174–8.

Karmer JF (1984) Ultrasound: evaluation of its mechanical and thermal effects. Archives of Physical Medicine and Rehabilitation 65: 223–7.

Kazis LE, Meenan RF, Anderson JJ (1983) Pain in the rheumatic diseases: investigation of a key health status component. Arthritis and Rheumatism 26(8): 1017–22.

Kitchen SS, Partridge CH (1991) A review of low intensity laser therapy: Parts 1, 2, 3. Physiotherapy 77(3):166–70.

Kumar VN, Redford GB (1982) Transcutaneous nerve stimulation in rheumatoid arthritis. Archives of Physical Medicine and Rehabilitation 63: 595–6.

Lehmann JF (1990) Therapeutic Heat and Cold, 4th edn. Baltimore, MD: Williams & Wilkins.

Lentall G, Hetherington T, Egan, Morgan M (1992) The use of thermal agents to influence the effectiveness of low-load prolonged stretch. Journal of Orthopaedic and Sport Physical Therapy 16 (5): 200–1.

Levy A, Dalith M, Abromovici A, Pinkhas J, Weinberger A (1987) Transcutaneous electrical nerve stimulation in experimental acute arthritis. Archives of Physical Medicine Rehabilitation 68: 75–8.

Lorig K, Konkolk L, Gonzalez V (1987) Arthritis patient education: a review of the literature. Patient Education and Counselling 10: 207–52.

Low J, Reed A (1990) Electrotherapy Explained. Oxford: Butterworth-Heinemann.

Lyngberg K, Danneskiold-Samsoe B, Halskov O (1988) The effect of physical training on patients with rheumatoid arthritis: changes in disease activity, muscle strength and aerobic capacity. A clinically controlled minimised cross-over study. Clinical and Experimental Rheumatology 6: 253–60.

Magee JD (1992) Orthopaedic Physical Assessment. Philadelphia: WB Saunders.

Meenan RF, Gertman PM, Mason JH (1980). Measuring health status in arthritis : the arthritis impact measure scales. Arthritis and Rheumatism 23: 146–52.

Merritt J L, Hunder CG (1983) Passive range of motion, not isometric exercises, amplifies acute urate synovitis. Archives of Physical Medicine and Rehabilitation 64: 130–1.

Minor MA, Stanford MK (1993) Physical interventions in the management of pain in arthritis: an overview for research and practice. Arthritis Care and Research 6(4): 197–206.

Minor MA, Hewett JE, Webel RR, Dreisinger TE, Kay DR (1988) Exercise tolerance and disease related measures in patients with rheumatoid arthritis and osteoarthritis. Journal of Rheumatology 15: 905–11.

Minor MA, Hewitt JE, Webel RR, Dreisinger TE, Kay DR (1989) Efficacy of physical conditioning exercises in patients with rheumatoid arthritis and osteoarthritis. Arthritis and Rheumatology 32: 1396–405.

Nienhuis R, Hoekstra A (1984) Transcutaneous electronic nerve stimulation in ankylosing spondylitis. Arthritis and Rheumatism. 27: 1074–5.

Nordemar R (1981) Physical training in rheumatoid arthritis. A controlled long term study ii: Functional capacity and general attitudes. Scandinavian Journal of Rheumatology 10: 25–30.

Nordemar R, Edstrom L, Ekblom B (1976a) Changes in muscle size and physical performance in patients with rheumatoid arthritis after a short-term physical training. Scandinavian Journal of Rheumatology 5: 70–6.

Nordemar R, Berg U, Ekblom B (1976b) Changes in the muscle fibre size and physical performance in patients with rheumatoid arthritis after 7 month physical training. Scandinavian Journal of Rheumatology 5: 223–38.

O'Driscoll SL, Jayson MV, Badley H (1978) Neck movements in ankylosing spondylitis and their responses to physiotherapy. Annals of the Rheumatic Diseases 37: 64–6.

Partridge REH, Duthie JJR (1963) Controlled trials of the effect of complete immobilisation of the joints in rheumatoid arthritis. Annals of the Rheumatic Diseases 37: 64–6.

Robinson HS, Haldeman J, Imrie J et al. (1980) Evaluation of a province wide physiotherapy monitoring service in arthritis control program. Journal of Rheumatology 7: 387–9.

Rosen NB (1994) Physical medicine and rehabilitation approaches to the management of myofascial pain and fibromyalgia syndromes. Baillière's Clinical Rheumatology 8 (4): 881–916.

Shipley M, Newman SP (1994) Psychological aspects of rheumatic diseases. Baillière's Clinical Rheumatology 7(2): 215–19.

Simon L, Blotman F (1981) Exercise therapy and hydrotherapy in the treatment of rheumatic diseases. Clinical Rheumatic Diseases 7: 337–47.

Skevington SM (1993) The experience and management of pain in rheumatological disorders. Bailliere's Clinical Rheumatology 7(2): 319–35.

Stenström CH (1994). Therapeutic exercise in rheumatoid arthritis. Arthritis Care and Research 7 (4): 190–7.

Trock DH, Bollet AJ, Dyer RH, Fielding LP, Miner WK, Markoll R (1993) A double-blind trial of the clinical effects of pulsed electromagnetic fields in osteoarthritis. Journal of Rheumatology 20: 456–60.

Viitanen JV, Suni J (1995) Management principles of physiotherapy in ankylosing spondylitis – which treatments are effective. Physiotherapy. 81(6): 322–9.

Wall PD (1989) Introduction. In Wall PD, Melzack R (Eds), Textbook of Pain, 2nd edn. New York : Churchill Livingstone 249–58.

Wallston KA (1993) Psychological control and its impact in the management of rheumatological disorders. Bailliere's Clinical Rheumatology 7(2): 218–33.

Williams J, Harvey J, Tannenbaum H (1986) Use of superficial heat versus ice for the rheumatoid arthritic shoulder: a pilot study. Physiotherapy Canada 38: 6–13.

Ytterberg SR, Mahowald ML, Kurg HE (1994) Exercise for arthritis. Baillière's Clinical Rheumatology 8(1): 161–89.

Chapter 8
The role of the occupational therapist in rheumatology

SUSAN TROMANS

Introduction

Records show that 'occupation' as a treatment was first recorded in 2600 BC, when the Chinese taught that disease resulted from organic inactivity. The Chinese remedy was to use physical training to promote health. In the western world the use of 'occupation' as a treatment first emerged in the American territories during the sixteenth century as a treatment for the mentally ill. It continued to develop in the USA with the emergence of occupational therapy (OT) in its earliest form, in 1914. In 1915 the first professional training school was opened in Chicago. By 1928 there were six schools in the USA, and by 1931 the National Registry of qualified occupational therapists was established.

In Great Britain the profession took a little longer to emerge. It was introduced as a concept in 1919 though the first qualified occupational therapist did not begin to work until 1925. She had been trained at the Philadelphia school in the USA and commenced work in the field of psychiatry at the Royal Cornhill Hospital in Aberdeen. The first training school opened in the UK in 1930 in Bristol, with the first diploma examination being held in 1938.

In 1960 the Professions Supplementary to Medicine gave official recognition to occupational therapy, since when all occupational therapists practising in the National Health Service in the UK have had to be state registered.

Originally, training schools were owned privately or allied to hospitals but, since 1971, they have become increasingly part of the higher education system, being based in polytechnics and then universities. The training course has subsequently developed through diploma to degree status (Creek, 1990; Jay, Medez and Monteath, 1995).

Originally the profession began life in hospital wards and workshops, working mainly with individuals with psychiatric disorders. Today, the breadth of the profession is enormous with occupational therapists working in hospitals, in prisons, and also frequently in the community covering a wide variety of clinical conditions. The one factor that has remained the same throughout is the firm belief that 'occupation' is a necessary and therapeutic part of treatment. This can be summed up by the following definition taken from *Occupational Therapy – an Emerging Profession in Health Care*:

> Occupational therapy is the assessment and treatment, in conjunction and collaboration with other professional workers in health and social services, of people of all ages with physical and mental health problems, through specifically selected and graded activities, in order to help them reach their maximum level of functioning and independence in all aspects of daily life, which include their personal independence, employment, social, recreational and leisure pursuits and their interpersonal relationships. (Blom-Cooper, 1990)

The aim of this chapter is to outline the role of the occupational therapist within the field of rheumatology and to describe the assessment and treatment process.

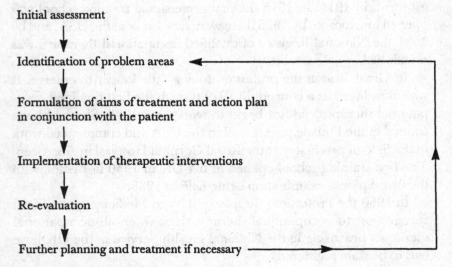

Initial assessment

↓

Identification of problem areas ◄

↓

Formulation of aims of treatment and action plan
in conjunction with the patient

↓

Implementation of therapeutic interventions

↓

Re-evaluation

↓

Further planning and treatment if necessary ──────►

Figure 8.1. Assessment and treatment process

The Assessment and Treatment Process

Assessment is the first and most important step in the treatment process for any therapeutic intervention. Without a thorough assessment of need it is impossible to determine relevant and achievable treatment aims and objectives. Assessment should be a two-way process with the patients being encouraged to identify their own strengths and limitations.

A comprehensive initial assessment needs to identify the following information.

Physical assessment:

- How long has the patient had the condition/symptoms?
- Which joints/muscles/soft tissues are currently affected?
- Which cause most trouble to the patient?
- Has any other joint, etc. been troublesome in the past?
- How long does morning stiffness last?
- Is the patient better at certain times of the day than at others?
- Are the symptoms worse after any particular activity?
- Does the patient have any deformities?
- Are these fixed or correctable?
- Are they recent or long-standing?
- Do they inhibit function?

The answers to the above questions may be gained by direct questioning, observation or actual physical examination. This information gives the therapist background information as to the history and progression of the condition and the effects that it may have on overall function.

Social situation:

- Does the patient live alone?
- Does the patient have a supportive family or friends living with them or nearby?
- Is the patient responsible for the care of anyone else, i.e. children or older relatives?
- What type of accommodation does the patient live in, i.e. house, bungalow, flat?
- Is it privately owned, council, rented?
- Are there steps to the main access?
- Does the patient receive help from Home Care, Meals on Wheels or a private agency?

- Does the patient attend a day centre, luncheon club or support group?

This information enables the therapist to gain a broad outline of the support that the patient has at home and the scope of the activities that he or she may need to be independent in.

Mobility:

- Does the patient use certain equipment to mobilise, i.e. a stick, walking frame, elbow crutches?
- Is this normal or a recent development?
- How far can the patient walk on a good day and on a bad day?
- How easily can the patient go up and down stairs?
- Does the patient drive?
- Can the patient use public transport?
- Does the patient have a wheelchair?
- If so which type and when is it used?

This information gives the therapist an insight into how easily the individual patient can move about and may indicate problems in mobility that are the key to other functional difficulties.

Transfers – can the patient:

- Move on and off a chair?
- Move from lying to sitting while in bed and from sitting to standing beside the bed?
- Get on and off the toilet?
- Get in and out of the bath or shower?

It is important for the therapist to ascertain whether or not the individual can complete all of the above activities independently or whether the assistance of another person or a piece of equipment is required. It is also important to note whether the patient is happy with the status quo, for there is no point in carrying out copious assessments and trials of bath equipment if the patient is perfectly content to strip wash!

If the initial assessment takes place in hospital then it is important to determine whether or not the patient is carrying out the above activities easily because of being in hospital, in which case would more difficulty be experienced at home? This may give some indication as to possible problem areas which may exist in the home. In the ideal world it is better to observe all the above activities as they are carried out, but in reality it is not possible to visit every patient at home. One way of circumventing this difficulty is to ask the relatives or friends of the patient to measure the furniture at home so that a similar situation can be re-created in the hospital setting.

Personal care:

- Can patients reach their feet to wash and dress?
- Can they reach above and behind the neck for the same reasons?
- Can they wash and style their hair?
- Can they shave or apply make-up?
- Can they manipulate items such as toothpaste tubes and aerosol cans?
- Can they use knives and forks independently?
- Can they hold cups or mugs?

This information can be gained either by direct questioning or by observation of the patient while in hospital. The therapist will then have an idea of the scope of the individual's abilities and the possible areas for intervention.

Domestic activities:

- shopping;
- cleaning;
- laundry and ironing.

Can the patients carry out these activities independently or do they require assistance?

Cooking – can the patient:

- open jars, tins and packets?
- peel and chop vegetables?
- strain pans?
- reach items from cupboards?
- carry plates?
- fill and pour a kettle?
- make a snack?
- make a full meal?

It is important to ascertain patients' normal eating habits and whether these are the result of the limitations placed on them by their condition. It is important to work with the primary nurse and dietician when identifying possible problems in this area.

Orthotics:
Orthotics is the correct name for describing splints.

- Does the patient wear any splints?
- If so, what kind are they, are they in good repair and are they still meeting the need that they were originally provided for?
- If the patient has had splints in the past and does not wear them is there a reason?

All splints should be reviewed and the wearing regime reinforced on a regular basis. This part of the initial assessment serves as an indication to the therapist of the patient's attitude towards splintage. Assessment should include an examination of how well the splint fits and a demonstration by the patient of how it is applied. This, of course, will depend on whether or not the patient has brought along the splint!

Work and leisure activities:

- Does the patient work?
- If so, what does the job involve?
- Is he or she experiencing any difficulties at present?
- How supportive is the employer?
- If the patient is unemployed is he or she seeking to return to some kind of work?
- What hobbies/leisure interests does the patient have?
- Is he or she looking for a new pastime to replace one that can no longer be done?

This gives the therapist a wider picture of the responsibilities and abilities of the patient.

Psychological factors:

- How does the individual feel he or she has coped with the illness?
- Does he or she ever feel stressed and unable to cope?
- How much does he or she know about the illness and how to cope with it?

- In general, how does the patient feel?

This is a very important part of the assessment and may take many sessions to explore fully. Although rheumatic conditions tend to be dominated by physical symptoms, the effects that these symptoms can have on the individual's psyche can be great and far reaching. Often patients need to be given the opportunity just to say when they feel they are not coping with their illness in order to take the first step towards coping better. This section also gives the therapist some insight into the knowledge base of the patient. If we are aiming to empower patients in order to help them to function better, it is important that they understand the information that we are giving them.

What do the patients identify as their main priorities?

Often patients will identify activities which are their main priorities and it is important that these are incorporated into the treatment plans. The priorities may concern areas that have not been covered in the previous sections. For example, on initial interview a patient may identify an important future event, e.g. a family wedding, which he or she is concerned about and wishes to find a solution to before other identified areas are tackled. If this priority, at least in the patient's eye, is ignored then the patient is less likely to trust and cooperate with the therapist on other issues.

Further in-depth assessments

From the initial assessment problems may be identified which require further assessment to take place in specific areas. The following is a list of more in-depth assessments that may be carried out and the reasons for doing so.

Hand and upper limb assessment

This may be requested by the rheumatologist or the orthopaedic surgeon prior to surgery. The purpose of this assessment is to determine whether patients will benefit from surgery or whether they are fully functional within their limitations. Hand assessments involve measuring range of movement in the joints of the upper limb, measurement of power and pinch grip, as well as a functional assessment of activities of daily living (ADL). Patients' perceptions of their abilities and feelings about surgery are important parts of assessments. Standardised assessments also exist which are useful tools when carrying out research or quantitative studies. The most well known of these is the Jebsen Hand Function Test (Jebsen et al., 1969) which is reliable, valid and standardised. It consists of a series of tasks that patients carry out while being timed. This assessment stands as a good indicator, over time, of the progression or remission of the disease.

Workplace assessment

This may be requested by the consultant, other health professional or identified by the patient and therapist. The purpose of the assessment is to examine any difficulties that may be occurring in the workplace or to look at any work practices that may be exacerbating symptoms. A common example of this is when looking at seating and workstation design in those patients suffering a repetitive strain disorder. Often a simple piece of equipment or a change in the way in which an activity is carried out can resolve a major problem. Part of the assessment may include offering advice of a more general, ergonomic nature to the employers. Workplace assessment can only take place with the consent of the employer and the patient. As a result it is not always possible to address problems in the workplace (see Chapter 11).

Occupational therapy interventions

As part of the treatment process OT interventions can be many and varied. The following is a list of interventions that may be carried out with rheumatology patients and the reasons for doing so.

Joint protection

This information forms the basis for all treatment carried out with rheumatology patients but is particularly important for those with rheumatoid arthritis.

The aims of joint protection are as follows:

- to provide patients with information relating to their condition which is understandable and realistic, and which also provides a base for understanding additional information which may be given in the future.
- to encourage patients to take an active part in the management of their condition;
- to encourage patients to lead as fulfilling a life as they wish using energy-saving principles;
- to prevent or reduce deformity by reducing strain and stress on the joints by encouraging patients to use the joints in their most stable positions;

- to reduce pain and inflammation in affected joints;
- to maintain functional independence.

It is important to remember that there are very few activities that people with rheumatoid arthritis must not do – it is the way in which they perform them that counts.

The above aims are translated into the following nine basic principles. These are introduced to the patient on a general basis and then reinforced in specific situations during further treatment sessions.

Principles of joint protection

(1) *Distribute the strain over as many joints as possible:* By using many joints to carry out an activity the stress and strain which ensues will be distributed throughout each joint, therefore the risk of moving the joint out of alignment is greatly reduced. Example: using both hands to carry an object, instead of trying to do so with only one hand or two or three fingers, reduces the strain throughout each individual joint, e.g. holding a cup with two hands instead of just the finger and thumb.

(2) *Use the largest joint possible:* The larger the joint, the better it can take the strain. Sometimes it may not be possible to use a larger joint, therefore a larger surface area may be better utilised instead. This way the load is spread over a greater surface area and therefore less strain is placed on individual surfaces. Example: using the hips and knees to rise from a chair instead of pushing the body forward using only the knuckles. An example of using a larger surface area is to carry a pile of books or a bag on the forearm instead of trying to grasp them in the fingers.

(3) *Avoid gripping objects tightly:* The smaller an object is the tighter someone with arthritis will tend to grip it. When an object is gripped tightly the forces acting on the joint increase and are therefore more likely to push the joint into a potentially deforming position. An easy way of combating this problem is to increase the size of any objects that need to be grasped. Example: choosing a larger pen with a fibre tip, or a fountain pen. Both will help to reduce the grip required to write.

(4) *Avoid holding the joints in one position for too long:* Holding the joints in one position for too long can result in increased pain and stiffness. It is better for the patient to try and change activities and joint positions frequently to avoid the build-up of deforming forces around the joints. Example: sitting down for a rest when

out shopping or walking can enable the person to continue shopping for longer, without increasing pain and stiffness.

(5) *Avoid forcing joints into deforming positions:* The inflammatory process of rheumatoid arthritis can lead to unstable joint capsules and weak muscles. This can result in joint deformity if excess strain is placed on the joints. Some of the common deformities seen in rheumatoid arthritis are outlined below.

- Ulnar deviation: this occurs at the metacarpal joints and results in the phalanges being pushed towards the ulnar border of the hand. Initially this may not cause the patient any functional problems but can result in a poor grip if allowed to develop to the extreme. Often it is the physical appearance of the hands that causes the patient most distress, rather than the limited hand function. Activities that encourage the development of ulnar deviation include any movement which forces the fingers towards the ulnar border of the hand, e.g. when opening a jar the patient will normally hold the jar with the right hand and turn the lid with the left. A solution to this is to use the opposite hand – this reverses the movement and pushes the fingers in the opposite direction, which is acceptable.

- Boutonniere deformity: this is caused when the proximal phalanx becomes hyperextended and the distal phalanx flexed. It can be aggravated by placing pressure on the tips of the fingers when turning lights on or when writing. One way of reducing this pressure is to use a pen with a larger barrel.

(6) *Maintain a healthy balance between rest and activity:* One of the most common symptoms of rheumatoid arthritis is fatigue. It is important for individuals to realise that this is a recognised part of the disease and that by pacing themselves they can achieve those things which they have to do while saving energy for the things that they would most like to do. Example: teaching energy conservation techniques (discussed later)

(7) *Use labour-saving gadgets and methods where possible:* If there is an easier way of carrying out an activity, it is worth the patient finding out about it. It could save pain, energy and time in the long run. Example: using ready prepared meals or vegetables; using an electric screwdriver instead of an ordinary one.

(8) *Wearing orthotics (splints) if they have been recommended:* Splints are designed to support, protect and rest the joints. They should be fitted correctly and issued with instructions and contraindications for use. There are many types of splints that can be used by people with arthritis; they are described in detail later in this chapter.

(9) *Listen to your body:* Patients know better than any professional how
     their bodies feel, and they should be encouraged to take notice
     of when they are tired or when they are in pain. Often they will
     carry out certain activities and suffer more pain later. They need
     to be aware of this and also to be encouraged to think how they
     could tackle the activity to prevent problems occurring again.

Energy-conservation techniques

Fatigue and loss of energy are problems often highlighted by patients
with arthritis. These symptoms can be the most debilitating aspects
of the disease. Not being able to carry out everyday roles can lead to
unhappiness, frustration and even depression.

Energy-conservation techniques encourage patients to look at the
activities which they carry out each day, and in doing so it helps them
to decide if there is a more efficient and energy saving way of carrying them out. By employing energy-saving steps patients can make
the most of the energy they have; this in turn will allow them to
accomplish those activities which are most important to them. The
techniques can be divided into four categories:

- *Pacing:* This involves spreading tasks evenly: changing activities
  from one set of joints to another and making the most of regular
  breaks. It may be necessary for patients to keep an activities
  diary, noting the tasks that they have to do and how tired or
  otherwise they feel after carrying them out. It may then be possible to look at how those particular activities could be spread
  more evenly.
- *Prioritise:* This requires patients working out for themselves
  which activities are important to them. They must set the priorities, not the professionals – whose priorities may be completely
  different!
- *Posture:* Energy can be wasted by a poor posture when carrying
  out certain tasks. The height of the workstation or furniture is as
  important as correct lifting and handling techniques. The physiotherapist may also give specific advice on posture that should
  be carried over into everyday activities.
- *Efficiency:* Some activities are carried out in a certain way for no
  reason other than being the way the patient has always done
  them! Often there is an easier method or a piece of equipment
  that can reduce the energy used to complete the task. Patients
  should be encouraged to carry out a time and motion study on

themselves – they may be surprised how often they walk from place to place simply because of poor planning. Reduction in the number of times an individual needs to go up or down the stairs can save energy to be used in a more pleasurable way!

Stress management and relaxation techniques

Stress is a common phenomenon in the life of everyone today. However, the physical changes imposed on someone with arthritis can be an additional source of stress, which may occur for a variety of reasons: frustration at not being able to carry out daily activities easily, having to ask for help, watching roles being taken over by others and of course pain.

Elizabeth Kubler-Ross describes five stages of emotional response to loss. It is thought that a similar process is experienced by those suffering from a chronic illness. Therefore we may see our patients denying their illness, being angry with those around them, bargaining with themselves and others, being depressed and finally coming to some degree of acceptance (Altschul and Sinclair, 1986). During these stages the approach that we take with them and their families may have to change several times in order for treatment to be effective. It is important for patients to understand that having arthritis does take time to come to terms with, and that admitting to having difficulty does not mean that they are 'going mad' or are weak-willed. With arthritis it is important that patients, and therapists, give consideration and thought to how they feel and cope psychologically as well as physically.

Arthritis obviously affects all of those involved with the patient, therefore time and consideration should also be given to carers and to the partners involved. Carers often feel obliged to cope with all difficulties, and fear a display of any inability to cope will be seen as a weakness. The team involved with the care of the patient should also be involved with the care and support of the carer.

Intervention in this area may be as simple as making the time to allow patients to air their worries and frustrations. Listening is often a forgotten and under-used skill. For some patients more formal counselling may be necessary and the therapists involved should ensure that they have the skills to carry this out competently.

Stress management can take the form of discussing the effects of stress and illness in a small group or on a one-to-one basis. Patients should be encouraged to identify how they feel when they are stressed and the situations in which stress occurs. It is then useful for them to identify those actions that relieve stress, and to look at how all three can interact to decrease the effects of stress. Formal relaxation may also be taught, but it is worth remembering that for it to be effective it must be practised regularly and not just when the patient is on the ward or attending for treatment.

The psychological effects of chronic illness are often forgotten in the busy world of medicine, and yet how individuals cope psychologically can have a tremendous effect on their level of physical ability. Patients should be given every opportunity to maximise their psychological as well as physical function.

Activities of daily living

Intervention in this area closely mirrors the categories used during the initial assessment: these may include observing how someone carries out specific activities such as washing and dressing, feeding or preparing a meal. All activities consist of a complicated series of sub-activities. When the activity is analysed it may be that only one part of the process is preventing the patient from completing the whole activity. If this is the case then by concentrating on solving the one step you can alleviate the total problem. Occupational therapists work with a problem-solving approach that is illustrated throughout the assessment and treatment process.

ADL can be used as a treatment technique for a variety of reasons:

- *to build up strength and stamina:* for example, the activity of getting washed and dressed. If the activity is carefully graded over a succession of sessions then an individual's exercise tolerance can be increased along with the level of functioning;
- *to reinforce joint protection and energy conservation principle:* often theoretical principles make more sense when translated into practical activities. An activity such as making a meal may be used as an exercise for the patient to practise and/or learn new skills. The patient is more likely to adopt new behaviours if given the opportunity to compare old methods with new methods;
- *to solve particular problems:* if an individual is having difficulty with a specific activity then carrying out the activity and applying a problem-solving approach may help to solve the problem. This may involve trying out pieces of equipment not used by the patient before, e.g. a bath board and seat to get in and out of the bath, or trying a new method or technique, e.g. making a cup of

coffee in the microwave instead of using the kettle or producing a one-off gadget to solve an individual problem, e.g. fabricating a holding device for an inhaler from splinting material for some-one with severe hand deformities who is unable to grasp and squeeze an ordinary inhaler;

- *to assess whether additional services or assistance may be required:* for example a series of graded kitchen activities may be carried out to ascertain whether an individual requires Home Care Services to provide full meal cover or assistance with a main meal only. Such activities can also help patients to clarify for themselves the extent of the assistance they require.

Orthotics

Splints may be made by occupational therapists, physiotherapists or the appliance department depending on the history of the hospital and the preferences of the medical team! As occupational therapists are constantly evaluating the daily functional activities of the patient they are often in the best position to provide or manufacture a splint that meets the medical needs while serving the functional needs of the patient.

Splints are designed to support, protect and rest vulnerable joint structures. They can act as an aid to decreasing inflammation, reducing pain and assisting function and should always be part of a total treatment programme. There are three main categories:

- *Resting splints:* these are to wear at night, or, as the name implies, while at rest, and may be for the hands or the knees. Their purpose is to rest inflamed or painful joints in a position that is least likely to cause extra stress and strain to vulnerable struc-tures. If a person has two resting splints for night use then he or she would be advised to wear one at a time – preferably on the joint that is most painful. Resting splints are usually made from a thermoplastic material that becomes soft when exposed to hot air or water. A pattern is made for the splint and cut out of the material. Once it has gone soft it can be moulded to the patient to achieve the desired position. The splints are held in place with strapping which must be appropriate to the patient's skin condi-tion and is easy to apply and remove. Obviously, each splint is custom-made for a particular person only and should therefore not be given to another patient to wear!

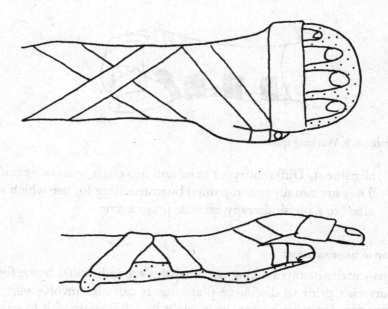

Figure 8.2. Resting splint

- *Working splints:* these are to wear when extra support is needed during an activity, for example ironing. Their purpose is to take the strain through the splint rather than through the joint. It is important for this type of splint to be removed regularly and also when exercises performed on the advise of the physiotherapist are carried out. If the splint is worn continuously then the muscles around the joint will become weaker. Most working splints (braces) are of the commercially produced type, with the metal support running along the palmar aspect of the wrist. These splints must be fitted correctly with the metal bar moulded to each individual patient if the splint is to do its job properly. Because of this splints should only be worn by the person they are fitted to. Working splints can also be made from thermoplastic materials. This can be very useful where the patient has pronounced deformities or requires a wrist splint to be moulded around an object such as a stick, to allow support at the wrist when attempting to mobilise.
- *Lively or dynamic splints:* these are designed to be worn after surgery, e.g. metacarpophalangeal joint replacement. The splints allow graded movement while maintaining joint

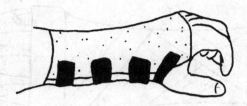

Figure 8.3. Working splint

alignment. Different types exist and are often hospital-specific. They are usually accompanied by instructions for use which are allied to a physiotherapy exercise programme.

Home assessment

This usually involves taking patients who are in hospital home for a short visit prior to discharge planning. It can also involve visiting outpatients in their homes, or it might be a follow-up visit to either category.

The purpose of this assessment is broadly to examine how an individual carries out specific activities in familiar surroundings. As previously mentioned it is not always possible to re-create a suitable environment for assessment in a hospital setting. If the patient is an inpatient a home assessment may be necessary, and particularly so if there has been a significant and potentially lasting change in either functional capability or social support. For example, a home assessment would be indicated where a patient is experiencing difficulty with transfers and climbing the stairs. Similarly, a visit may be carried out with someone who has previously lived with a partner who assisted them in most activities and is now returning to live alone.

Inpatients

It is often better to observe someone carrying out an activity in familiar surroundings. In this way problems become easier to identify and solve in the setting in which they normally occur. So, for instance, it may be necessary to carry out a home assessment if an individual is struggling with transfer problems while on the ward or reports that the furniture is much lower at home. Similarly, if a patient's method of mobilising has changed, i.e. the patient now walks with a frame instead of a stick, then a visit would be necessary to ensure there was enough room at home to enable the patient to walk about safely. Uncertainty about a person's safety on steps and stairs may be another reason for carrying out a visit. This may result in the provision of assistive equipment, e.g. extra stair rails or referral to the local authority for major adaptations such as a stair-lift or perhaps a recommendation that the patient reside downstairs on discharge from hospital.

The ultimate aim of a pre-discharge home assessment is to identify and solve any potential problems before discharge, hence preventing early readmission. It is vitally important that the reason for the assessment is explained clearly to patients as often they believe it is some kind of 'test' they must 'pass' before they are allowed to go home!

Outpatients

Often it can make more sense to arrange to visit at home people who are referred from the outpatient department in order to assess their needs and difficulties in their own surroundings. This usually involves the therapist carrying out the previously outlined initial assessment while asking the patient to demonstrate specific activities which he or she finds difficult. This would be the preferred environment for therapists to see all their patients in but it is obviously costly in terms of time and has safety implications for therapists working alone.

Follow-up visits

Patients with a rheumatological condition tend to have been patients of the rheumatology team for many years. Often they receive tremendous support and help in hospital and then once discharged can feel isolated. Follow-up visits can be carried out to monitor function and provide support over varying periods of time. Changes in function can be identified and responded to in a timely fashion instead of the necessity arising to respond to a crisis situation. From a psychological standpoint the patient can derive support knowing someone can be asked to call if necessary.

Occupational therapy intervention with the pregnant patient

There are three fairly common rheumatological conditions which affect young women, and as a result they may become pregnant during the course of their illness. These are rheumatoid arthritis (RA), systemic lupus erythematosus (SLE) and ankylosing spondylitis (AS). In addition, the young woman who develops juvenile chronic arthritis (JCA) as a child may well have deformities of certain joints which will be disadvantages should she become pregnant, and as a result such patients also will require a great deal of support.

During pregnancy many patients with rheumatoid arthritis go into remission, their symptoms disappearing completely or being significantly reduced. Unfortunately, after giving birth a similarly high proportion experience a return of their inflammatory symptoms, often with a vengeance!

Conversely, patients with AS may well develop more back problems as the maternal bulk grows larger and they will therefore need a great deal of support throughout their pregnancy. Patients with JCA may have many more mechanical problems than a patient with RA and will therefore benefit greatly from OT intervention.

Ideally the occupational therapist would aim to see the patient during her pregnancy and to follow her quite closely afterwards. During pregnancy there can be a tendency to forget how bad the inflammation has been and for the patient to be lulled into a false sense of security. During this time the patient and her family are likely to be making decisions about how the baby will be cared for and about purchasing the relevant equipment. It is at this stage that the patient needs to consider carefully how she will cope if her joints become inflamed and painful once again. Careful decisions need to be made when choosing prams, car seats and cots. Lightweight, easily manoeuvrable prams and pushchairs are preferable to the large, heavy traditional prams. Car seats should be light to lift and easy to secure. Cots should have maximum adjustability at the base so that the need to bend down into the bottom of the cot is avoided as much as possible. The release mechanism on the side of the cot should be easy to use with either hand.

One of the most useful steps a pregnant patient can take is to talk to someone else with a similar condition who has already had a child – it is easier to learn from someone else's mistakes! Young Arthritis Care Contacts, the midwife or health visitor, specialist nurse or therapist may be able to arrange this.

As well as general information the patient may also need specific advice in the following areas:

- *Joint protection and energy conservation:* it is useful spending some time before the baby arrives making plans. It may be better to have a carrycot or Moses basket downstairs for the baby to sleep in during the day instead of having to go up and down stairs to a cot in the bedroom. Similarly a supply of clean clothes, nappies and changing equipment downstairs will limit the need for endless trips upstairs. Obviously, not all eventualities can be planned for, but a little thought beforehand does help.

- *Orthotics:* carpal tunnel syndrome is common in pregnant women whether they have arthritis or not and may result in the need for wrist splint. If the patient already has wrist splints then the fit should be checked and altered if necessary. If the patient is worried about lifting the baby while wearing her splints then it may be appropriate to make a pair of thermoplastic wrist splints prior to the birth. These have the advantage of being slightly softer to the touch and are water resistant.

- *Psychological aspects:* having a baby and not having arthritis can be a daunting experience in itself. Pregnant women with arthritis also have the uncertainty of their disease pattern to cope with too. They should be encouraged to talk through their worries with their therapist, specialist nurse, doctor or midwife. Again it can help greatly to talk to someone else who has been there and survived! It is important that partners should also be involved in the care and planning from the earliest stages – they may not be giving birth or have the arthritis but will be involved in the care of the new baby. They should also be given the opportunity to express their worries and fears.

Availability of assistive equipment in the UK

Today, most assistive equipment is supplied by the local authority social services department. Hospital-based occupational therapists may have access to this equipment but do not usually hold a store of such equipment for issue themselves. Each local authority may have different types of equipment and has different priority systems and criteria for its issue. As a result it can be very confusing to know what is available or what the patient is entitled to! The best source of information is usually the occupational therapist, who has to deal with the community services on a regular basis and usually has a good working knowledge of the local system. If the equipment is not available from social services then the occupational therapist will be able to advise patients on where to purchase it privately, if they wish to do so.

Conclusion

This chapter has briefly outlined the role of the occupational therapist within rheumatology. The role is as diverse as the nature of the conditions associated with it. However, for the patient to receive a comprehensive, effective package of care it is necessary that all members of the rehabilitation team work closely together. Because of this, providing hospital contracts allow it, most OTs are happy to receive referrals from any health professional whether based on the ward, in outpatients or in the community.

Case Study

Helen is a 30-year-old single nurse, living alone and working in a sterile environment. She has recently been diagnosed with RA and was referred by the clinical nurse specialist, from the OPD clinic, for an opinion on wrist braces and work assessment.

Problems identified at initial interview

(1) wrist pain during activity at home and at work;
(2) difficulty carrying out routine tasks at work, and a non-supportive manager;
(3) difficulty coming to terms with her illness;
(4) difficulty with some activities of daily living;
(5) little knowledge of her condition, joint protection or energy conservation;
(6) difficulty with driving.

Occupational therapy intervention

(1) Provision and fitting of 'off the shelf' wrist braces for use at home and when driving; manufacture of thermoplastic wrist braces for use at work: As these were washable Helen was able to clean them with sterile spray. They were monitored by infection control and to date have not presented an infection problem.
(2) Work assessment visit to identify specific problems and possible solutions in conjunction with the patient's manager. Some problems were addressed by changing work methods slightly whilst others required specialised equipment.
(3) Time was built into treatment sessions to allow Helen to express her feelings and frustrations in a supportive environment. This was particularly important for her as she felt that she had to appear to cope at work and as she lived alone had no one to offload to once she left work.
(4) Assessment and provision of small pieces of equipment to enable Helen to remain independent at home without increasing her pain: e.g. tap turners and jar openers.
(5) Information about RA and advice on joint protection and energy conservation techniques: This was related to work as well as home and was discussed in more detail during and after the work assessment visit.

(6) Helen was provided with wrist braces for use during driving and advised to contact the Disabled Drivers' association for information on insurance. This was an area with which she was particularly concerned with.

Conclusion

Helen will continue to be monitored and supported by the OT team. At present she is coping well at work with the help of the suggestions made on the visit. Her manager is now more supportive as solutions to many of her anticipated problems were also resolved during the visit. Helen's splints will continue to be reviewed every six months to ensure a good fit and that they are still appropriate. This will also give her the opportunity to discuss any new problems as they emerge.

References

Altschul A, Sinclair H (1986) Psychology for Nurses. London: Baillière Tindall 211–12.

Blom-Cooper L (1990) Occupational Therapy. An Emerging Profession in Health Care. Report of a commission of inquiry. London: Duckworth.

Creek J. (Ed) (1990) Occupational Therapy in Mental Health. Edinburgh: Churchill Livingstone.

Jay P, Medez A., Montreath H (1995) The diamond jubilee of the professional association, 1932–1992: an historical review. British Journal of Occupational Therapy 55(7): 252–5.

Jebsen RH, Taylor N, Trieschamnn RB, Trotter MJ, Howard LA (1969) An objective and standardized test of hand function. Archives of Physical Medicine and Rehabilitation 50: 311–19.

Recommended reading

Brattstrom M (1987) Joint Protection and Rehabilitation in Chronic Rheumatic Disorders. London: Wolfe Medical Publications.

Chapter 9
The role of the podiatrist in rheumatology

CLARE WIDDOWS

Introduction

The foot is a highly complex organ of balance and propulsion. It acts not only as a foundation for the rest of the body but its function can also affect every other motion in the body. As any patient who suffers from foot problems will tell you, pain on weight-bearing has a significant effect on one's general well-being and can lead to severe lifestyle restrictions. Pain assessment literature has also consistently shown that acute and chronic pain can lead to severe depressive states which further exacerbate the patient's condition (Moldofsky and Chester, 1970).

Unfortunately, the feet are commonly involved in a number of rheumatological conditions and may indeed be the site of presenting symptoms. As the alleviation of pain is one of the major goals in the treatment of any rheumatological condition and because of the high incidence of foot problems, the podiatrist should be a key member of the multidisciplinary team (Chapman, 1996; Wolfe and Cathey, 1991). This chapter will therefore explain the common rheumatological manifestations which present in the foot and explain the podiatrist's contribution to the care of this group of patients.

State registered podiatrists are specialists in the assessment and treatment of the lower limb and its associated pathologies. To obtain state registration a three-year degree course must be completed. State registration is essential for work within the National Health Service. Unfortunately, the terms 'podiatrist' and 'chiropodist' are not protected and therefore care must be taken when referring patients for treatment in the private sector to ensure that the practitioner is state registered.

An increasing number of state registered podiatrists are now undertaking extensive postgraduate training to become surgical podiatrists. A surgical podiatrist is able to carry out ambulatory foot surgery. This is invasive forefoot surgery, which is carried out under local anaesthetic on a day-case basis. An example of the work they may carry out is hallux valgus surgery or straightening a hammer toe. A surgical podiatrist must serve an extensive pupillage under an orthopaedic surgeon, which then allows the individual to carry out the surgical procedures in his or her own right.

Foot Examination

In order to assess the feet, the podiatrist asks the patient to stand barefoot, without socks or shoes. The feet are then observed.

(1) The medial longitudinal arch extends from the heel (calcaneum) to the base of the first toe (first metatarsophalangeal joint (MTP)). In the normal foot this arch is not in contact with the ground except at the heel and the first toe.
(2) The toes should all lie flat against the floor and there should be no evidence of dorsal corns/callosities.
(3) From behind, a bisection (a line drawn down the centre of the muscle bulk) of the lower leg and a bisection of the heel (a perpendicular line dividing the back of the heel in half) should be straight and perpendicular to the floor. The feet should also be slightly turned out (abducted 10–15 degrees).

The feet are then examined with the patient sitting.

(4) The plantar surface (bottom) of the foot should be free from callosities/hard skin. The presence of corns and callosities is a reason for referral to the podiatrist.
(5) Next the nails are examined: are they normal, thickened (onychauxis) or deformed (onychogryphosis)? Can the patient reach his or her feet and manage nail care? If not, refer the patient to the podiatrist.
(6) Finally, footwear: is it suitable? Unsuitable footwear is often a major cause of increased foot pain. Certain criteria must be followed when selecting footwear:

- Will it be wide enough and deep enough to allow room for toe deformities?
- Has it got laces or straps to hold the foot securely in position during walking?
- Is there enough room to allow an insole or orthosis if necessary?
- Is the upper soft enough to reduce pressure on the top of the toes?
- Has the sole got good shock-asorbing qualities?

If the patient has severe foot deformity, it may be necessary to refer the patient to an othotist for extra-depth or custom-made footwear (Moncur and Shields, 1983; Stewart, 1996). An orthotist is a medically trained individual who is involved in the prescription and manufacture of specialist footwear.

What Happens When the Foot Fails to Function Normally?

To understand the changes that occur in the foot and the impact such changes have on the gait cycle of rheumatological patients it is essential to have a basic understanding of normal foot function. Each foot consists of 26 bones and as such has many joints and articulations. However, there are several major joints which are important when walking, i.e. during the gait cycle. These joints are:

(1) the *subtalar* joint, which consists of the three articulations between the superior surface of the calcaneum and the inferior surface of the talus. This joint can be considered the keystone of the foot and a good range of motion is essential for shock absorption when walking; see Figure 9.1.
(2) the *ankle* joint, which consists of the talar trochlear surface and the distal end of the tibia and fibula; see Figure 9.2.

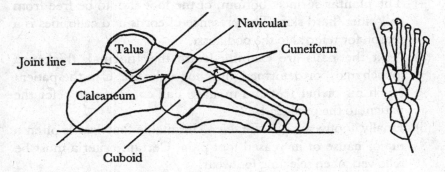

Figure 9.1. The subtalar joint (STJ)

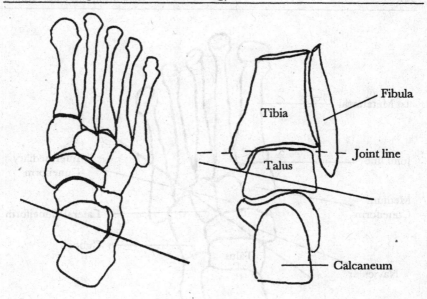

Figure 9.2. The ankle joint

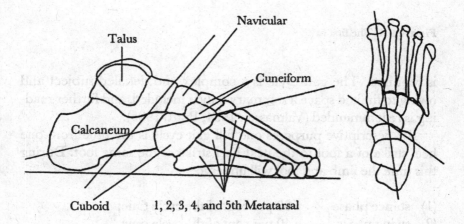

Figure 9.3. The midtarsal joint (MTJ)

(3) the *midtarsal* joint, which is the most complex joint in the foot. It consists of two joints which act as one functional unit. The two articulations are the talonavicular and the calcaneocuboid joints. See Figure 9.3.

(4) the *first ray*, which is a functional unit consisting of the first metatarsal and the medial cuneiform. See Figure 9.4.

It is not sufficient to understand the static foot in isolation. An appreciation of the foot in motion and also the effect of walking on the foot

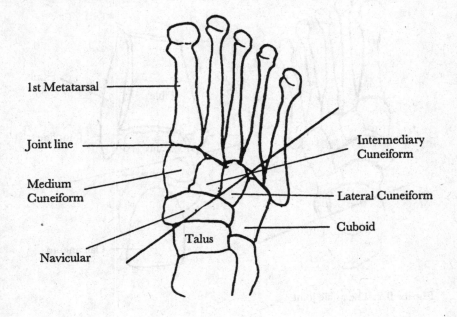

1st Metatarsal

Joint line

Intermediary
Cuneiform

Medium
Cuneiform

Lateral Cuneiform

Cuboid

Talus

Navicular

Figure 9.4. The first ray

is required. The gait cycle is a complex and detailed subject and owing to limited space a summary only is included, and further reading is recommended (Valmassey, 1994; Pratt, 1995).

For descriptive purposes one full gait cycle is the time from one heel strike of a foot to the next heel strike of the same foot. During this time the limb and foot will undergo:

(1)   stance phase   60 per cent of the cycle time;
(2)   swing phase   40 per cent of the cycle time.

It is the stance phase of the gait which is of particular importance to podiatrists. It can be sub-divided into the (1) contact phase; (2) midstance phase; (3) propulsion, as shown in Figure 9.5.

Any alteration to or limitation of normal joint motion, which frequently occurs in rheumatological conditions, severely alters the dynamic stresses in the foot on weight-bearing. As a result shock absorption is lost and the body weight and ground reaction forces become transmitted to parts of the foot and lower limb which are not accustomed to absorbing these forces and pain and further joint destruction can occur.

0%			60%	100%
Stance phase			Swing phase	
Contact	Midstance	Propulsive		
27%	40%	33%		

0%			100%	
Heel strike	Forefoot loading	Heel lift	Toe off	

Figure 9.5. Gait cycle divisions

Podiatrists examine the gait of individual patients by carrying out a biomechanical examination. The aims of a biomechanical approach to patient management are:

(1) to try to establish the primary causes of abnormal foot function;
(2) to realign the foot with the use of functional foot orthoses (see below) so that the foot will function as closely to normal as is possible for that patient, providing joint destruction is not established.

Foot orthoses are moulded devices which are worn in the shoes. Their purpose is to control abnormal motion. Podiatrists may be able to provide accommodative or supportive insoles which help in pain relief by dissipating stresses and cushioning the forefoot and/or rearfoot. It is important, therefore, that the patient has adequate footwear to accommodate insoles or devices comfortably.

Rheumatoid arthritis: the rheumatoid foot

One of the major rheumatological conditions to affect the foot is rheumatoid arthritis. With the increasing success of hip and knee arthroplasty the effect of RA on the foot is assuming greater importance as the dominant cause of pain on weight-bearing. A recent study found the foot overwhelmingly the most important cause of difficulty in walking (Kerry, Holt and Stockley, 1994)

Changes in the foot

RA is a systemic inflammatory disease which is also described as a collagen-vascular disease as all the collagen tissues are affected by the disease. In the foot these tissues include blood vessels, ligaments, tendons, dermal tissue and cartilage. Initially there is inflammation of the soft tissues around the joints which is due to synovitis and often the synovial membrane of the joint becomes thickened. As the disease progresses there is destruction of the articular cartilage, which leads to disorganisation of the joint architecture and secondary subluxation or even dislocation.

The patient classically complains of pain, stiffness and swelling of the feet, particularly first thing in the morning. In the foot characteristic changes take place.

(1) The MTP joints become painful, stiff and tender. Patients often complain of a feeling of walking on pebbles (Young et al., 1995). This is often due to ligament weakening and rupture caused by inflammation and destruction of the ligaments. As the patient weight-bears the foot continues to deform.

(2) Dorsal subluxation of the toes at the MTP joints occurs due to the rupture of the plantar ligaments leading to overriding or retracted toes. Hallux valgus (bunion) deformity can occur.

(3) The fibrofatty padding, which normally bears weight across the metatarsal heads, migrates forwards and therefore the metatarsal heads become inflamed. Loss of connective tissue in the fat pads also occurs which may be due to direct enzyme attacks of the collagen or secondary to steroid treatment. Corns and callosities tend to develop over the metatarsals and can be extremely painful.

(4) Rheumatoid nodules commonly occur on the plantar surface of the heels, under the metatarsals and on the tops of the toes. They are subcutaneous inflammatory granulomatous lesions which may ulcerate either spontaneously or due to trauma and therefore provide a portal of entry for infection.

(5) The tendons in the foot weaken and rupture. The most commonly affected is the posterior tibialis tendon which causes excessive sub-talar joint pronation, i.e. a valgus deformity occurs. Early treatment with an orthosis is indicated (Brown, 1987).

(6) The ankle joint itself may also be severely affected with a marked restriction of movement which causes the patient to lean forward producing further stress in the knees, hips and lumbar spine (Klenerman, 1995). A retrocalcaneal bursa often occurs between the calcaneus and the tendo Achilles. This bursa is fixed and filled with viscous fluid and the area is extremely painful to touch or on moving the ankle joint. Pain is often relieved by aspiration and/or injection of the bursal sac with a

mixture of steroids and local anaesthesia. In these cases, the patient must be referred to a doctor.
(7) The patient is at risk from ulceration of the feet and legs due to vasculitis, steroid therapy, increase in plantar pressures and loss of sub-dermal connective tissue.

Goals of the podiatrist

(1) to improve the comfort of the patient via reduction of callosities and corns;
(2) to redistribute body weight away from the metatarsal heads and keep the weight moving forward over the foot by the use of orthoses or insoles;
(3) to make sure all bony prominences are protected;
(4) to help prevent lesser toe deformities;
(5) to decrease the shock to the feet and legs, i.e. to try to promote a gait which is as normal as possible;
(6) to reduce the risk of ulceration;
(7) to give advice on footwear which promotes shock absorption and prevents dorsal toe problems.

Osteoarthritis is one of the most common clinical rheumatological problems. It is a degenerative joint disease, which is characterised by wearing out of the joint and the initial changes occur in the articular cartilage. It is not, however, usually a serious problem in the foot, except in the instances of hallux valgus and hallux limitus.

The symptoms tend to be of gradual onset and occur initially after walking. However, as the disease process continues, pain at rest may become more common. Stiffness of joint motion is particularly common and tends to be worse after periods of sitting and immobility.

Hallux valgus is a common abnormality of the first MTP joint, which involves an adductus (varus) deformity of the 1st MT and an abductus (valgus) deformity of the great toe. The first MTP joint undergoes bony enlargement and is often covered by a bursa. This bursa that covers the area often becomes inflamed and damage to the skin may also occur. The deviation of the great toe also puts pressure on the adjacent toes and causes them to hammer. Tight-fitting shoes are thought to exacerbate the condition. Treatment in the early stages is education of the patient regarding footwear and separation of first and second toes. Severe cases may require surgery (Mann and Coughlin, 1981) and must therefore be referred to a surgeon or surgical podiatrist for assessment.

Hallux limitus is a common podiatric problem and refers to a condition in which there is a limitation of motion at the first MTP joint. The severity of the patient's symptoms depends on the activity of the patient and the degree of joint degradation present. Patients may complain of painful joint motion or pain on wearing high heels. Signs of hallux limitus will also vary but may include the presence of a dorsal bunion, crepitus/pain on passive movement of joint and a callus on the plantar aspect of the first toe.

Several theories exist concerning the causes of hallux limitus and include a long first metatarsal, previous trauma to the joint and abnormalities in gait pattern. The podiatrist's role in the treatment of this condition is directed towards conservative care and focuses on the biomechanical causes. Orthoses serve two purposes in the treatment of hallux limitus. In the early stages the devices are designed to improve the mechanics of the first metatarsal joint and in the later stages they limit motion to prevent further irritation of the joint. In severe cases, when conservative care is not sufficient to reduce pain, surgical intervention may be necessary to correct the underlying joint pathology (Crawford, 1992).

Seronegative Arthropathies

Reiter's syndrome is described as the combination of non-specific urethritis, conjunctivitis and arthritis. The arthritis typically affects the lower limb and is asymmetrical. The knee, ankles and feet are most commonly affected. Digital involvement of the toes is often accompanied by diffuse swelling referred to as dactylitis (sausaging) and footwear changes may be needed. Some 50 per cent of patients complain of severe heel pain on weight-bearing and this heel pain is often the most disabling symptom of this condition. The pain is due to the inflammation/tension on the insertion of the plantar aponeurosis on the calcaneum and is often linked to tight calf muscles. The soleus/gastrocneumis and plantar aponeurosis work as one functional unit during the gait cycle. The podiatrist can help with advice about footwear, insoles and calf-stretching exercises. In acute cases, the severe heel pain may be helped by special strapping to the area.

Other foot manifestations commonly seen are:

(1) *Keratoderma blennorrhagia:* a skin rash occurring on the soles of the feet or the palms of the hands. The lesions are clinically indistinguishable from pustular psoriasis. Podiatrists can help by providing cushioning insoles to relieve pressure and increase comfort.

(2) *Nail changes:* the nails become yellow or white and are frequently thickened and detached from the nail bed. Regular podiatry treatment can help in the management of such nails, by reducing and drilling the nails.

Ankylosing spondylitis is a chronic inflammatory arthritis which mainly affects the spine with inflammation and ossification of the ligaments resulting in a marked limitation of movement. The peripheral joints are also commonly affected. The synovitis is non-specific and often progresses to bony ankylosis. Enthesopathy frequently occurs at the sites of ligamentous attachments, e.g. insertion of the plantar aponeurosis producing heel pain similar to that experienced in Reiter's syndrome and the insertion of the Achilles tendon at the heel. Podiatry treatment involves advice about footwear, insole therapy and calf-stretching exercises.

Psoriatic arthritis is a seronegative arthropathy which may occur in association with the skin condition psoriasis. It is a rare condition as only 5 per cent of patients with psoriasis go on to develop arthritis. The onset of arthritis is usually preceded by the skin condition in the majority of cases and there is no correlation between the activity of the psoriasis and the activity of the arthritis. The psoriatic skin lesions typically occur on the scalp, elbows or knees but may also be seen on the soles of the feet. Nail changes of the hands and feet occur in 80 per cent of patients with the arthropathy and these changes include multiple pitting, onycholysis (lifting of the nail from its bed) and thickening/discoloration of the nail. Once again podiatry treatment can help in the management of such conditions by reducing painful, thickened nails and removing psoriatic plaques.

Gout is an inflammatory arthritis resulting from elevated serum uric acid levels and urate crystal deposits in and around joints. The classic clinical picture of gout is the sudden onset of intense pain, swelling and redness in the affected joint which is commonly the first metatarsophalangeal joint. The joint is hot and often so painful that the patient cannot even bear the weight of bedclothes on it. Other joints frequently affected by acute gout are the ankles, knees, fingers and elbows. An attack may settle within a few days or it may take weeks before the joint slowly returns to normal. Often the outer layers of the skin will peel away from the area that was most severely affected. Once the joint has settled to normal there may be no signs of gout until a further attack occurs in the joint. This second attack may be precipitated by a period of trauma to the area and can occur weeks or years after the initial attack.

A definite diagnosis of gout is essential before beginning any treatment therapy. When treatment commences the aim of the treatment is to manage the acute attack and prevent long-term complications by decreasing serum urate levels. In the days before effective treatment was available acute attacks commonly led to a chronic polyarthritis. Urate crystals damaged the joint cartilage and the tophaceous deposits caused permanent joint destruction. The podiatrist's role is limited but advice can be offered on pressure relief.

As can be seen from this chapter, there are many rheumatological conditions which present in the foot and the podiatrist has a role to play in the care of all such patients.

Case History

A female patient aged 49 with a 15-year history of rheumatoid arthritis was referred to the podiatry department following ulceration to the top (dorsum) of the right second and left third toes. The ulceration was directly related to the dorsal subluxation of her lesser toes rubbing on the narrow and shallow toe box of her footwear. The patient had a 8-week history of ulceration and had been struggling to manage the lesions on her own at home. The patient's current medication was methotrexate.

When the patient arrived for assessment at the podiatry clinic she was wearing high-heeled court shoes and both lesions were covered with sticking plasters. The lesions were intensely painful and frequently bled. The patient had never been offered any previous footwear or footcare advice and she was unaware that she was entitled to NHS podiatry treatment. This highlights the lack of understanding of the role of the podiatrist in the rheumatological team, as early advice might have prevented the problems that occurred. The patient was also unaware that because of her medical condition that she could have directly referred herself to her local community podiatry/chiropody clinic.

Actions of podiatry department

(1) Treatment of the ulcerated sites with debridement and the use of appropriate wound-care products. The department liaised with the patient's practice nurse to have the dressing changed.

(2) Advice about footwear was given to the patient. One week later the patient had changed her shoes to a pair with a deep toe box, which were more suitable and accommodated the subluxed toes. A marked improvement of the lesions was visible and the patient

was already noticing a decrease in pain. Six weeks later the ulcers were fully healed and the patient was very pleased with the outcome.

(3) The joint function of the foot was assessed and it was discovered that there was a marked limitation of subtalar and ankle joint range of motion. As a result her gait cycle was severely affected, resulting in overloading of the metatarsals. This overloading of the metatarsals was producing callus over the area and the patient was beginning to complain of forefoot and ankle pain. Supportive and accommodative insoles were therefore prescribed to redistribute pressure and cushion the feet in an attempt to limit further joint damage and increase comfort on walking.

(4) The patient was seen regularly for podiatry treatment as she was experiencing increased difficulty in reaching her feet and also, because of impaired hand function, nail cutting was becoming a major problem. The patient was also finding increasing problems with callus formation over the metatarsals, which required regular reduction.

Outcome

The ulcers had healed within six weeks of initial referral. However, the patient still attends the clinic every six weeks for regular treatment during which her disease progression can be assessed and appropriate advice given. Regular treatment also significantly reduces the pain experienced by the patient.

Conclusion

This patient's case history highlights the role of the podiatrist. If the patient had been referred to the podiatry department for footcare/footwear advice the painful ulceration could have been prevented.

References

Brown P (1987) Rheumatoid flatfoot. The Foot 77(1).

Chapman C (1996) Developments in pain assessment and pain management that are relevant to podiatry. Journal of Podiatric Medicine 51(5): 71–3.

Crawford M (1992) Hallux limitus etiology and treatment. Lecture presented at Podiatry Association Seminar.

Kerry R, Holt G, Stockley I (1994) The foot in chronic arthritis: a continuing problem. The Foot 4: 201–2.

Klenerman L (1995) The foot and ankle in RA. British Journal of Rheumatology 34(5): 443–9.

Mann RA, Coughlin MJ (1981) Hallux valgus: etiology, anatomy, treatment and surgical considerations. Clinical Orthopaedics and Related Research 157: 31.

Moldofsky H, Chester WJ (1970) Pain and mood patterns with rheumatoid arthritis: a prospective study. Psychosomatic Medicine 32: 309–18.

Moncur C, Shields MN (1983) Clinical management of metatarsalgia in patients of rheumatoid arthritis. Clinical Management and Physical Therapy 3: 7–13.

Pratt DJ (1995) Functional foot orthoses. The Foot 5(3): 101–9.

Stewart J (1996) Patient satisfaction with bespoke footwear in people with rheumatoid arthritis. Journal of Podiatric Medicine 51(2).

Valmassey R (1994) Clinical biomechanics of the lower limb. St. Louis, MO: C.V. Mosby.

Wolfe F, Cathey MA (1991) The assessment and prediction of functional disability in rheumatoid arthritis. Journal of Rheumatology 18: 1298–306.

Young M, Coffey J, Taylor P, Boulton A (1995) Weight bearing ultrasound in diabetic and rheumatoid patients. The Foot 5: 76–9.

Chapter 10
Surgery in rheumatic disease

SARAH LOUKES

Introduction

This chapter is about surgical intervention for those people who suffer a rheumatic disease. Surgery, whilst not a cure, can help by relieving pain and increasing mobility, thereby helping the patient to maintain independence. The outcome usually demonstates an improvement in the patient's quality of life. The first part of this chapter classifies the synovial joints, then briefly describes the two most common diseases which call for surgical intervention. Part 2 describes the different surgical options currently in general use, and Part 3 deals with the patient pre-admission, the stay in hospital and finally ensuring a safe discharge home following surgical intervention for a total hip replacement.

Part 1: Classification of Joints

Freely moving synovial joints involved in rheumatoid disease are characterised by:
- the ends of bone being covered in cartilage;
- the whole joint being enclosed in a fibrous capsule;
- the capsule of the joint being lined with synovial membrane. See Figure 10.1.

The synovial cavity contains the synovial fluid required for lubrication. Freely movable synovial joints are divided into sub-types:

- gliding, e.g. carpal and tarsal bones in the wrists;

257

- hinge, e.g. elbow, ankle, knee;
- pivot, e.g. atlas, axial bones;
- ellipsoidal, e.g. between radius and wrist;
- saddle, e.g. trapezium and metacarpal bones in the hand;
- ball and socket, e.g. hip, shoulder.

Synovial joints have a space between the articulating bones described as the synovial cavity. Due to the arrangement of the articular capsule and accessory ligaments, these articulating bones are freely movable. It is the various movements of the body that create friction between these moving parts. The movement of the synovial joint is limited by the shape of the articulating bones, the tension of the ligaments, and the arrangement and tension of the muscles. To reduce this friction, sac-like structures called bursae are situated in the bodily tissue.

The two most common diseases involved in orthopaedic surgery as a result of rheumatoid disease are rheumatoid arthritis and osteoarthritis.

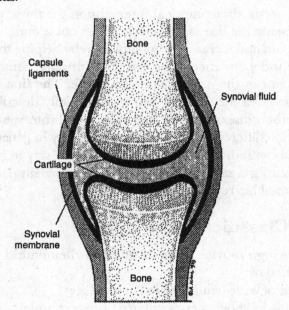

Figure 10.1. Synovial joint. Reproduced with permission of Arthritis Care

Rheumatoid arthritis (RA)

This is thought to be an auto-immune disease in which the body attacks its own cartilage and joint linings, causing inflammation, swelling, pain and loss of function. The main symptom is inflammation of the synovial membrane. If left untreated the membrane thickens, the synovial fluid increases, and the resulting pressure causes pain and tenderness. The membrane then produces abnormal granulation tissue (pannus) which adheres to the surface of articular cartilage allowing fibrous tissue to adhere to the exposed bone ends. The tissue ossifies and fuses the joint so that it becomes fixed. The range of motion of the joint is greatly restricted. The growth of the membrane causes joint distortion. It is this which gives the clinical appearance of RA. Removal of the pannus reduces its growth, helps to prevent deformities, and improves joint function. Ligaments and tendons also become inflamed, leading to shortening, stiffening and scarring, resulting in contractures and subluxation (partial dislocation) of the joint.

Osteoarthritis (OA)

This is more common than RA. It is a degenerative disease which may or may not be inflammatory. The articular cartilage becomes thinned and in order to compensate for lost bone surface the adjacent bones develop outgrowths known as osteophytes. This reduces space in the joint cavity and restricts movement of the joint. The synovial membrane is rarely destroyed and other tissues are unaffected.

A significant difference, as far as surgery is concerned, is that OA usually strikes the large joints of the knee or hip, whereas RA is first seen to affect the small joints of the feet and hand.

Part 2: Surgical Intervention

It is worth pointing out at this juncture that all surgical procedures involve risk, and joint replacements are no exception. The main danger is *infection of the new joint*; the result, should it happen, could mean its removal. To avoid this all patients are screened pre-operatively for any source of infection, e.g. urinary tract infection, leg ulcers, broken skin, chest infections, etc. Also, patients are routinely given prophylactic antibiotics for 24–48 hours post-operatively. In addition, because an artificial object is being inserted into the body there is a small risk of an *allergic reaction*. A common post-operative complication is blood clots, and in lower limb surgery the incidence of *deep vein thrombosis* is great. Many patients are routinely anticoagulated to prevent this occurring. Anti-embolic stockings are worn immediately post-operatively, and gentle movement of the lower limbs is encouraged as soon as the patient is awake. Early mobilisation also helps to avoid this condition. *Pulmonary embolism* is another complication, but is less common. Physiotherapy, deep breathing, anticoagulation and early mobilisation are ways to avoid some of these side-effects.

Common surgical procedures

Arthroplasty is the surgical reconstruction of a joint. There are two types of arthroplasty :

(1) *Excision arthroplasty:* This is the where the ends of one or both articulating surfaces are excised leaving a gap which subsequently fills with fibrous tissue. An example of this is a Girdlestone arthroplasty of the hip. It is used to restore movement to a stiff hip deemed unsuitable for total hip replacement (THR) because of infection. The femoral head and proximal femoral neck are removed. Relief of pain will result but the joint may remain unstable. Another very common example is known as a Fowler's operation. Here the joints involved are the metatarsophalangeal joints of the foot. The metatarsal heads are trimmed and the base of the proximal phalanges are excised. The toes and forefoot are then realigned giving the foot a more normal appearance.

(2) *Replacement arthroplasty:* This is the replacement of the whole or part of the joint with an artificial joint known as a prosthesis, as for example with total hip or knee replacement. Today we are fortunate in that other joints can also be replaced either totally or partially, i.e. the shoulder, the elbow and the metocarpophalangeal joints of the hands.

Total hip replacement (THR)

This is the most common orthopaedic operation performed on older people. It is performed to reduce pain and to improve overall physical function. Professor John Charnley performed the first successful operation in 1962 at Wrightington Hospital, Lancashire, and it was the forerunner of all orthopaedic intervention ever since. It is a ball-and-socket joint, and its insertion involves replacing the femoral head with a metallic prosthesis and inserting a high-density polyethylene cup into the acetabulum. The femoral prosthesis may be cemented or uncemented.

Cemented procedure: Bone cement is used to secure the prosthesis in the correct position and alignment as required by the surgeon. This putty-like material, often methymethacrylate, sets rock hard in 8–10 minutes after preparation. The advantage of cement is that it is an instant, firm method of securing the prosthesis. Post-operatively the patient may start weight-bearing the next day. The disadvantage of cement is that, in time, with continued use of the joint, the cement may crack and weaken allowing the joint to loosen, thus wearing away the bone stock. This process may eventually lead to another operation to replace the loosened prosthesis and is known as a 'revision'. Revision of an artificial joint is a long surgical procedure requiring the patient to be anaesthetised for a longer period. The removal of the prosthesis is more traumatic than the initial replacement, requiring the cement to be chipped out, often causing damage to the remaining bone. For this reason cemented joint replacements are commonly used in elderly people who will cause less wear and tear on the new prosthesis, and as a result are less likely to require joint revision.

Uncemented procedure: Uncemented joints are used on younger people where the likelihood of joint revision is very high because of their life expectancy. This method means the post-operative period is longer, with more restrictions on weight-bearing. Often patients may need crutches for several months post-operatively. The most common uncemented joint to be replaced is the hip, for which many surgeons develop their own prosthesis. One recent development is the 'Norwich Hip', an uncemented femoral prosthesis developed by orthopaedic surgeons at the Norfolk and Norwich Hospital. This prosthesis has a fin-like structure, with holes at the top of the shaft, which allows the patient's own bone eventually to grow into the spaces, thus making the prosthesis secure. Revision of the joint is easier, and therefore less surgically traumatic to the patient.

Total knee replacement (TKR)
The knee joint is a complex weight-bearing joint that rolls, rotates and glides. In a TKR the femoral condylar surfaces are replaced with a metallic and high-density polyethylene prosthesis.

Total shoulder replacement
The shoulder is the most flexible joint in the body and is also a ball-and-socket joint. A metallic prosthesis is placed in the humeral shaft following removal of the head of the humerus and a high-density polyethylene prosthesis is inserted into the glenoid area of the shoulder prosthesis and normally cemented into place.

Total joint replacement for wrist, elbow or ankle
Wrist replacement involves the insertion of a metallic implant in to the radius and the metacarpal bone following removal of the carpal bones. This operation can restore motion and relieves pain.

Elbow replacement prostheses are inserted into the humerus and radius to correct degenerative changes.

With an *ankle replacement* the joint surfaces can be replaced with metallic and polyethylene devices. As with wrist and elbow replacement, the operation is still undergoing further study looking at the revision of prosthetic materials. Wrist and ankle joint replacement operations are not as commonly done as hip, knee and shoulder replacements, and the outcomes are still being evaluated.

Silastic implants

These are small, radio-opaque artificial joints, used mainly to replace the metacarpophalangeal joints in the hands to correct deformity and reduce pain. They do not, however, improve muscular power. They are now regarded as being second to the hip replacement in terms of success.

Osteotomy

This literally means cutting through bone. It is done primarily to change the position of the bone for more effective weight-bearing. It also provides greater stability. A wedge or slice of bone is removed from the medial or lateral surface of the bone. The two cut surfaces are then brought into alignment and held in position by plates or with staples.

This procedure is used on several bones: In the *pelvis* the iliac bone is cut so that the roof of the acetabulum will more fully cover the femoral head to make the joint more stable. In the *femur* the shaft is cut below the trochanter to create a false joint to correct long-standing congenital dislocation of the hip. It is also cut below the trochanter as treatment for OA of the hip. In the *tibia* an osteotomy is performed to improve the weight-bearing properties of the knee joint, to delay replacement of the joint. *Spinal* osteotomy is commonly done as a spinal fusion, to straighten abnormal spinal curvature, to strengthen joints damaged by ruptured discs and for correction of spondylolisthesis (dislocation of a vertebrae). Finally, osteotomy is used in the *metatarsal bones* for certain foot deformities such as hallux valgus.

Synovectomy

This involves removal (excision) of the synovial lining of a joint for overgrowth associated with rheumatoid arthritis. All of the lining or just portions of the lining may be removed. It is most frequently carried out on the small joints of the fingers (MCPs) when the disease has progressed despite intense medical treatment and before the joint is irreparably damaged. Synovectomy will relieve joint pain, corrects deformity and also provides stability to the joint. It can help to restore muscle balance and so increase mobility. It is also performed on the elbow and knee joints but with less success on the ankle, wrist and interphalange joints. Post-operative physiotherapy is very important for this operation to prove beneficial.

Tendon repairs

These may be carried out for the release of ruptured tendons or contracted ligaments The removal of subcutaneous rheumatoid nodules is occasionally performed, though they tend to recur.

Arthroscopy

This is a diagnostic procedure, used to identify musculoskeletal disorders and also to assess the condition of ligaments, tendons, cartilage or synovium inside the joint. It usually requires a general anaesthetic as it is a painful procedure, though a local anaesthetic can be used. It is regularly performed as a day case in a day procedure unit. It involves making two or three small incisions in the skin so that the arthroscope can be inserted to gain different views of the joint. The procedure allows for the complete examination of the synovium, menisci and joint cartilage. In reality it is an endoscopy of a joint. Arthroscopy allows for soft tissue surgery to take place, such as the repair of cartilage. It can also reveal the existence of tears in ligaments and can identify and possibly remove loose bodies. It is most frequently performed on knee, elbow and shoulder joints, though smaller arthroscopes have now been developed which allow for similar examinations to take place on tiny finger joints. Complications of the procedure include bleeding into the joint, oedema and infection. Patients need to be aware of these possible complications so they can contact medical help after discharge if necessary. The stitches are removed by the practice nurse at the GP's surgery.

Arthrodesis

This is the fixation of a badly damaged and painful joint. The diseased joint is excised and fusion of the bone ends takes place. The end result means the joint will be pain free but will no longer have the capacity to flex. It was previously carried out on hip and knee joints but is a rare procedure nowadays because other options are available, as already described, to reduce pain. Quite often the only option open for a badly damaged ankle is fusion of the ankle and tarsal bone. Eventually a suitable prosthesis will be developed. Arthrodesis is mainly used on badly damaged radiocarpal joints of the wrists to provide pain relief and stability. It is a very successful operation for this joint, resulting in a pain-free, stable joint together with improved grip strength. Some patients will refuse the operation because they are warned they will no longer have the option of wrist flexion.

Part 3: The Patient

Because surgical intervention plays such an important role in the treatment of patients with rheumatic disease, many rheumatologists now run a combined clinic with an orthopaedic surgeon. It is at this stage that the rheumatologist and the patient will have decided that surgery may be a viable option and will therefore be seeking the advice of the surgeon to this end. In this instance surgery will be an elective procedure, carried out for a combination of the following symptoms :

- joint destruction, deformity;
- pain;
- incapacity;
- loss of joint function;
- poor quality of life;
- loss of independence.

There is no age limit for surgery but the patient needs to be as fit as possible within the limits of his or her disease. Because a prosthesis (artificial joint) has a limited life, surgery is usually delayed for as long as possible. Once the surgeon, the rheumatologist and the patient have decided on surgery, the patient is assessed by those members of staff of the multidisciplinary team who will eventually be involved in the patient's care.

Most hospitals now run a *pre-assessment (admission) clinic* to assess the patient prior to admission for surgery. This is to prevent operations from being cancelled. Pre-assessment clinics are normally nurse led. They often last a full day, and patients are seen by the appropriate members of the rheumatology/surgical team. The assessment by the physiotherapist is very important, as patients will be taught exercises which will help them post-operatively. The patient will also be seen by the phlebotomist and ECG technician for blood and heart tests respectively, and the radiologist will take X-rays of the appropriate joints. If necessary access to an anaesthetist, a dietitian and a doctor is available if the nurse feels this is appropriate. These team members allow for the provision of vital information and in addition provide an opportunity to answer any questions about the procedure which the patient may have.

Certain routine tests are carried out :

- *Blood tests:* These include full blood count, urea and electrolytes, random blood sugar, cross-matching and an antibody screen. These are to exclude anaemia, renal and cardiac problems and diabetes. All patients for large joint replacement require two units of blood to be available prior to their surgery. Some hospitals offer patients the opportunity of autologous blood transfusion. This is a scheme where patients pre-deposit one or two units of their own blood prior to surgery. It is important that the date of surgery is not altered once given as blood, once deposited, has a limited life.
- *Mid-stream specimen of urine* to exclude urinary tract infection.
- *Electrocardiogram* to provide a baseline for each patient, and also to exclude any anomalies. Many hospitals have age restrictions on this procedure, whereby only patients over 50 years of age will be tested unless there are other medical reasons.
- *X-rays* of the joint to be replaced. In the case of hip replacement, the pelvis is X-rayed. To avoid unnecessary exposure of the patient, X-rays taken within 6 months of the procedure are usually acceptable. Chest X-rays are confined to patients with specific chest problems. Patients who have involvement of the cervical spine may have restricted neck movement and may need cervical spine films.

If the patient is identified as at risk from the anaesthetic, they will be assessed by an anaesthetist in the pre-admission clinic. Otherwise, they will be seen on the ward pre-operatively on admission. Information, both written and verbal, is given to the patient at the clinic and covers the following:

- date and time of admission to hospital.;
- pre-operative fasting;
- premedication;
- anaesthesia;
- pain control;
- position in bed and of 'tubes';
- immediate and subsequent post-operative care;
- length of hospital stay;
- discharge home.

Ideally, patients will be admitted to a rheumatology unit for their surgery; otherwise to an orthopaedic ward. Usually the procedure is elective (planned).

The following are certain areas worth highlighting:

- *Anaemia* is a common condition in rheumatoid arthritis. Many patients are on iron supplements, either oral or intramuscular. Even so, some may need a pre-operative blood transfusion to restore their haemoglobin to an acceptable level prior to surgery. An acceptable haemoglobin depends on the individual patient's average level. Most anaesthetists like patients to have an Hb of 10 gd/l or above.

- *Medication:* As the patient may be on toxic drugs or steroids it is important to be aware of drug interactions, increase or decrease of doses, or even consider omission for a few days pre- and post-operatively. The rheumatologist needs to be actively involved in the care of patients waiting for surgery.

- *Non-steroidal anti-inflammatory drugs (NSAIDs):* The majority of patients with rheumatoid arthritis and some with osteoarthritis will receive NSAIDs. These may cause gastric irritation which can lead to gastric bleeding post-operatively. As a result NSAIDs are often given in conjunction with a prostaglandin analogue such as misoprostol. This drug can help to prevent NSAID-associated ulcers.

- *Steroids:* Patients taking steroids systemically will need a boost of hydrocortisone to prevent collapse from adrenal insufficiency. This is given either intramuscularly or intravenously depending on the surgeon's and anaesthetist's instructions. Normally the patient will be given an intravenous injection of hydrocortisone 100 mg at the start of the anaesthetic. They will then be given an IM injection six-hourly for 24–48 hours, depending on instructions. Once the patient is able to take oral medication, oral steroids are normally restarted with a reduction in the IM hydrocortisone.

- *DMARDs:* Some patients will be taking DMARDs, e.g. gold, penicillamine or methotrexate. Though these drugs are not normally stopped for surgery the rheumatologist will need to be consulted as some surgeons consider methotrexate to compromise healing. Others are happy to leave the patient's DMARDs alone. Routine blood tests to monitor the general blood picture are continued if required while the patient is in hospital. Many rheumatology departments have drug protocols for DMARDs which are useful for staff not familiar with such procedures.

- *Antibiotics* are routinely given prophylactically as infection can lead to the removal of the new prosthesis. The dose, duration and frequency are decided upon by the surgeon concerned.
- *Anticoagulants* are given routinely by some surgeons to prevent deep venous thrombosis and pulmonary embolus. They can be administered orally or subcutaneously. Patients taking NSAIDs and salicylates need to be monitored for excessive bleeding. In some cases the NSAIDs may be omitted for a few days.
- *Immobility:* Patients with rheumatoid arthritis are usually less mobile and so at greater risk of developing post-operative complications. Immobility can increase the risk of developing a chest infection, deep vein thrombosis or pulmonary embolism. The skin of the patient taking steroids is usually fragile, so very careful handling of these patients is important. In addition, special care of all pressure areas is paramount.
- *Painful joints* need to be protected with pressure-relieving aids, e.g. special mattresses and bed cradles, and here the occupational therapist can play a leading role.

Total Hip Replacement (THR)

The following account is of a total hip replacement but much of the information relates to a total knee replacement also, whether the patient has RA or OA.

The visit to the pre-assessment clinic is the time to give specific information and to find out what the patient and his or her family's expectations are of the impending surgery. As no joint replacement is as good as a fully functioning natural joint, outcomes will depend upon the patient's general health, muscle tone and the condition of all other joints. He or she should therefore be made aware of the following facts. The range of movement will be less in the replaced joint and also the joint will have a limited life. Nonetheless, the patient should experience less pain and have improved mobility. The post-operative period is recognised as an interval of hard work for the patient, as it involves a great deal of physiotherapy. Videos of hip and knee replacements pre- and post-operatively are available and can be invaluable in getting the above message across. Although the patient is discharged home after approximately one to two weeks, it will be several months before he or she is fully recovered from the surgical procedure.

After admission of the patient to the ward immediately pre-operatively, the nurse should involve the patient in compiling the care plan. Some hospitals have multidisciplinary care plans so as to avoid repetition of questions.

Admission is also the time to consider discharge planning, as potential problems can be avoided with foresight. If the patient lives alone, a period of rehabilitation might be suitable. It may also be necessary for the occupational therapist to visit the patient's home for the installation of specific aids such as hand rails. Many of these problems are highlighted at the pre-assessment clinic but if not there is still time to organise them.

Routine pre-operative tests and checks are performed over the following 24–48 hours, adhering to the following timetable:

- repeat blood tests;
- consent and marking of affected area;
- shaving of area if required taking great care with fragile skin;
- urinary catheterisation if requested by surgeon;
- measuring patient for anti-embolic stockings;
- information on time of surgery and pre-operative fasting;
- premedication, if given;
- journey to theatre;
- tubes and position in bed post-operatively;
- pain control;
- intravenous fluids and drugs.

Theatre nurses are available to talk to patients if they are apprehensive. The anaesthetist should visit the patient the day before surgery. He or she will explain the type of anaesthetic to be given and methods of pain relief. The options for anaesthesia are general anaesthesia or some form of regional anaesthesia, e.g. spinal or epidural. The advantages of the latter are improved post-operative pain control. The effects of *spinal* injections diminish over a period of an hour or so but, if given in conjunction with diamorphine, pain relief can last several hours. *Epidural* anaesthesia is often continued post-operatively with a continuous 'top up' of a solution of diamorphine or methadone given via a syringe pump. This may continue for up to 48 hours if necessary. Careful monitoring of vital signs, especially respiration, will continue until the epidural catheter is removed. Most anaesthetic departments have their own protocols for these procedures. Regular anti-emetics are given to control nausea. *Patient-controlled analgesia* (PCA) is commenced in the recovery ward. It is an intermittent intravenous injection of a diamorphine solution self-administered via a syringe pump by the patient in pre-set doses with a 'lock-out' time-interval pump. Again, intramuscular anti-emetics need to be given to control nausea and a strict protocol for recording vital signs and the doses administered must be followed. Pre-operative patient teaching is also given once a patient has been selected for this form of pain control. *Intramuscular injections* of an opiate or NSAID can be given when needed if the patient has had a general or 'one off' spinal anaesthetic. They take 20–40 minutes to work and therefore are not as effective for controlling pain as a continuous epidural anaesthetic or PCA. *Rectal suppositories* of diclofenac can be administered in the recovery ward or on the general ward to control pain. These should not be given if the patient is asthmatic or receiving anticoagulant medication. Many wards have patient information literature on pain control, anaesthesia and pre- and post-operative regimes. Patients and their families can discuss pre-operatively any aspects of care which they are concerned about. The multidisciplinary team, which consists of the rheumatologist, surgeon, anaesthetist, nurses, house surgeon and registrar, physiotherapist, occupational therapist, social worker, dietitian, phlebotomist, ECG technician, chaplain and radiographer, will visit the patient at various times during their hospital stay.

Following a total hip replacement, the patient will be lying supine in bed with either an abduction pillow between their legs, or a (yellow leg) foam trough. Intravenous fluids are commenced at the start of the procedure and the first dose of prophylactic intravenous antibiotics is given at the induction. There may be one or two suction drains in the wound, but some surgeons do not use any. Intermittent, pulsating foot pumps are in regular use during surgery to improve circulation to the patient's lower limbs. Anti-embolic stockings are applied on returning to the ward. Once the patient's vital signs are stable, he or she may be gradually sat up in bed. A posterior surgical approach is more unstable than an antero-lateral one, leaving the patient more vulnerable to dislocation. The patient should not sit higher than 45° for several days. The dorsalis pedis pulse on both feet needs to be monitored regularly to ensure adequate circulation to the extremities until the regional anaesthesia has worn off, when the patient is then encouraged to dorsiflex both feet. The patient may start to drink when thirsty. All surgeons have different routines but in general the care is similar.

First post-op day

Check haemoglobin. If patient adequately hydrated, not anaemic and tolerating oral diet and fluids, remove intravenous infusion.

Blood transfusion is given if necessary to restore the haemoglobin levels.

First or second post-op day

Remove suction chains. Remove epidural catheter or PCA infusion. Mobilise patient initially with a zimmer frame. Remove urinary catheter. Discontinue antibiotics.

Third day onwards

Increase mobilisation until walking independently with crutches or stick. Adjust analgesia, usually oral, to keep patient as pain-free as possible.

Complications following total hip replacement

Possible complications are:

- dislocation of hip;
- deep venous thrombosis;
- pulmonary embolism;
- urinary retention;
- foot drop, due to compression of nerve;
- chest infection.

Restrictions

Following a total hip replacement, patients are vulnerable to dislocation until the muscles surrounding the hip joint return to normal tension after approximately 6 weeks. They are instructed:

- to sleep on their backs;
- not to cross their legs;
- not to bend down to pick anything up, instead to use a 'helping hand' aid;
- not to bend the operated leg to put on socks or tights, instead to use a dressing aid;
- not to sit on low chairs or toilets, instead to use high chairs and raised toilet seats;
- to learn how to get in and out of bed safely.

In addition, advice on resuming sexual activity is given. The main advice is not to abduct the hip. Patients resume sexual activity when they feel comfortable, usually after six to eight weeks.

The physiotherapist and occupational therapists are closely involved in patient teaching and the provision of aids to make life easier and safer. If necessary the social worker is involved to arrange the provision of home care on discharge. Some patients require physiotherapy after discharge home, as an outpatient at the GP surgery or on a domicilliary visit. If the occupational therapist is concerned about home conditions, she or he will also provide a follow-up visit.

Most patients are loaned a raised toilet seat on discharge. They may also be supplied with blocks to raise their chair and also the bed, should this be required. Many patients buy 'helping hands' and dressing aids. A post-operative X-ray is performed before discharge.

The patient and his or her family or carer are given the discharge date in advance so that transport and domestic arrangements can be made. Sutures are normally removed 10–14 days post-operatively by the district nurse. If patients are undergoing anticoagulation therapy with warfarin, regular monitoring of their blood is arranged with the GP or anticoagulation clinic. Patients are seen in the outpatients' clinic six weeks post-operatively and they will also be reviewed by the rheumatologist. Patients are discharged home with information leaflets concerning the surgical procedure.

Conclusion

Though already stated, it is worth repeating that surgery is not a cure for rheumatic conditions but it is a valuable part of the overall treatment of the disease. Just as the disease is multifaceted, so is the care given whilst the patient is undergoing surgery. The multidisciplinary team are involved in the physical and emotional care of the patient and they are also available to family and carers for help and support. Any surgical intervention can be frightening but, with support and encouragement, the surgical outcome should be successful.

Recommended Reading

Tortora J, Anagnostakos P (1990) Principles of Anatomy and Physiology, 6th edn. New York: Harper & Row.
Mourad LA (1991) Orthopaedic Disorders. Toronto: Mosby.

Chapter 11
Arthritis and employment

ELIZABETH M. BARRETT

> My body is chained to me – a dead weight. It is my warder. I can do
> nothing without first consulting it and seeking its permission. I jeer at its
> grotesqueness. I chafe at the thongs it binds on me. On this bully I am
> dependent for everything the world can give me. (Barbellion, 1919)

What is the Problem?

The development of any chronic illness, such as rheumatoid arthritis
(RA), presents an individual with a plethora of problems, setting off a
chain reaction of changes, not only in the body, but also in the
already complex range of social relationships. The individual is faced
with a range of stresses including adjustment to medical treatment
and uncertainty about the course of the disease as well as his or her
ability to fulfil social and work roles.

To understand fully the impact of a disease like RA, it has to be
considered in the wider context of the contemporary working society
– a society in which there is a strong emphasis on striving and achieving. This does not sit comfortably with chronic illness and 'failing'
due to illness. Being temporarily sick is socially acceptable. To be
chronically sick and therefore permanently unable to work is something else entirely. We work not just for money, important though
that is, but because it gives a purpose to our lives as well as a sense of
achievement, a structure to our day, social contact – a way of meeting people and making new friends – and it also gives us social status.

....it's important for men to work... it's what men do – support their families. (male, aged 54)

I needed to work. I needed an income but I enjoyed it too. I liked the orderliness of it all. I liked the people (or most of them!). The status is important too. We are pigeon-holed according to what we do. It makes us what and who we are. I still miss it. (female, aged 59)

We also have to add into the equation the fact that people have certain perceptions and beliefs about some illnesses and disabilities. For instance, rheumatism is commonly thought to be a painful, crippling disease of old age. Given this perception, it is hardly surprising that young people, in whom RA is not unusual, find this difficult to equate to their particular situation and the age element itself can add yet another stress factor to an already difficult situation. This disruption of the normal or usual sequence of life events can leave people feeling they have aged prematurely or, as Singer (1974) suggests, that 'stages of the individual's biography may be felt to be lost'. Patients frequently comment that they feel they are 'too young' to have arthritis and will often describe a feeling of having 'missed out' or fear that they will not have the same life experiences or opportunities as their contemporaries. There is also a very strong feeling, bordering on fear in some patients, about how they will be perceived by others once their diagnosis becomes common knowledge. Many will deny their illness or seek to disguise or hide its manifestations and their growing disability.

The mismatch between reality and expectation is picked up by Hewlett (1994) who, in a group of 45 RA patients, looked at expectations of future disability and compared this with a self-report questionnaire to assess their actual level of disability at baseline and 6 months later. Only 50 per cent of expectations were correct and incorrect expectations were almost twice as likely to be pessimistic as optimistic. If, as Hewlett asserts, only 10 per cent of patients actually become severely disabled, yet 40 per cent expect to be, any consideration of future employment must be biased – in many instances needlessly. This disruption of life plans, expectations and aspirations, whether real or perceived, is a recurring theme for people in the early stages of RA.

I feel I can't plan ahead because I don't know what is coming next. It's almost like a bereavement. It's the end of what I had thought would happen. I can't see the future. I just know it won't be what I had in mind. I have no career left. I can't do that any more and I'm not the same person to my family. I can't even do what normal Mums do. (teacher, aged 34)

Given the nature of RA, those who develop it are right to be concerned about the future but that concern must be used in a constructive and useful way to maximise potential and minimise the effects of the disease. It seems clear from the literature and from those people with RA that in developing a chronic illness their lives are changed and disrupted in all aspects, including employment. They find themselves much more likely to have to stop work permanently than those who do not have RA. In much of the literature this phenomenon is termed 'work disability'. There is no one single accepted definition of work disability but it has been variously described as:

...a limitation in the kind or amount of work lasting more than six months which has resulted from a chronic health condition or impairment. (Haber, 1971)

Not working due to illness. (Yelin and Katz, 1991)

... the inability to perform work due to physical, mental or other health conditions. (Straaton et al., 1996)

... complete cessation of work. (Meenan et al., 1981)

It is recognised that people with disabilities face added problems in employment and that they are one of the groups who are over-represented amongst the unemployed. A study carried out by the Manpower Services Commission (Colledge and Bartholomew, 1980) showed that more than one-third of those who were unemployed long term had some handicap or illness and 13 per cent were registered as disabled. Clearly, many factors including economic, environmental and personal, and not just disease itself, influence the ability to work. Added to this is our very individual reactions to similar situations – we have all observed people with similar levels of disease activity who have differing limitations and residual disabilities. This would seem to suggest that disability and the resultant ability to work, or not, is dependent on the interaction between many variables including personality.

Undoubtedly, there are those with arthritis who, against the odds, continue to work, adapting to accommodate their disease, changing jobs or reducing the number of hours they work. Regrettably, others are unable to continue in employment.

The literature on work disability in RA spans two decades and the factors researchers have found to be most influential in causing it can be summarised as follows:

Demographic factors

Older females with RA, particularly if they are less well educated, are more likely to become work disabled. (Yelin et al., 1980)

Those who are married or are in a stable partnership are more likely to stop work. The probability of stopping work is 0.61 in the married and 0.33 in the single. (Reisine, McQuillan and Fifield, 1995)

Education factors

Low levels of education are associated with a greater chance of developing arthritis or with developing the disease more severely, but there is a need to consider income and occupation too. (Callahan and Pincus,1988; Leigh and Fries, 1991)

Patients with lower levels of educational attainment are more likely to be work disabled. Medical treatment was found to have no positive effect on employment status. (Doeglas et al., 1995)

Disease factors

The chances of stopping work on health grounds increase with time from onset. (Yelin et al., 1980)

The greater the number of deformities and disease flares and the greater the perceived level of pain, the greater the risk of stopping work. (Reisine et al., 1995)

Functional factors

Poor function as measured by the Health Assessment Questionnaire (HAQ) is one of the best predictors of work disability. (Reisine et al., 1989)

Physical capacity, especially hand function, increases the risk of stopping work. (Minor and Hewett, 1995)

...decreased mobility. (Straaton et al., 1996)

Social/environmental factors

Women who occupy multiple roles in working and homemaking report fewer symptoms and have fewer disability days. (Verbrugge, 1983)

Poor mobility combined with difficulties in transport prevent people getting to and from work and stop them returning to work. (Straaton et al., 1996)

Work factors which work against the employee

...lack of control of the pace of work. (Yelin et al.,1980)

...those employed in service industries, as opposed to white collar workers, i.e. more manual work. (Yelin et al., 1986; James et al., 1995)

...lack of autonomy in the job. (Reisine et al., 1989)

...the need for manual dexterity in the job. (Reisine et al., 1995)

The fewer the hours worked the greater the likelihood of work disability. (Reisine et al., 1995)

The problem, then, is trying to maintain employment when so many factors, including the variability of the disease itself, actually militate against those who wish to work.

The estimates of the number of people with all types of arthritis who have to stop working vary widely up to a maximum of 85 per cent (Pincus et al., 1984). Observation within my own clinical area specifically in RA indicates levels of around 30 per cent ceasing work permanently due to their RA within 5 years of onset in both men and women. In a cohort of 160 RA patients who had been working at onset, 535 potential working years were lost – a mean of 10.9 years per person.

Table 11.1 shows how, in 15 years, the total number of people claiming Invalidity Benefit rose from 559 000 in 1977–78 to 1,438,000 in 1991–92 (Social Security Statistics: HMSO, 1993). The proportion claiming benefit on the basis of having arthritis or rheumatism increased from 54 000 to 184 000 over the same period. Berthoud (1994) maintains that 29 per cent of the extra cases are actually people of pensionable age, who because retirement pensions are taxable and invalidity benefit is not, chose to remain on the latter for as long as they could. The second cause he states is that 16 per cent of the extra cases are due to women in the labour market, paying national insurance contributions and therefore being eligible for benefits. Another 13 per cent he attributes to the gradual increase in the number of people of working age, with long-term illness or impairment resulting in 42 per cent of 'genuine growth' in the number of claimants whilst there is no evidence of a comparative increase in the numbers of people with disabilities. The difference is the number of people *claiming*, not those eligible to do so. It is impossible to know the proportion of disabled people who, because of their

Table 11.1. Invalidity Benefit claimants incapacitated at end of statistical year – all causes (thousands)

	1977–78	1987–88	1991–92
Males	462.00	808.00	1063.00
Females	97.00	240.00	375.00

Source: Social Security Statistics (HMSO, 1993).

disabilities, are unable to work and, of these, what proportion are claiming benefits given the apparent vagueness of some individuals in regard to registering as disabled (BLAR, 1994) and in addition the reluctance of some people to put in a claim or the unfamiliarity of others with what benefits are available.

Various explanations could account for the increase in claimants. It has, perhaps, become more socially acceptable to be seen to be claiming benefits and therefore more people claim for their disabilities. The system might, of course, be being abused with individuals exaggerating their problems and thus claiming benefits they are not entitled to, especially during a period of economic recession when unemployment is high and there is an incentive to make a claim for a benefit paid at a higher rate than, for example, unemployment benefit or where low paid or part-time work would not be 'topped up' to the same level. Equally, it could be that there are more people with disabilities but that data-gathering systems have lagged behind. Certainly, current statistics do not indicate a concomitant rise between 1977 and 1992 in the number of people with disabilities, and the number of new claimants each year has remained static. It appears that people are not leaving the system; they are not moving on to other benefits or back into employment.

Given the choice between two equally qualified applicants for a specific post, employers are less likely to choose one whose disabilities may potentially require him or her to have frequent spells off work, require time off for doctors' and hospital appointments and render their work attendance unpredictable and patchy in addition to the problems of morning stiffness and constant fatigue. Who can blame the employer? Berthoud (1994) refers to the result as a 'ratchet effect', with the number of claimants rising when unemployment rises but not falling when unemployment falls – leaving people marooned on benefit because employers want fit, able and reliable employees.

The practical problems of trying to maintain employment in the face of RA are best described by those who have had to cope.

> My job was lifting bales of wire netting and dipping them in acid. I had to lift them out and move them on to the next man. It was heavy, hard work before I had arthritis. It was impossible to adjust. The conveyor belt just kept bringing the rolls of netting. I had to keep the spindles going. You couldn't stop or have a break. If I slowed down the blokes either side of me lost money. There was no way you dared to slow down – other people depend on you. Some days I felt I couldn't keep going but you have to. The only way was to keep going to the toilet for a 10-minute sit down. They couldn't argue with that.

> There was no way of adjusting. I couldn't alter the pace much. I have a strong personality – I did what I could but it wouldn't have made much difference – even doing it slowly hurt. It was not so much the pace as the type of job.

> I 'flex' my hours. I go in very early and build up hours so that if I don't feel well enough to work I just ring up and tell them I am taking some time owing and don't have to take time off sick.

What Statutory Help is Available?

Access to and information on the benefits relating to sickness, disability and employment is extremely complex and presents a tortuous pathway for those who need to seek help and advice. The fact that many people with a severe disability (BLAR, 1994) do not claim their entitled benefits is perhaps indicative of the perceived complexity of the system.

The financial benefits are subject to constant review and changes. The exact details of current benefits and the amounts payable are available from the Department of Social Security and leaflets widely available from post offices, libraries, etc.

One benefit which does warrant mentioning specifically is the Incapacity Benefit introduced in April 1995 which has replaced Sickness Benefit and Invalidity Benefit. It encompasses a new system of assessing an individual's ability to work: the 'all work' test.

Incapacity for work is defined as being 'by reason of some specific disease or bodily or mental disablement' (Robertson, 1995). An individual has to show he or she is incapable of work either through the 'own work' test (ability to do *usual* work) or the 'all work' test (ability to do *any* work). Voluntary work of less than 16 hours per week is allowable and reasonable expenses for that work can be claimed. Therapeutic work can also be carried out for up to 16 hours per week and is defined as helping to 'improve, or to prevent or delay deterioration in, the disease or bodily or mental disablement which causes the incapacity for work'. The work must be on the advice of a doctor and the earnings less than £44 per week.

Some individuals will be deemed incapable of work, for example:

- those in receipt of the higher rate Disability Living Allowance or constant attendance allowance;
- the terminally ill who are not expected to live beyond 6 months;
- those registered blind;
- anyone who is tetraplegic, paraplegic, demented or in a persistent vegetative state.

Others will be exempt from being required to undergo the all work test if a DSS doctor certifies:

- severe learning difficulty;
- a severe and progressive neurological and muscle-wasting disease (e.g. multiple sclerosis);
- active and progressive inflammatory arthritis;
- progressive impairment of the cardio-respiratory system which limits effort tolerance;
- dense paralysis of the upper limb, trunk and lower limb on one side of the body;
- multiple effects of impairment of the function of the brain or nervous system causing severe motor, sensory and intellectual deficit;
- severe mental illness;
- severe and progressive immune deficiency states.

The 'own work' test is applicable where someone has been recently employed and is now claiming to be unfit to work and the 'all work' test applies after 28 weeks of incapacity or where someone has not recently been in employment. As listed above, people with active and progressive inflammatory arthritis, certified by a DSS doctor, are exempt from the 'all work' test. The decision to exempt someone is made only where there is sufficient information. Where there is not, the 'all work' test will be applied and the individual will complete a questionnaire about his or her medical condition and its effects on his or her capacity to do any work. The questionnaire covers the ability to carry out a range of tasks and a medical statement from the general practitioner is also submitted. A points system operated by the DSS determines whether the test is 'passed'. The decision is made by the adjudicating officer and a right to appeal exists. A further medical examination may be required before the final decision is made.

> I get invalidity benefits. They keep changing what they call it. When I changed to invalidity benefit I cried all day – the word upset me so much. What was wrong with sickness benefit? It took me a long time to get over it.

> I had to fight for the Orange Badge because I could walk 100 yards – but I can't carry anything.

> I only got the Disability Allowance a few months ago – when all my savings had gone. No one told me what I could get.

> I found out about all the benefits by chance. I didn't know these things existed until I went for my gold injection and happened to ask the nurse about the Orange Badge.

> The offer of voluntary redundancy came and it seemed like the answer. I didn't have to go through all the hassle of going on health grounds – I just took my money and went. Then I began to run into problems claiming benefits.

Who Benefits?

The disability employment adviser (DEA) has a specific role in helping and advising people with a disability who wish to continue in, or return to, work. They work alongside the Client Advisers at the job centre and are part of the placing, assessment and counselling team (PACT), providing professional advice and support in assessing abilities and employment potential. The team can carry out a full assessment, contact local employers to discuss an individual's problems and suitability for a given vacancy, organise the trial of either a particular post or equipment to help in a particular job. They might also assess and advise on ways of making a current job easier to maintain. Advice on further training might be applicable, or even sheltered employment. Anyone with a disability should have access to help and advice.

It appears that, despite the potential benefits consulting a disability employment adviser might bring, relatively few people do so (Helliwell, 1995). A survey conducted in Norfolk in 1993 as part of a larger research study (BLAR, 1994) looking at access to services amongst people with a range of rheumatic conditions resulting in severe disability also found that many were unaware of the existence of the DEA.

From June 1994 a range of services available to people with disabilities and their employers was extended and simplified under the 'Access to Work' programme. It provides practical help and advice for people who have disabilities and also for their employers, by contributing towards:

- a support worker if someone needs practical help either at work or for getting to work;
- equipment (or adaptations to existing equipment) to suit individual needs;
- adaptations to a car, or taxi fares or other transport costs if someone cannot use public transport to get to work;
- alterations to premises or a working environment so that an employee with a disability can work there.

It would appear that a comprehensive system is available to those people who develop a chronic disabling illness, a system that will allow them to remain gainfully employed, assessing and meeting their needs in the workplace and advising and supporting both the individual and the employer.

Where continuation of employment is no longer feasible despite aids and advice, a benefits system offers financial assistance.

> I saw the DEA – the office was upstairs. He will come down and see you in the reception area but it's pride – you have to ask them to come down. I explained what was involved in RA and he told me there was nothing really I could do. If somebody had left work and gone there it would have knocked them straight back and left them with no hope.
>
> I found myself a part time job in the local shop.

People with newly diagnosed RA seem to be facing particular problems in that the assumption is made that current aggressive medical treatments will prevent joint damage and that they as individuals will, in due course, resume their normal occupation. Whilst this may be the case for some it is a sweeping assumption to make and every case should be considered on its own merits. Many never make contact with the DEA and few know of the Access to Work scheme. The whole subject of financial assistance and the new incapacity benefit highlights the problem of whether everyone should be entitled to long-term benefits unless proved otherwise – or the converse with everyone being entitled to work unless proved to the contrary.

There are countless anecdotes of those whom the system has failed, where the reality does not always tally with the rhetoric.

> I used to employ blokes in the garage and would always go for the ones I could rely on. The job needed doing. It didn't matter how sympathetic I felt – if they couldn't keep going they were no use to me. Then I got it [RA] and then I knew what it was like from the other side. I just couldn't do the job any more so I went off sick and then I registered as unemployed. I looked for a job for 2 years but no one would take me on and I don't blame them – I knew what their problems were. You spend your life going to the doctor's or the hospital for appointments and X-rays and blood tests. I'm never at home and when I am I'm shattered. The job people suggested I went off long-term sick because it would be easier for all of us but I didn't like it. I still thought there was something I could do. They told me I couldn't see the special employment chap [DEA] because I was long-term sick. What are they for? Eventually they sent me on a computer training course. I stuck it for 2 weeks. They wanted me to work and learn on the job for £10 a week just for the experience. I don't need that sort of experience. I used to have YTS lads. I know all about cheap labour. (male, aged 49)

It could be argued that if, in addition to the current statutory assistance available, discrimination in the workplace were to be banished then those people with chronic disabling illnesses would find getting and keeping work easier. One of the areas addressed by the 1995 Disability Discrimination Act (HMSO, 1995), due to be introduced over a number of years, is that of employment. The stated aim of the Act is to end the discrimination faced by people with disabilities and, in employment terms, it will apply to employers who employ more than 20 people. Smaller firms will be expected to follow good practice guidelines. The Act does not apply to operational staff employed in the armed forces, the police, the prison service, the fire service or to anyone employed on board ships, hovercrafts or aeroplanes.

The specific measures covering employment will mean that:

- Employers will have to take reasonable measures to ensure that they are not discriminating against disabled people. It will be against the law for an employer to treat a disabled person any less favourably that anyone else on the basis of their disability unless there is a good reason and this will apply to all employment matters: recruitment, training, promotion and dismissal.
- Employers will have to consider what changes they could make in the workplace or the job to help a disabled person actually do

the job. They will then be expected to make those changes but can consider the costs and benefits in deciding what steps it is reasonable to take.

- Trade unions, trade associations and professional bodies will also have to treat disabled people no less favourably than others.
- Employers will still be able to recruit or promote the best person for the job.
- Employers will not be expected to make any changes which would break health and safety laws.

Where people with disabilities feel themselves to have been discriminated against they will be able to have their complaint heard by an industrial tribunal. They will no longer have to register as disabled and employers will not be required to employ a quota of registered disabled people.

The impact of such legislation will be closely scrutinised.

Asking the Right Questions

For the person with newly diagnosed RA the first few weeks and months after diagnosis can be anxious ones. The way ahead may seem unclear; no one can predict precisely how or if their disease will progress or gauge the likely level of future disability; well-meaning friends and relatives offer their homespun advice; decisions have to be made about courses of treatment, the potential side-effects of which can be frightening; employers want to know about the future.

Not everyone feels able to be outspoken at work about their arthritis, fearing it could have a detrimental effect on their future employment

> We knew they were looking for redundancies. You didn't dare go off sick because of all the redundancies coming. You never knew who was going to be laid off next. I got laid off in spring 1990. It's possible the arthritis had something to do with it but I couldn't prove it.

Others feel able to discuss their problems and anticipate a positive response.

> I tell everybody. It's easier if they know. They can't help if they don't know. I tell them I can't do it – they must help me. It's easier to be straight about it.

Patients will often experience their most disabling episodes early on, before they have had time to adjust and adapt and, thinking this will be their permanent state, opt out of the workforce even before full treatment has been instituted.

> I finished work one lunchtime – I wasn't well. Then I came into hospital and haven't been back to work since.

Patients should be encouraged to ask questions about continuing to work at a very early stage, before taking any irrevocable decision. They need to discuss with their doctor the possible course of their disease in the light of the treatment instituted and how long it will be before the chosen treatment reaches its optimal effect.

They must also discuss the interaction between their arthritis and the demands of their employment:

- Is the work manual or sedentary?
- What level of manual dexterity is required?
- Is the job very physically demanding?
- Can the hours of work be altered (e.g. starting late to accommodate early morning stiffness)
- Can certain elements of the job be delegated?
- Can they plan more changes of activity during the day?
- Are there times for rest?
- What is the exact pattern of the joint involvement? (e.g. hands or feet)
- Is fatigue a particular problem?

The individual needs to decide just how important work is, first in terms of finance:

- Are they supporting a family?
- Are they the main income earner in the family?
- Is their income essential to the family finances?

The second consideration is the psychological benefits – the rewards and status. These factors may help determine whether or not patients wish to continue in work or whether they would prefer not to work at all. Some may feel that, on balance, working fewer hours would improve their overall ability to cope both inside and outside work.

The issue of employment has to be seen within the context of a review of the whole family which involves not just financial considerations but also the change in family dynamics. A change in the prime earner may be acceptable in some families but not others. Some well partners might be willing to increase their working hours to counterbalance a decrease in the hours of the ill partner because of the RA. There are no 'right' answers but it is essential that individuals have at their disposal all the information they need on which to base their decision and that the final decision is one which they can feel comfortable with even though it may not be ideal.

Discussing future employment with an employer or immediate manager is not always easy and much will depend on the manager's understanding of RA and how accurate and realistic that understanding is.

> The boss's father has RA. I felt he understood because he had seen it. He was prepared to keep the job open for 12 months. The boss understands how variable it is.

Although personal experience can be invaluable there is the danger that it is biased and too pessimistic leading to inappropriate decisions or even discrimination.

Patients admitted to a rheumatology department for assessment early in the course of their disease have the advantage of ready access to specialist staff who can help answer the detailed questions necessary to make the decision about work. They are also able to talk to other patients, some of whom will already have been through the same process. At this stage joining a self-help group or taking part in an arthritis education programme can give the opportunity to confront the issues involved in a supportive environment.

As has been described earlier in this chapter, the disability employment adviser is available to discuss and offer assistance. Many patients will not have had reason to be in contact with a Job Centre and will therefore not be aware of the existence of the DEA, but making contact with the PACT team should prove beneficial to both employee and employer. Where financial concerns exist, or where a change in employment status is being considered, it is vital that advice is sought from the Department of Social Security before any decision is made.

The nurse who comes into contact with patients suffering from any form of arthritis, and in whatever setting, has the responsibility along with other health professionals to ensure that patients know where to seek advice and information and even, when necessary, to help formulate the questions to be asked. Any newly diagnosed chronic illness gives rise to stress because the future suddenly becomes uncertain. Making fundamental decisions at such a time is not ideal, particularly when only limited information is available on which to base the decision. It may not be the right time to take decisions about employment but sadly many patients often find themselves pressured into doing so at this point. Reassuring patients that a final decision does not have to be made so early is very important: such decisions can and should be delayed. The level of disability may alter, for better or worse, in a few short months and they may then feel very differently about working or not, as the case may be.

It may, on occasions, be appropriate to prompt or act as the patient's advocate in introducing the topic of employment into a consultation or discussion. It may simply be a case of suggesting the topic is raised at the next clinic appointment or, alternatively, helping the patient to write a list of questions to ask or giving telephone numbers of agencies to contact. The ultimate decision is clearly the patient's but it is essential that the nurse is satisfied that the decision is an informed one and that all possible sources of information and help have been utilised and the appropriate questions asked.

Work is fundamental to a large proportion of people. A disease which strikes at a time when many would expect to be employed and which brings into question the continuation of employment has to be confronted. Nurses are involved with patients throughout their illness and as such are in a central position to guide and direct questions and concerns appropriately.

Case Study

Mrs C, aged 53, was an accounts clerk for over 20 years. She was diagnosed as having RA in January 1992. She was finding it difficult to make the decision about giving up work and had been advised by a social worker to make notes about how she felt as well as the advantages and disadvantages of continuing to work. She found his exercise very beneficial. She kept the notes she made at the time.

On giving up work

1. For staying at work

- Earning money.
- The company (not always good).
- Being employed and feeling some status.

- Job satisfaction.
- Keeping the brain active and busy.
- The dignity in life of being employed.

2. Against staying at work

- Long days – an early start at 8 a.m.
- Total lack of energy after 2 to 3 hours' work – MUST sleep but nowhere to rest or sleep. Plus, stiff and aching joints after rest – slow to get started again.
- Problems climbing stairs – need to do stairs at work plus long walk from car park.
- Sitting for long hours at desk, followed by problems moving about.
- Pressure and stress when busy – can I cope?
- Long periods of writing causes major aches and pains in arm and wrist.
- Could I use a computer keyboard for up to 6 hours a day?
- Problems lifting and moving files, books, boxes, etc.
- Holding phone for long periods.
- Could I cope on bad days? Would I need to go off sick? (NEVER off sick.)
- Could I put up with Radio 1 all day?!
- Could I cope with the draught from the open windows which others will not allow me to close?
- Lack of heating in the office.
- Use scooter to go to work – could I ride it again and get warm when I get to work?
- Could I be ready to leave home at 7.45 a.m. every morning? I can't get going in the mornings.
- Could I ride my scooter in bad weather and can I control it in all hazards?
- I would need to rest/sleep ALL weekend to get ready to go back to work on Monday.
- I would have NO social life.
- I never feel well.
- Once I get worn out I cope less well with the aches and pains.
- I wouldn't have the energy to do any housework or meals. I would be exhausted in the evenings.
- No time for my grandchildren and animals (fingers hurt after writing this).
- Would I become as stressed and worried as before if I couldn't

cope? Would I start to make mistakes? Would I suffer from lack of concentration again?

- I would always be struggling to catch up.
- I don't want to be a liability to other staff on bad days or have to take time off.

Notes

I have now found peace of mind in leading life at a slower pace. Making a decision on my job is a problem that won't solve itself.

My right hand especially keeps giving me my answers but I won't recognize them.

May 1992

The boss has been to see me and given me notice of dismissal on 14 August. He said I would become a burden to workmates and a liability to him or his colleagues. He felt I would become as ill again as I was in the last weeks at work. He was most kind. I feel great sadness.

References

Barbellion WNP (1919) The Journal of a Disappointed Man. Guernsey, Channel Islands: Guernsey Press.

Berthoud R (1994) Incapacity Benefit: How Will the New Medical Assessment Work? London: Policy Studies Institute.

British League Against Rheumatism (BLAR) (1994) Disability and Arthritis. London: BLAR.

Callahan LF Pincus T (1988) Formal education level as a marker of clinical status in rheumatoid arthritis. Arthritis and Rheumatism 31: 1346–57.

Colledge M, Bartholomew R (1980) A Study of Long-term Unemployed. Sheffield: Manpower Services Commission. Cited in Smith, R (1985) A doctor's guide to the facts and figures of unemployment. British Medical Journal 291(19 October).

Doeglas D, Suurmeijer T, Krol B, Sanderman R, Leeuwen M, Rijswijk M (1995) Work disability in early rheumatoid arthritis. Annals of the Rheumatic Diseases 54: 455–60.

Haber LD (1971) Disabling effects of chronic disease and impairment. Journal of Chronic Diseases 24: 469–87.

Helliwell PS (1995) Employment status of patients in rheumatology outpatients clinics. Letter to the editor. British Journal of Rheumatology 34(7): 693.

Hewlett S (1994) Patients' views of changing disability. Nursing Standard 8(31): 25–9.

HMSO (1993) Department of Social Security Statistics. London: HMSO.

HMSO (1995) A brief guide to the Disability Discrimination Act. London: HMSO.

James D, Cox N, Davies P, Devlin J, Dixie J, Emery P, Gallivans S, Gough A, Prouse P, Williams P, Winfield J, Young A (1995) Major life events as a result of rheumatoid arthritis. A comparison between nine centres in 446 patients in the first three years of disease. British Journal of Rheumatology 34 (Suppl.2): 9.

Leigh J, Fries J (1991) Education level and rheumatoid arthritis: evidence from five data centres. Journal of Rheumatology 18(1): 24–34.

Meenan RF, Yelin E, Nevitt M, Epstein W (1981) The impact of chronic disease. Arthritis and Rheumatism 24(3): 544–9.

Minor MA, Hewett JE.(1995) Physical fitness and work capacity in women with RA. Arthritis Care Research 8(3):146–54.

Pincus T, Callahan LF, Sale W, Brooks AL, Payne L, Vaughn WK (1984) Severe functional declines, work disability, and increased mortality in seventy-five rheumatoid arthritis patients studied over nine years. Arthritis and Rheumatism 27(8): 864–72.

Reisine S, Grady K, Goodenow C, Fifield J (1989) Work disability among women with rheumatoid arthritis. Arthritis and Rheumatism 32(5): 538–43.

Reisine S, McQuillan J, Fifield J (1995) Predictors of work disability in rheumatoid arthritis patients. Arthritis and Rheumatism 38(11): 1620–7.

Robertson S (1995) Disability Rights Handbook. London: Disability Alliance.

Singer E (1974) Premature social ageing: the social-psychological consequences of a chronic illness. Social Science and Medicine 18: 143–51.

Straaton K, Maisiak R, Wrigley M, White M, Johnson P, Fine P (1996) Barriers to return to work among persons unemployed due to arthritis and musculoskeletal disorders. Arthritis and Rheumatism 39(1): 101–9.

Verbrugge LM (1983) Multiple roles and physical health of women and men. Journal of Health and Social Behaviour 24: 16–31.

Yelin E, Katz PP (1991) Labour force participation among persons with musculoskeletal conditions 1970–1987. Arthritis and Rheumatism 34(11): 1361–70.

Yelin E, Henke C, Epstein W (1986) Work disability among persons with musculoskeletal conditions. Arthritis and Rheumatism 11: 1322–33.

Yelin E, Meenana R, Nevitt M, Epstein W (1980) Work disability in rheumatoid arthritis: effects of disease, social and work factors. Annals of the Rheumatic Diseases 95(3): 551–6.

Chapter 12
Osteoporosis: its significance in rheumatoid disease

MARGARET-ANN VOYCE

Introduction

Osteoporosis is recognised by the World Health Organisation (WHO) as a major worldwide health-care problem. An imbalance between bone resorption (removal) and bone formation (replacement) eventually results in osteoporosis. Osteoporosis is 'characterised by a low bone mass and a micro-architectural deterioration of bone tissue leading to an enhanced bone fragility and a consequent increase in risk of fracture' (WHO [1994] definition). The word 'osteoporosis' means porous bones. The bones maintain their shape but contain less calcium in a network of collagen fibre. They become thinner and more brittle and consequently often fracture with a minimum amount of trauma. The calcium phosphate mineral gives strength and hardness to the bones and the collagen fibres give a certain amount of flexibility. Bones also contain fluoride, sodium, potassium and magnesium citrate.

Osteoporosis is a silent insidious disease which does not cause symptoms until a fracture occurs. It accompanies the ageing process. Patients with this condition present at the rheumatology department with a chronic disease causing disability, much misery and pain and a resulting loss of independence. Though this disease can be prevented and treated, it cannot be cured.

Epidemiology

As the population ages, one in three postmenopausal women, mostly over the age of 65, and one in two women, mostly over the age of 70 are affected. According to the National Osteoporosis Society (NOS, 1993) literature, the disease causes 60 000 hip fractures, 50 000 wrist fractures and 100 000 other fractures annually, 40 000 of which are clinically diagnosed vertebral fractures, and only one-third of vertebral fractures are clinically apparent. Two million people in the UK suffer from this bone disease by the age of 65. Osteoporosis cost the National Health Service approximately £742 million in nursing and social care in 1994, according to the DHSS (1994) Report of the Advisory Group on Osteoporosis, and it has a significant impact on the mortality and the morbidity of the nation.

Bone Growth and Remodelling

Bone is a living tissue constantly being renewed throughout life. This allows one to grow and the skeleton to be repaired if it is fractured, damaged or weakened, and to respond to any physical stress which may occur. The skeleton is made up of 206 separate bones which support and protect the body; 20 per cent of the skeleton is trabecular meshwork bone and 80 per cent is cortical tubular bones, the proportion varying from site to site.

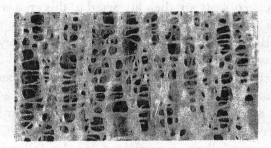

Normal Bone

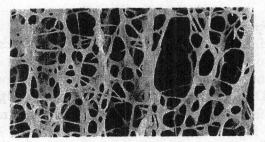

Osteoporotic Bone

Figure 12.1. Showing the difference between normal bone and osteoporotic bone. Reproduced with kind permission of the National Osteoporosis Society

The active cells involved in bone remodelling are known as osteo-clasts. These are multinucleate and they resorb calcified bone and cartilage and remove degraded material by dissolving the mineral out of the bone; subsequently the collagen, which is the matrix within the bone, breaks down. If these cells become overactive then the bone will be lost and osteoporosis results.

Osteoblasts form new bone by laying down the matrix of collagen fibres into which calcium salts are then deposited. These strengthen the bone. The osteoblasts are more active in the growing phase of life. Normally bone resorption and formation are balanced and bone mass is maintained, but if the osteoblasts are relatively inactive then not enough new bone will be laid down and osteoporosis results.

Osteocytes are more mature osteoblasts. They are trapped within the calcified bone and they lie on the surface. These detect and respond to information about local stresses applied to the bone and they modify bony absorption and formation. They regulate the amount of calcium between the bone and the blood and are impor-tant in the nutrition and maintenance of normal bone.

Bone remodelling starts with a period of resorption lasting approximately two weeks when osteoclasts invade and erode an area of bone. Osteoblasts are then attracted to this area where new bone matrix is being deposited and mineralised over the next three months. Bone resorption and formation is delicately balanced and bone mass is maintained, reaching its peak around 30 years of age after which there is a slow decline at 0.3 per cent per year until the menopause when it is estimated women experience a rapid period of bone loss at approximately 3 per cent per year. Women have usually lost 30 per cent of bone mass by the age of 70 (Woolf, 1994).

Bone remodelling is regulated by the following circulating hormones:

- *Parathyroid hormone:* This regulates the amount of calcium in the blood. If there is a deficiency of this hormone then vitamin D cannot be converted into an active form and consequently it cannot be absorbed by the intestine from the food. Without vita-min D new bone cannot be mineralised properly, therefore if the level falls too low extra parathyroid hormone is made, if the level is too high then more calcitonin is made.
- *Calcitonin:* Calcitonin is released by the thyroid gland to balance the effects of parathyroid hormone and activated vitamin D so as to maintain constant levels of calcium in the blood. Men have higher circulating levels of calcitonin than women.

- *Growth hormone:* This is especially active in the early years and is produced by the pituitary gland. The effect of this hormone is controlled by hormones in the liver and conveyed by the blood-stream to the growing areas.
- *Oestrogen and progesterone:* Oestrogen is produced in the first part of the menstrual cycle and progesterone in the second half. Oestrogen slows down the resorption of bone and it aids the absorption of calcium from the food in the intestine. Oestrogen is essential for full bone-cell health. Oestrogen protects the bone against parathyroid hormones and raises the level of calcium. Following the menopause, levels of this hormone fall dramatically. All that is formed in post-menopausal women is from the conversion of androgen in the fatty tissue so therefore the adipose tissue protects women against osteoporosis. Premature deficiency of oestrogen leads to osteoporosis.
- *Testosterone:* This is produced by men in the testes and protects and maintains the strength in the bones in males. Testosterone production in men is only lost slowly over the years. Any premature deficiency leads to osteoporosis.
- *Adrenal glands:* Corticosteroids are made in these glands. Without these hormones the body cannot respond to stresses of infection. An increase of this hormone produces an illness called Cushing's syndrome. Corticosteroids are used therapeutically in inflammatory diseases. An excess results in osteoporosis and fracture. This is through the action of various mechanisms, direct and indirect, on the bone cells.

Types of bone tissue

- *Cortical bone:* This is dense and solid and forms the tube of long bones.
- *Trabecular bone:* This is the filigree-like structure inside many bones. It looks like a honeycomb and is more porous and found mostly in the vertebrae, pelvis and at the ends of long bones. It has a greater surface area and is therefore metabolically more active, the turnover rate being approximately ten times greater than in the cortical bones. Trabecular bone is lost rapidly during the female menopause, whilst both men and women lose cortical bone slowly after the mid-life.

The bone matrix contains protein called collagen, which takes the form of fibres. These are very strong and form a quarter of the bone structure. Other proteins in the bone help to keep the bone mineral crystals of calcium, phosphate and water attached to the fibres of the collagen within the bone. The deposition of the minerals in the bones is called mineralisation.

Types and Causes of Osteoporosis

Bone mass at any age results from peak bone mass achieved during growth and adolescence, the age at which onset of loss begins and the rate at which bone is lost. 80 per cent of peak bone mass is genetically determined, but the achievement of this peak is also influenced by factors such as diet, physical exercise and each individual's hormonal environment. Low peak bone mass, early onset of loss or rapid rate of loss can all lead to osteoporosis (Bhalla, 1993).

Primary idiopathic

Postmenopausal women 10–15 years after the menopause experience fractures of the distal radius and vertebrae. This relates to the rapid loss of bone mass at the menopause which may be as great as 5–6 per cent per annum due to oestrogen deficiency. The earlier the menopause, the more years of postmenopausal bone loss and the greater the risk of low bone mass and fracture in later life.

Senile osteoporosis

Men and women experience vertebral and hip fractures in later life. This relates to a gradual age-related bone loss, which in women is on top of their rapid postmenopausal bone loss.

Secondary causes

Secondary causes are those associated with other disorders. These include:

- endocrine disorders;
- connective tissue disorders;
- immobilisation;
- liver, bowel and kidney disease;
- drug related, e.g. corticosteroids, heparin;
- malignancy;
- gastric surgery; post-transplantation.

Endocrine disorders: These include hyperthyroidism, hyperparathyroidism and, particularly in men, hypogonadism (reduced male sex hormone levels), Turner's and Cushing's syndrome.

Connective tissue disorders: These include rare conditions such as Marfan's syndrome, Ehlers-Danlos syndrome, and osteogenesis imperfecta.

Immobilisation: This can be due to illness such as a stroke, multiple sclerosis or local immobilisation due to limbs being in plaster.

Liver, bowel and kidney disease: These conditions interfere with the absorption of calcium and vitamin D.

Drug related: This includes prolonged therapy with corticosteroids, heparin, anti-convulsants, thyroxine and alcohol.

Malignancy: For example, conditions such as myeloma, leukaemia and lymphoma.

Gastric surgery and post-transplantation: For example, cardiac or liver.

Risk Factors Contributing to Osteoporosis

Endogenous risk factors

- sex – women;
- race;
- genetic.

According to the recent report of the Advisory Group on Osteoporosis (DHSS, 1994) 45 per cent of women have strong risk factors, but only 20 per cent think they are at risk. Women are generally more at risk than men because, on average, they live longer, are smaller-boned and they have extra demands on their calcium levels during pregnancy and lactation.

Caucasian and Asian populations suffer a higher incidence of osteoporosis than do Afro-Caribbeans who have denser skeletons (Campbell, Compston and Crisp, 1993). A family history of a mother or grandmother with osteoporosis also carries a risk.

Exogenous risk factors

- amenorrhoea;
- lifestyle;
- drugs;
- disease.

Amenorrhoea for more than six months in premenopausal women suffering from anorexia nervosa or bulimia, female athletes in training, ballet dancers and gymnasts, all have low oestrogen levels. Women who have had a premenopausal bilateral oophorectomy are at risk. Women who have experienced a late onset of menstruation (menarche) have a lower peak bone mass than those who have an early menarche (DHSS, 1994).

Lifestyle carries its own risk factors. Women who smoke sometimes experience an earlier menopause than non-smokers and they also tend to have a lower body weight. Passive smokers suffer the same disadvantage. Excessive alcohol intake, over 14 units per week for women and over 21 units per week for men, is associated with osteoporosis. Poor diet in childhood and during later life, particularly a deficiency in calcium and vitamin D, can precipitate osteoporosis. Slimmers often lack a nutritionally balanced diet. Lack of physical activity, especially in the elderly, can increase the risk of osteoporosis.

Drugs: A prolonged course of corticosteroids administered for conditions such as rheumatoid arthritis and asthma can cause osteoporosis. The damage done is related to the dose given and the duration of the treatment. It also depends on the age and sex of the patient. An 80-year-old patient with polymyalgia rheumatica taking 10 mg of prednisolone daily could be more at risk than a 30-year-old man treated for psoriasis on a dose twice as great.

Patients who have received heart and liver transplants and who are prescribed immunosuppressant drugs and corticosteroids are at risk of osteoporosis.

Patients on long-term maintenance doses of heparin are also at risk, together with patients receiving thyroxine on a long-term basis for hypothyroidism.

Anti-convulsant drugs can precipitate this disease as they can affect the metabolism and the absorption of oestrogen, and it can also arise when bone cells are destroyed following radiation treatment and chemotherapy.

Disease: Patients with diseases such as a chronic inflammatory bowel disease, kidney disease, chronic liver failure, myeloma, hypothyroidism and those who have had a gastrectomy are sometimes unable to absorb calcium and this has an effect on bone density. Rare conditions, such as Cushing's syndrome, osteogenesis imperfecta, hypogonadism in men or Crohn's disease, all carry the risk of osteoporosis.

Symptoms of Established Osteoporosis

Symptoms are related to a fracture. Most vertebral fractures are asymptomatic, but approximately one-third result in spontaneous severe back pain radiating around the thorax and abdomen. Chronic back pain sometimes results with pain often experienced on

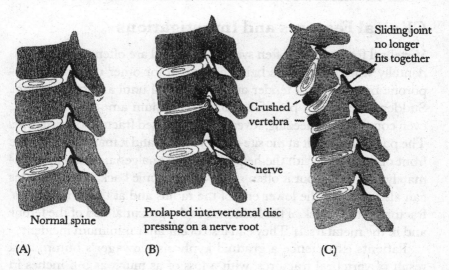

Sliding joint no longer fits together

Crushed vertebra

nerve

Normal spine

Prolapsed intervertebral disc pressing on a nerve root

(A) (B) (C)

Figure 12.2. Crush fracture

standing and resting. Chronic pain in the neck, due to hyperextension of the neck, occurs with chronic vertebral osteoporosis.

Breathlessness can occur due to the lungs being squashed inwards within the rib cage, with the result that the lungs are unable to expand. Patients can suffer from indigestion and acid reflux due to the stomach being moved upwards into the chest; this can also result in loss of appetite.

Patients complain of 'being fat' due to loss of space between the ribs and the pelvic brim causing the abdomen to protrude forward – the use of a corset makes the symptoms worse! In extreme cases patients complain of pain due to friction between the lower ribs and the pelvic brim. There is little room for the bladder in the pelvis and stress incontinence results.

Pain radiating from the spine to the chest affects the arms and this makes personal hygiene difficult as patients are unable to lift their arms. Communication is sometimes difficult due to extreme kyphosis, as the head may drop forward onto the chest and eye contact is then lost.

There can be loss of confidence, particularly following falls and fractures, which often results in reduced activity, insomnia and depression resulting in low self-esteem. Alteration in body shape causes embarrassment and distress. Because of their clothes not fitting properly, sufferers avoid going out and as a result they often lack vitamin D which makes their osteoporosis worse, and in addition they become isolated.

Clinical Features and Investigations

Vertebral fractures are often symptomless and are often revealed accidentally when X-rays are being examined for other reasons. Osteoporotic bones are not tender and feel normal until a fracture occurs. Sudden severe back pain following a minimum amount of trauma, even coughing or sneezing, reveals a compressed fracture of vertebrae. The pain may be felt at the site of the fracture and it may radiate to the front of the body. With the help of rest and analgesia, it lasts approximately 6–8 weeks but it often settles into chronic backache. Fractures can also occur at the lower end of the radius and at the wrist (Colles' fracture), at the neck of the humerus, at the proximal end of the femur and in the metatarsals. They can also occur after minimum incident.

Patients experience a gradual kyphosis (dowager's hump) as a result of vertebral fractures, with a loss of as much as 5-6 inches in height, plus progressive spinal deformity accompanied by gradual onset of backache.

Pain is often experienced when standing and resting. Because of poor posture the patient's head protrudes, and it is difficult for the patient to hold the head up and this causes complaints of painful neck muscles.

Investigations

Investigations are to confirm osteoporosis, to exclude other causes of bone pain and fracture and to look for causes of osteoporosis.

Imaging

- plain X-ray to confirm fracture;
- bone densitometry to confirm osteoporosis;
- bone scan to exclude metastases.

Biochemical markers for the assessment of bone turnover

There is a new assay to measure the urinary excretion of free deoxypyridinoline (Dpd) as an improved assessment of bone resorption rate. At present it is not generally available except at approved centres. It is said to be useful to identify and monitor patients at risk of significant bone loss. Timely intervention can then be provided with antiresorptive therapy, for example HRT, alendronate sodium and etidronate disodium. It is maintained that the assay will show patients' response as early as one month after the start of effective therapy (Robins et al., 1994).

Pathology

- alkaline phosphatase to exclude myeloma and metastases;
- calcium (corrected) plus alkaline phosphatase to exclude osteo-malacia or primary hyperparathyroidism;
- thyroid and liver function tests for underlying dysfunction;
- plasma biochemical profile to exclude metastases;
- serum testosterone in men, which may identify undetected hypogonadism;
- immunoelectrophoresis of serum and urine to exclude myeloma;
- ESR or plasma viscosity to exclude multiple myeloma or skeletal metastases.

Biochemical markers of bone formation and resorption are research tools at present.

Clinical Indications for Bone Densitometry

The bone mineral content in a bone should be measured in patients with:

(1) oestrogen deficiency due to amenorrhoea or early menopause (natural or surgical);
(2) vertebral deformity or low trauma fractures;
(3) osteopenia noted on X-rays;
(4) patients on long-term steroid therapy; and
(5) to quantify bone loss in other forms of secondary osteoporosis, e.g. anorexia nervosa or hypogonadism;
(6) to monitor therapy for osteoporosis; useful every 12–24 months;
(7) to identify those at risk such as those with a family history of osteoporosis;
(8) to diagnose osteoporosis when suspected.

The Various Types of Bone Density Measurement

Radiography (X-rays)

These are necessary to detect the presence of a fracture. Osteoporosis cannot be diagnosed with certainty as there are other causes of bones appearing porous on a plain X-ray such as osteomalacia. In addition, standard X-rays are not sensitive enough, as 30 per cent of bone mineral content can be lost from the bone before it is apparent. X-rays provide limited information and radiation exposure is high, which limits the frequency of measurements. Although it is the most readily available technique it is not good enough to assess osteoporosis.

Quantitative computerised tomography (QCT)

This is an X-ray technique which uses a computerised image processor to produce cross-sectional images of a slice through the bone. This gives a detailed examination of the bone and surrounding tissues. This method is expensive and patients are exposed to higher doses of radiation, and therefore the area scanned is restricted and the procedure cannot be repeated frequently. The scan is painless but patients must lie still in the tunnel of the machine.

Dual photon absorptiometry (DPA)

Useful for providing bone density measurements of deep sites of the hip and spine but this has been superseded by the DEXA.

Dual-energy X-ray absorptiometry (DEXA)

This is a safe, non-invasive procedure using a low dose of radiation. It is an accurate and reliable method of measuring bone density. This method is usually used to measure the bone density of the lumbar spine, usually the second, third and fourth lumbar vertebrae, and the proximal femur.

An X-ray tube emits an X-ray beam with two different energies. Detectors identify these two separate beams and can differentiate between bone and other tissues. The height and weight of patients are recorded. Patients lie on the couch and the radiographer scans the lumbar spine and the non-dominant hip. This takes approximately 20 minutes and uses one-sixth of the radiation level of a chest X-ray. During the scan the radiographer can ask patients about their lifestyle and diet, and advise accordingly. The results are compared with those from a normal population, and present and future risk of fracture can be estimated. Treatment recommendations can be based on this.

Results

These are quoted as BMC (bone mineral content). This is the actual amount of calcium, measured in grams, present in the area of interest. The BMD (bone mineral density) is the amount of calcium in grams/cm^2 (see Figure 12.3). This gives a measurement comparable between patients and their separate scans. The BMD is then quoted as a Z score and a T score. These can be expressed as a standard deviation or as a percentage. Z scores compare the result with the

BMD of scanned adults of the same age and sex. T scores compare the result with the BMD of young, normal and healthy adults aged between 22 and 30 years, of the same sex.

If the bone mass is 2.5 standard deviations below the expected peak bone mass (T score >2.5), then the patient has osteoporosis and treatment is recommended. The lower the bone mass is below the mean T score, the more likely the patient is to benefit from preventive therapy. (Young adult bone mass = T score 0). See Figure 12.3. This patient is not at risk of osteoporosis and therefore does not require treatment.

Ultrasound

This measures density of sound waves as they pass through bones. It is non-invasive, portable and relatively inexpensive. It is said heel ultrasound may well predict fracture at different sites as well as DEXA and in some cases better. This technique is still being evaluated, and is still considered a research tool. Its greatest value will lie in its use as a screening tool for use in general practice.

Osteoporotic Fractures

Osteoporotic fractures can occur when the bone mass is reduced enough to cause a fracture, either:

(1) through minimal trauma, sneezing, coughing, lifting or normal movement;
(2) spontaneously;
(3) as the result of a fall.

Osteoporotic fractures cause pain, disability and often loss of independence.

Spinal fractures

These usually occur between the ages of 50 and 70, often spontaneously, and are often not associated with pain. The incidence rate therefore cannot accurately be recorded. The spinal vertebrae are usually rectangular, separated by a 'cushion like' intervertebral disc. There are few nerve endings inside the vertebrae and none in the discs, but plenty on the surface. The vertebrae become porous, weakened and deformed. The front of the bone collapses and becomes wedged. With the weight of the body the spinal vertebrae totally collapse, eventually producing crush fractures. The rib cage often sits

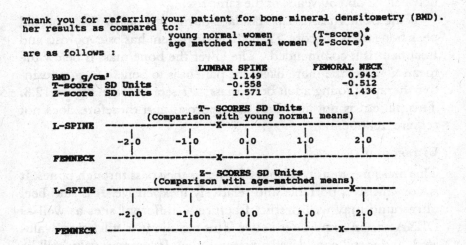

```
Thank you for referring your patient for bone mineral densitometry (BMD).
her results as compared to:
                         young normal women      (T-score)*
                         age matched normal women (Z-Score)*
are as follows :

                              LUMBAR SPINE          FEMORAL NECK
    BMD, g/cm²                   1.149                 0.943
    T-score  SD Units          -0.558                -0.512
    Z-score  SD units           1.571                 1.436

                         T- SCORES SD Units
                  (Comparison with young normal means)
    L-SPINE    ------------------------X------------------------------

                -2.0      -1.0       0.0       1.0       2.0

    FEMNECK    -----------------------X--------------------------------

                         Z- SCORES SD Units
                  (Comparison with age-matched means)
    L-SPINE    ----------------------------------------------X--------

                -2.0      -1.0       0.0       1.0       2.0

    FEMNECK    ---------------------------------------------X----------
```

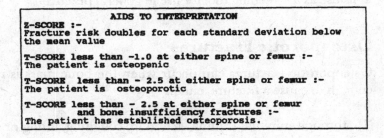

```
                     AIDS TO INTERPRETATION
Z-SCORE :-
Fracture risk doubles for each standard deviation below
the mean value

T-SCORE less than -1.0 at either spine or femur :-
The patient is osteopenic

T-SCORE  less than - 2.5 at either spine or femur :-
The patient is  osteoporotic

T-SCORE less than - 2.5 at either spine or femur
            and bone insufficiency fractures :-
The patient has established osteoporosis.
```

Figure 12.3. Sample result of BMD

on the hip bones at this stage. The spine curves outwards producing a kyphosis and the lower spine tilts inwards producing a lordosis. Patients complain of progressive loss of height and backache. Patients who suffer from a spinal fracture are five times more likely to experience another fracture. Acute vertebral fractures usually cause a sudden onset of severe back pain following minor trauma. The pain worsens with movement. Patients complain of muscle tenderness and spasm. Treatment is with rest and analgesia but mobilisation should start as soon as pain control allows. The severe pain usually improves after 3–4 weeks and the vertebral fractures heal in 3–4 months, but the shape of the vertebrae cannot be restored.

Wrist fractures (Colles' fracture)

These fractures are associated with the winter months, especially during the icy weather when classically a woman of 50+ puts her arm out to save herself from falling. Usually she breaks the neck of the humerus, the distal ulna and radius near the wrist, and a Colles' fracture occurs. Recovery is usually good after a couple of months, but some Colles' fractures cause persistent pain and loss of function. It is a warning that the bones are weak.

Shoulder fracture

Fracture of the proximal humerus is less common and it is difficult to fix, so patients are usually treated with a sling.

Hip fracture

This fracture occurs at the proximal end of the femur. It usually occurs in older people, especially women around 79 years of age, and the overall rate is four times higher in women than in men, but similar in both sexes below the age of 50. This fracture is much more serious and usually heralds a serious physical decline. Approximately 20–30 per cent die within six months and 50 per cent become disabled and unable to walk independently; 20 per cent lose independence (Woolf, 1994). These fractures usually follow a fall and are treated in hospital; either a new hip joint is fitted or the bones are pinned and plated. These patients, occupying orthopaedic beds, often require prolonged hospital admission as a result of the advancing age and post-operative complications.

Pelvic fractures

These are less common but many require prolonged bed rest which leads to loss of function long term.

Rib fractures

Cracked ribs are fairly common and they require little treatment except analgesia.

Male Osteoporosis

One in 10 men will suffer from osteoporosis and this will increase with the growth in an ageing population. By the age of 60, 3 per cent of men suffer from fractures and by the age of 80, 8 per cent of men suffer from fractures. Fewer men suffer from osteoporosis because they tend to have a higher bone mass, as much as 30 per cent greater in maturity, and therefore stronger bones, and they also have larger muscles. They do not have the sudden loss of sex hormones that women experience during the menopause and therefore they have a slower rate of bone loss with ageing. Men do not live as long as women. Many men with osteoporosis have underlying health problems such as hypogonadism, conditions needing long-term steroids, prolonged bed rest and paralysis, and they may have a low testosterone level. Excess smoking, high alcohol intake, little physical activity, low levels of vitamin D and poor calcium absorption can all contribute to osteoporosis. Sufferers complain of loss of height, which can be up to 5 inches, back pain as a result of curvature of the spine which often leads to difficulties in bending, standing and sleeping, and other symptoms include low levels of energy, poor mobility, lack of independence and depression. Among men who suffer from osteoporosis, 20 per cent have hypogonadism. For 45 per cent the cause is idiopathic, for 20 per cent it is steroid induced, and 10 per cent have other health problems. Finally, 5 per cent suffer as a result of excess alcohol or smoking (Frances et al., 1989).

Rare Forms of Osteoporosis

Idiopathic juvenile osteoporosis

This is quite a rare condition and occurs between the ages of 8 and 14 years in the pre-pubertal period. There is a sudden onset of pain in the back, hips and legs, and it is often associated with fractures in the spine and lower extremities. Deformities of the spine are common. The serum calcium and phosphate levels may be higher than those of a child of similar age. No specific treatment is given and both total immobilisation and excessive exercise should be discouraged. The condition is self-limiting and usually remits at puberty.

Osteoporosis in pregnancy

This condition is fairly uncommon during pregnancy. It is most commonly diagnosed during the first pregnancy, but can occur during the second or third pregnancy, the first having been unremarkable. Symptoms occur in the last few weeks of pregnancy and for up to 3 months after. The patient presents with acute pain in the spine and may be hips. The pain so severe that it restricts the ability to cope with a young baby. The treatment is gentle regular exercise plus a well-balanced diet rich in calcium. The condition resolves spontaneously over the course of some months and the women return to an active life.

One underlying condition may be osteogenesis imperfecta diagnosed during childhood, the cause of which is unknown, or the cause may be missed juvenile osteoporosis.

Immobilisation osteoporosis

Osteoporosis can occur as a result of local immobilisation following a fracture. A limb is immobilised in a plaster cast, and after a few weeks bone density is reduced. The bones slowly return to normal following physiotherapy. Similar changes occur in paralysed limbs as a result of poliomyelitis.

Osteoporosis can also occur as a result of prolonged bed rest; for example, in patients confined to bed for several months following a fractured hip.

Post-traumatic osteoporosis or Sudeck's atrophy occurs in a limb, usually a hand, a few weeks after a fracture. The hand becomes painful, stiff, warm and shiny. It usually resolves following active exercises, wax baths and elevation.

Treatment of Osteoporosis

Introduction

The aim of treatment is to prevent fractures from occurring, to reduce pain and disability once fractures have occurred, and to improve the quality of life.

Before treatment begins it is essential to exclude secondary osteoporosis. It is important to explain to the patient the cause and the underlying condition that lead to osteoporosis, which often reduces the fear and anxiety. It is also important to reduce the chronic pain cycle as this produces reduced activity, depression and a feeling of isolation. Regular analgesia may be necessary.

Drugs

Analgesia

Analgesics should be administered according to the severity of the pain. Paracetamol is effective and has few side-effects. Paracetamol plus codeine may be used. Non-steroidal anti-inflammatory drugs are sometimes prescribed, and opiates may be necessary if the pain due to a fracture is severe: fentanyl patches are effective. Local nerve blocks may also help to control the pain.

Hormone replacement therapy (HRT)

HRT, if taken at the menopause or after bilateral oophorectomy, is the most effective preventive therapy against osteoporosis, as once bone mass is lost it cannot be restored to the normal level. This treatment helps to prevent fractures once osteoporosis has developed. All patients, before commencement of HRT, should be told why they are taking it, what it is for, what the side-effects may be and how and when to take it. The benefits of oestrogen therapy have been recognised for 30 years. Epidemiology data show that if HRT is taken for at least 5 years the occurrence of fractures of the wrist, hip and vertebrae are reduced by 50 per cent (NOS, 1993). Bone loss is at its greatest in the early postmenopausal years – 3 per cent per annum – due to increased resorption rather than decreased formation. Loss rates decline to just over 1 per cent every year by 7 years after the menopause (DHSS, 1994). Anti-resorptive drugs play an important part at this time.

Oestrogen is an anti-resorptive agent and when the ovaries cease to produce this hormone at the menopause it is advantageous to replace it with natural oestrogen produced from animals or synthetic oestrogen which has been chemically engineered. There are a number of preparations containing oestrogen and progesterone, and there are different ways to administer it. It should be explained to the patient that finding the correct dosage and route may take a little time!

As a result of increasing life expectancy, women can expect to live over a third of their lives in a postmenopausal state. With HRT the quality of their life can be much improved.

Advantages

Oestrogen prevents atrophic changes in the genito-urinary tract, prevents cardio- and cerebrovascular disease and it is noted that, as a result of this, women live three years longer. It reduces the symptoms of the menopause: hot flushes, night sweats, vaginal dryness, tiredness and depression. Patients should be warned that menstruation may return, but if normal periods have ceased then the patient cannot become fertile.

Disadvantages

HRT can cause bloating, nausea, nipple and breast tenderness and fluid retention, all of which should disappear after a few months. If forewarned, these are usually coped with. Most side-effects resolve with the adjustment of the oestrogen dose, or with the type of progesterone used. HRT should be stopped if severe migrainous headaches or focal headaches are experienced for the first time. Medical advice should be taken if irregular vaginal bleeding occurs whilst taking HRT.

Contraindications

HRT is usually contraindicated in patients who have breast cancer, endometrial cancer or liver disease and those women who have had recent thrombosis. Malignant melanoma, known or suspected pregnancy, undiagnosed vaginal bleeding and endometrial hyperplasia are also reasons for not taking HRT.

Who should take hormone replacement therapy?

All women at risk of osteoporosis should take HRT. This includes those who have experienced an early menopause, whether natural or surgical; those with a history of anorexia or bulimia; women who have been treated with corticosteroids; those who have experienced numerous fractures over the age of 50, and women who have recorded a low bone density measurement following DEXA scan.

Before taking HRT all women should have their blood pressure recorded, a vaginal smear taken and a mammogram should be performed as for normal screening. HRT restores the oestrogen levels prior to the menopause and the therapy should continue for at least 5 years. It can be initiated at any time. The risk of breast cancer is not increased significantly within 5 years of treatment, but after more than 5 years of HRT treatment the risk rises by 25–50 per cent (Colditz et al., 1995). It should be noted that the risk of breast cancer has to be weighed against the risk of osteoporotic fracture, and the benefits have been shown to outweigh the risks.

Women who have not had a hysterectomy should take oestrogen and progesterone administered cyclically, as this prevents the risk of endometrial cancer: oestrogen to control the menopausal symptoms and to protect the bones, plus progesterone, for at least 12 days at the end of the cycle to remove the proliferate endometrium of the uterus, resulting in a menstrual bleed. The minimum of oestrogen to protect the skeleton is 0.625 mg of conjugated equine oestrogen or 2 mg of oestradiol. Now on the market are 'period-free' or 'menstruation-free' preparations of continuous oestrogen and progesterone which are very attractive to older women. These can be used in women a year after their last period.

Continuous oestrogen should be given to women who have had a hysterectomy in the same dose of natural oestrogens as mentioned previously. It should be stressed that natural oestrogens are used in HRT whereas larger doses of synthetic oestrogens are used in oral contraception. Oral preparations are usually well tolerated but some women prefer alternative routes of delivery. A transdermal patch, which is a waterproof hormone-laden patch, is attached to the buttock or abdomen, which allows its contents to be absorbed through the skin directly into the bloodstream. If the patch causes skin irritation it can be changed to a different site every day. Sometimes poor adhesion presents a problem though present patches are much improved on their predecessors.

An oestradiol pelleted implant can be inserted subcutaneously in the abdomen. This is effective for 6 months. Both these methods are beneficial to patients with malabsorption, and often avoid the problem of poor compliance.

An oestrogen gel is now available. It is applied to each upper arm and shoulder, or alternatively each inner thigh, once daily.

Regular monitoring of blood pressure, regular breast examination and, where appropriate, mammography is recommended. Unfortunately the fear of cancer, transient postmenopausal symptoms and menstruation are the main reasons why women only use HRT for a short term. Many believe they are too old and prefer to go through the menopause naturally. A double prescription charge on the combined pill is another disincentive to continue! Patients need information, support and encouragement from doctors and nurses at this stage.

Selective oestrogen receptor modulators (SERMs)

SERMs are a new and novel treatment option for those women who either are unable to take HRT or who would prefer not to, because of fear of developing breast cancer, or because of experiencing well known side effects. Raloxifene is the first agent of this kind and should be licensed in the UK during 1998. The important aspect of this drug, which is a close relative to tamoxifen, an earlier version of a SERM, is that it can protect against bone loss, and gives cardiovascular protection similar to HRT. As the drug does not appear to engage the breast receptors a woman is no longer at risk of stimulating breast cancer. Also, it has no effect on the womb, therefore no bleeding occurs and as a result there is less likelihood of uterine cancer developing. Unfortunately, it does not have a particularly beneficial effect on menopausal symptoms. Because of this, early menopausal women who are happy to do so, may still choose HRT. However, those older women who have no menopausal symptoms, but wish to protect bone density, and the cardiovascular system may well prefer a SERM.

Bisphosphonates

Bisphosphonates are powerful anti-resorptive agents. They inhibit osteoclasts by coating of the bone surfaces but allow osteoblasts to continue to form new bone. These drugs may increase bone density by about 5 per cent over 4 years. This form of treatment can be used for osteoporosis in men and women.

Etidronate disodium (Didronel PMO)

This is licensed to be used in patients suffering from established vertebral osteoporosis. It is generally well tolerated but poorly absorbed and should be taken with tap water on an empty stomach in the middle of a four-hour fast and away from other medications, in particular antacids or mineral supplements as these will reduce absorption. Cyclical etidronate is prescribed in three-monthly packs, that is 14 consecutive days of Didronel 100 mg followed by 76 days of calcium carbonate 500 mg. The calcium should be taken daily dissolved in water, with meals, though at any time of day. It should be taken long term. The contraindications are severe renal impairment, hypocalcaemia, hypercalcuria, pregnancy and lactation.

Alendronate sodium (Fosamax)

This drug is an amino-biphosphonate and is indicated when the bone mineral density is decreased at any skeletal site. It is a more potent agent than Didronel. It is well tolerated but cases of oesophagitis are reported because patients are going back to bed immediately after taking the dose and therefore irritating the lining of the oesophagus. Patients must therefore take a single dose of 10 mg when out of bed first thing each morning, half an hour before any food or drink other than a large (7oz/200 ml) glass of water. Antacids may affect the absorption of this drug, so they should be taken well apart. It is recommended that alendronate be taken long term.

Calcitonin

Calcitonin is a potent anti-resorptive hormone. This drug is a powerful inhibitor of osteoclastic absorption. It acts by blocking the stimulatory effects of the parathyroid hormone and as a result bones become stronger and are less likely to fracture. A form of calcitonin is derived from salmon or pork and therefore it is important that before the injection, which is given subcutaneously or intramuscularly, a test dose is administered. It is often used to reduce acute pain in spinal fractures. This treatment prevents cortical and trabecular bone loss in osteoporotic women. The side-effects are nausea, vomiting, dizziness and diarrhoea. Its main disadvantage is that it has to be given by injection, although intranasal sprays are available in some countries.

Calcium supplements

It is important to ensure that anyone at risk of osteoporosis takes adequate calcium in the diet or as a supplement. Adequate calcium is important at all ages. Calcium supplements are useful for patients with a dietary deficiency, for vegans, for those with lactose intolerance and in patients where other treatments are unacceptable. They are an excellant choice for the elderly housebound. They can be purchased in chemists or health food shops and they may be swallowed whole, chewed or acquired in a soluble form. The usual supplement is 500 mg to 1 g to ensure a total intake of 1–1.5 gm/day. Vitamin D is required in addition to calcium to aid the absorption of calcium in the intestine and it has been proved beneficial for people over 75 years. Calcium with vitamin D will increase the bone density, reduce cortical bone loss, reduce hip fractures by 43 per cent and non-vertebral fractures by 32 per cent in this particular age-group. Many older patients have a poor diet and lack fresh air and sunshine.

Vitamin D metabolites

Patients with established osteoporosis have lower calcium absorption from the gut, especially the elderly owing to reduced sunlight exposure and low renal function. Low doses of vitamin D help to overcome this. Calcitriol, a vitamin D metabolite, is more potent and can reduce the number of vertebral fractures.

Testosterone

This hormonal supplement is beneficial for men with established osteoporosis. Caution is used with long-term therapy because of effects on the prostate and lipids. This is given intramuscularly. One form is Sustanon.

Anabolic steroids and fluoride

These are little used for osteoporosis in the UK.

Those women for whom HRT is inadvisable because of medical history should be advised that prevention depends on a healthy diet, and exercise, if appropriate, particularly in the early postmenopausal age-group. Whilst prevention remains paramount, attaining this may be more difficult if access to HRT is denied. A baseline BMD scan could be sought and repeated 1 or 2 years later to judge whether a deterioration in bone mass has occurred.

Physiotherapy

Physiotherapy can be beneficial in the overall management of osteoporosis for the education and active prevention of the disease by encouraging exercise. Exercise has a significant effect on the bone density. Mechanical strain through weight-bearing and muscle contracture is a major factor in maintaining skeletal structural integrity. Active people have a higher bone mass when compared with sedentary people. Regular weight-bearing activity will increase bone mass by stimulating osteoblast activity. Exercise helps to alleviate pain, prevents deterioration of the condition, reduces stiffness of the shoulders, neck, chest, spine and legs, and prevents a worsening posture. Exercise should be done frequently within the limits of pain.

Physical activity and exercise, especially in the elderly, should be encouraged as it keeps patients agile, helps with balance and coordination, and reduces the risk of falls. It is often helpful to involve the carers in the exercise regime.

In established osteoporosis there may be vertebral collapse resulting in pain and deformity. Exercise should then be directed at encouraging general mobility and maintaining good posture. As mentioned earlier, the stooping posture that occurs in severe osteoporosis can result in problems with breathing, and stress incontinence due to increased pressure from the abdominal contents on the pelvic floor muscles. Therefore it will be important to include breathing exercises and pelvic floor strengthening excercises in the programme. These should ideally be performed every 2–3 hours!

Pain relief

Following acute vertebral collapse, patients will often be in very severe pain requiring strong analgesia. Fentanyl patches can be of great benefit in helping to control pain. The doses available are 25 mg, 50 mg and 70 mg. Physiotherapy can also play an important part in pain control. Heat can be beneficial – heat pads may be purchased from a chemist, or often a hot water bottle wrapped in a towel and placed on the aching area for 15–20 minutes, two to three times a day, can provide relief. The application of cold is also beneficial (see Chapter 7) if applied to the painful area for 5–10 minutes two to three times a day. Transcutaneous electrical nerve stimulation (TENS) is a small electrical unit with two to four pads which are applied to the painful area for 1–2 hours. These machines, if proved to be beneficial, can usually be provided on a short-term loan from a physiotherapy department and, if found successful, may be purchased.

Acupuncture

This is a technique long practised in China. Some physiotherapists provide this treatment in conjunction with advice on posture and a suitable exercise regime.

Yoga, megapulse and ultrasound

These are all treatments patients have found to be useful in relieving pain.

Hydrotherapy

When the acute pain has settled, exercise therapy in warm water of approximately 98°F, provided there are no contraindications, can relieve pain and muscle spasm, enable mobilisation and strengthen the spine. Swimming, although a good general exercise, is not always the best exercise as it is a non-weight-bearing activity but it is beneficial in improving muscle strength and general fitness.

Physiotherapists are able to monitor the progress of the disease through measuring the spinal mobility of sufferers by recording height, posture, chest expansion and flexibility on a regular basis. These measurements can be used as a baseline to measure the outcome of exercise programmes and to tailor an exercise regime to the patient's needs.

Patients can help themselves by brisk walking at least three times a week, cycling, playing golf, attending keep-fit sessions, and good posture at home and at work. Posture can be checked by standing facing a wall with a firm wedge between the head and the wall to check that the head is not tending to poke forwards. Exercise should continue as part of life's pattern, as bone loss is resumed once exercise ceases.

People who suffer from osteoporosis are often nervous about exercising because they are afraid of causing fractures by too much exercise. It is important, therefore, that the physiotherapist educates them about their condition and encourages confidence in being able to exercise safely and effectively, therefore improving the quality of their lives.

Prevention

The aim of prevention is to maintain peak bone mass and bone strength throughout life and also to prevent falls.

Primary

The management of osteoporosis lies in prevention and education. A healthy lifestyle should begin at school, especially during adolescence. Advice concerning the dangers of smoking, alcohol abuse, slimming diets, diet neglect, anorexia nervosa and bulimia, and the dangers of over-exercising should be stressed, together with the benefits of sensible exercise. It is important that expectant mothers have an adequate calcium intake, and recognise the symptoms of osteoporosis during pregnancy. During the menopause, middle-aged women should be given information, help, advice and support regarding HRT and osteoporosis and the need for a healthy lifestyle. Appropriate booklets, which may be acquired from the National Osteoporosis Society, are very useful and informative. It is important to encourage exercise in the form of walking, swimming or dancing at least three times a week. There is an increasing need for the education of the nursing and medical professions.

Secondary

Postmenopausal women should be encouraged to take HRT and continue for at least five years as it not only reduces the risk of osteoporosis but also the risk of strokes and coronary heart disease. Regular height, weight and blood pressure checks are advisable.

Elderly women should be encouraged to exercise, have plenty of fresh air and a good balanced diet. Poor nutrition often leads to low body temperature which encourages hypothermia with subsequent lack of coordination. It is important in winter that the elderly be kept warm and if they venture out that they take a walking stick to prevent falls, especially if the pavements are icy and wet. Loose carpets, rugs, stair coverings and trailing flexes should all be checked. Good lighting and regular eye and hearing tests are important. Bifocals are often the causes of falls. Tranquillisers and sleeping pills should be prescribed with care as they often produce drowsiness in the elderly which reduces the sense of balance and encourages falls. Those in this age-group often have reduced sensation in their feet and their muscles are weaker. It is important, therefore, that they do not wear slippers but have good, comfortable, well-fitting shoes. Advice from the chiropodist and orthotist is welcome. Their physical condition will often precipitate falls; for example, a low blood pressure will often produce fainting and blackouts. The elderly often have poor postural control and a slow reaction time.

Tertiary

Treatment should consist of HRT, bisphosphonates, and for patients over 75 years, calcium and vitamin D. At diagnosis a special exercise programme should be devised to be practised regularly at home, and tailored to the patient's needs. Ways of preventing further fractures should be considered. The expertise of an occupational therapist is very helpful, including advice on activities in the kitchen. The provision of long-handled dustpans and brooms, trolleys to carry plates around, cupboards lowered to avoid straining and reaching up, and perching stools to take the strain of standing are often very useful and acceptable. Advice should be offered regarding chair height, as too low a chair can put stress on the back when attempting to rise from it. Checking the height of the bed and replacing the blankets with duvets avoids bending when making the bed. Grab rails are often of benefit on the stairs. The National Osteoporosis Society gives advice on clothes specially designed for the use of the disabled and infirm so as to prevent twisting and stretching. They suit all ages, all tastes and all capabilities.

Diet

Hippocrates once said 'Thy food shall be thy cure'. If not exactly a cure, then food does help to prevent many illnesses and conditions. A well-balanced diet, rich in calcium and vitamin D, is very important for normal healthy bones. This is necessary from childhood and throughout life, though especially during adolescence, pregnancy and lactation, in order to ensure peak bone mass is attained and maintained. Diet should be moderate in quantity and of good quality.

Calcium

Calcium crystals and bone minerals are deposited around the fibres of the collagen within the bone. If there is too little collagen then there is nowhere for the calcium to be deposited and it is excreted in the urine. If there is too little calcium then the bones become brittle and fracture easily.

The normal daily intake of calcium should be between 800 and 1000 mg, but postmenopausal women need approximately 1500 mg. Most diets include only about 500 mg per day.

Calcium absorption rate decreases during illness and in later life. High-fibre and low-calorie diets are frequently low in calcium. Calcium is found in the non-fat part of milk. A pint of skimmed milk a day is recommended. Low-fat yoghurt, cheese and green vegetables, especially spinach and broccoli, canned sardines and salmon, especially when eaten with the bones, are all beneficial.

Vitamin D

This facilitates the absorption of calcium from the small intestine into the bloodstream. It is important to get enough but not an excessive amount. Ultraviolet light is converted in the skin to vitamin D and this is then converted in the liver and the kidneys to calcitrol which is necessary to maintain blood calcium levels. After the age of 50 the skin gradually loses this ability. The elderly and the housebound are at risk from a deficiency of this vitamin, and require 1000 units a day. Vitamin D is sold as cod liver oil and halibut oil, or as vitamin pills, often in combination with calcium. In the diet vitamin D has been added to cereals, margarine and low-fat spreads. It is naturally obtained from liver, cheese and oily fish such as herring, salmon and sardines. It is also found in milk. A good mid-life diet can help prevent osteoporosis and should include vegetables and fresh fruit, fibre enriched with calcium (too much fibre reduces calcium absorption), dairy products such as skimmed milk and yoghurt, a minimum amount of salt used in cooking and at the table because this can result in calcium being excreted from the kidneys, and a reduction of sugar such as in cakes, biscuits and jams. Plenty of fluid should be encouraged in the form of water and fruit juice but only 14 units of alcohol per week.

Education

Education 'from the cradle to the grave' is most important and nurses are among the best educators, as they are often able to provide opportunistic counselling! It is important that they dispel all myths, correct misunderstandings and advise patients on the appropriate course of action based on their own knowledge.

- The midwife should advise pregnant, lactating and weaning mothers on the importance of good nutrition, plenty of calcium and a healthy lifestyle.
- The health visitor should advise mothers, especially of children from the age of one onwards, on the importance of adequate calcium in a healthy diet, plus the importance of exercise.
- The school nurse, the practice nurse and the health visitor can all advise schoolchildren on diet and exercise. The early years of the developing child are critical in determining the peak bone mass.

The school nurse, the practice nurse and the family planning nurse can advise adolescents on the dangers of smoking and excessive drinking, anorexia and bulimia, poor diet, lack of weight-bearing exercise and over-exercise. During adulthood the midwife, practice nurse, family planning nurse, occupational health nurse (she in particular sees men and women who do not attend the GP's surgery) can all offer appropriate advice on lifestyle, diet, exercise and the importance of recognising the risk factors of osteoporosis.

For the middle-aged, the family planning nurse, health visitor and practice nurse are all able to offer advice on appropriate lifestyle, diet and weight-bearing exercise, and give information on the short- and long-term benefits and risks of HRT. They can assess those people at risk from osteoporosis and offer advice on preventive therapy. It is important that this group does not experience a rapid bone loss during the menopause.

For those in old age, the health visitor, practice nurse, district nurse and the rheumatology nurse specialist all play an important part in education, advising patients on appropriate lifestyle and diet, and suggesting with the help of a physiotherapist a suitable exercise programme. These nurses can recognise the risk factors of osteoporosis and advise on drug intervention for prevention, or on bone density measurement if the patient is suffering fractures following minimal trauma. They can also refer to the occupational therapist for advice on activities and aids to daily living and how to prevent falls. They can also advise on the effectiveness of treatment once osteoporosis has been diagnosed and drug treatment commenced. This age-group often requires support and counselling because body image has been altered and independence lost. They are often reluctant to take analgesics.

It is important that all nurses in the primary health care team should have regular study days and seminars to keep them informed of current treatments and research.

Nurses in accident and emergency departments can play a valuable role in preventing future fractures due to osteoporosis by alerting patients to the various treatments available and by discussing with them the nature of the disease. They also can alert the medical staff as to whether there is an underlying condition present. Orthopaedic nurses should also have a sound knowledge of osteoporosis, its prevention and treatment. Patients often need encouragement because their confidence has been lost due to repeated falls. Frequent study days and seminars on osteoporosis would be beneficial to all nurses in the acute hospitals. GPs as well as nurses need a continual update on osteoporosis, its prevention and treatment. Educational packs, such as those provided by the National Osteoporosis Society, should be readily available. Doctors over the past decade have become more aware of osteoporosis and preventive treatment has been initiated early, especially for those patients at risk. It is important that the medical profession keeps up to date with research so they can provide unbiased opinions.

The public

It is important to raise public awareness. Many patients remain undiagnosed until substantial bone loss has occurred and fractures have been experienced. Open days and meetings are important at which the public can meet the professionals on an informal basis, seek help and advice, and collect material relevant to research to read at home. Patients can then make informed decisions about their treatment and the management of their disease, and perhaps adjust their expectation.

Support groups, educational and group sessions play an important role. Not only do patients gain encouragement and support but they can also share their learning and experiences. Carers also gain valuable support and information from these groups.

Community pharmacists play an important part in compliance with treatment. They are the most easily accessible health professionals and can discuss with patients their fears and anxieties, the importance of taking the drugs and the side-effects.

Conclusion

Osteoporosis is a major health and socioeconomic problem in the western world. The cost of human suffering and the financial implications are considerable. It is therefore important that primary and secondary health-care teams, the public and other health professionals work together to prevent, advise, treat and follow up patients at risk and those suffering from the disease. It is also important that the public and health professionals know where to get help and advice. The rheumatologists and their health care teams should possess the current knowledge about osteoporosis and have the skills to help control pain, assess disability and formulate a rehabilitation programme. Rheumatology nurses in particular should not only be able to identify those at risk so that treatment can be initiated early, but should assist in the management of the disease, encouraging a healthy lifestyle, a balanced diet and adequate exercise. Steroid-sparing agents, such as azathioprine and methotrexate, are often used in arthritic conditions. Osteoporosis and the liability to fracture are features of inflammatory joint disease, including rheumatoid arthritis, ankylosing spondylitis, psoriatic arthropathy and lupus, as well as being connected with the use of steroid treatment, immobility due to pain and the disease process. The risk is greater in postmenopausal women undergoing treatment with corticosteroids. This may not be a consideration if the steroids are given orally in doses below 7.5 mg (research has yet to prove this with absolute certainty), or in small doses directly into painful arthritic joints. The damage to bones due to steroids relates to the dose and duration and how strong the bones were before the treatment. It is important that patients confined to a wheelchair because of arthritis should still be able to exercise. It is important that rheumatology nurses liaise with the multidisciplinary team – occupational therapists, physiotherapists, chiropodist and orthotist – as osteoporosis produces physical suffering and emotional strain, as well as possible financial hardship. It is therefore vital to take lifelong preventive measures. Adjustment to chronic illness takes time and requires considerable encouragement, support and a positive approach from the whole team. Patients with osteoporosis will also need psychological and social support.

Case Study

- Woman aged 38.
- Nulliparity. Lives alone. Small stature.
- Alcohol – 20 units a week. Smoker.
- Anorexia nervosa.
- Amenorrhoea.
- Asthma – high dose of steroids.
- Complained of backache for a time. Unconfirmed diagnosis of rheumatism.
- Sudden onset of excruciating chest pain radiating around the chest towards the spine.
- Diagnosed vertebral crush fracture.

Treatment

- Rest, initially in bed, to help vertebral fracture to heal.
- Fentanyl patches 25–50 mg commenced for pain. HRT also started.
- Slow rehabilitation, hydrotherapy plus gentle exercise.
- Advice on improving lifestyle.
- Reduce smoking and alcohol intake.
- Encourage patient to join eating-disorder group.
- Reduce steroids slowly.
- Provide patient with information from National Osteoporosis Society.
- Provision of social support to improve self-confidence.
- Start treatment with a bisphosphonate.

Useful Addresses

National Osteoporosis Society
PO Box 10
Radstock
Bath BA3 3YB
Tel: 01761 471771

Women's Health Concern
83 Earls Court Road
London W8 6EF
Tel: 0181 780 3916

Amarant Trust
Grant House
56–60 St John's Street
London EC1 4DT
Tel: 0171 490 1644

British Menopause Society (for health professionals only)
36 West Street
Marlow
Bucks SL7 2NB
Tel: 01628 890199

Disabled Living Foundation
346 Kensington High Street
London W14 3NS
Tel: 0171 289 6111

References

Bhalla A (1993) Genetics, bone mass and early intervention in preventing osteoporosis. Osteoporosis Review 1(4): 1–3.

Campbell G, Compston J, Crisp A (1993) The Management of Common Metabolic Bone Disorders. Cambridge: Cambridge University Press.

Colditz GA, Hankinson SE, Hunker DJ, Willett WC, Manson JE, Stampfer MJ, Hennekens C, Rosner B, Speizer FE (1995) The use of oestrogens and progesterones and the risks of breast cancer in post menopausal women. New England Journal of Medicine 332(24): 1589–93.

DHSS (1994) Advisory Group on Osteoporosis. Osteoporosis Report November 2(8): 13.

Francis R (1993) National FHSA/HA Symposium. The role of the specialist managing osteoporosis in a cost constrained environment, Café Royal, London, 8.

National Osteoporosis Society (1993) Menopause and Osteoporosis Therapy (Booklet), Practice Nurse Manual. Wells, Somerset: St Andrews Press.

Robins SP, Henning W, Hesley R, Ju J, Seyedin S, Seibel MJ (1994) Direct, enzyme-linked immunoassay for urinary deoxypyridinoline as a specific marker for measuring bone resorption. Journal of Bone and Mineral Research 9(10): 1643–9.

Woolf AD (1994) Osteoporosis. London: Martin Dunitz Ltd.

World Health Organisation (1994) Technical Report Series 843. Geneva: WHO.

Index